Minor Illness
or Major Disease?

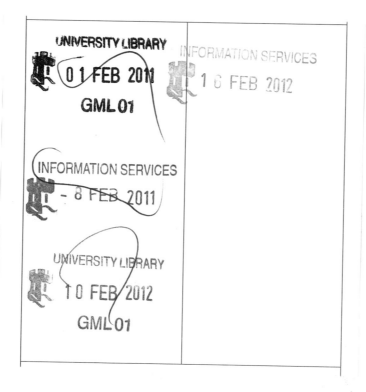

Minor Illness or Major Disease?

The clinical pharmacist in the community

FOURTH EDITION

Clive Edwards
BPharm, PhD, MRPharmS, Hon FICR
Prescribing Adviser
Newcastle upon Tyne, UK

Paul Stillman
BA, MB, ChB, DRCOG
General Practitioner,
Crawley, West Sussex, UK

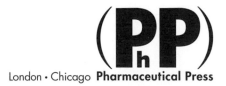

London • Chicago **Pharmaceutical Press**

Published by the Pharmaceutical Press
An imprint of RPS Publishing

1 Lambeth High Street, London SE1 7JN, UK
100 South Atkinson Road, Suite 200, Grayslake, IL 60030-7820, USA

© Pharmaceutical Press 2006

$(\mathbf{P_hP})$ is a trade mark of RPS Publishing

RPS Publishing is the publishing organisation of the Royal Pharmaceutical Society of Great Britain

First edition published 1982
Second edition published 1995
Reprinted 1995, 1997
Third edition published 2000
Reprinted 2002, 2003, 2004
Fourth edition published 2006
Reprinted 2009

1005914915

Typeset by J&L Composition, Filey, North Yorkshire
Printed in Italy by Rotolito Lombarda SpA

ISBN 978 0 85369 627 8

A catalogue record for this book is available from the British Library

To Pat and Joy

Contents

Preface

The title of this book originates from a series of articles written by the authors which were published in *The Pharmaceutical Journal* between 1979 and 1981. This series coincided with a period of renewed interest in responding to symptoms by pharmacists. The articles were published as a book by the Pharmaceutical Press in 1982, and after another series in *The Journal* and two further editions, the present book is the fourth edition of *Minor Illness or Major Disease?*

This latest edition, like the first, is written at a time of great interest in the role of the pharmacist outside the dispensary. The new pharmacy contract, the appearance of Minor Ailments Schemes and the continuing deregulation of prescription-only medicines to OTC status give the pharmacist new opportunities to advise on self-treatment of self-limiting illness, to reduce health risks and foster healthy lifestyles in an expanding public health arena.

The enhanced role of the pharmacist gives him or her a more prominent profile in the primary healthcare team and allows a closer collaborative working relationship with general practitioners and other health professionals.

Indeed, we believe that the teaming up of a pharmacist and a doctor to become joint authors of this book over 25 years ago is testament to the fruitful outcome that is possible when the complementary skills of the two professions are combined.

This edition follows the familiar format of previous ones. Signs and symptoms are explored, following a system of questioning used by the medical profession to obtain a medical history that allows the pharmacist to decide whether the patient has a minor illness and can self-treat, or whether there is a need to seek a medical opinion.

In most chapters there is a new section, 'Second opinion', which provides the reader with a brief insight into the action the doctor might take when a patient presents for advice. Advice on the treatment options of minor symptoms for pharmacists is given in each chapter, together with a summary of conditions that could be responsible for the symptoms described, and warning signs and symptoms which signal that referral to a doctor is appropriate.

The new edition includes more herbal remedies than previously, and a small bibliography appears at the end of most chapters focusing particularly on reviews and evidence of the efficacy of over-the-counter medicines.

These bibliographies are merely tasters for a larger library of publications, but give some useful background to the enthusiastic student who may wish to pursue a particular topic. (With respect to this, we would also recommend that the reader refer to *Prodigy*, a publication from the Sowerby Centre for Health Informatics at Newcastle, published on the website www.prodigy.nhs.uk, for further and more detailed information on individual conditions and treatments.)

The book is divided into two parts. Part A, Responding to symptoms, constitutes the major portion and deals with the diagnosis and treatment of minor illnesses that present to the pharmacist. Part B, Preventative self-care, contains new chapters that focus on the interventions pharmacists can make to reduce health risks and to protect the public against ill health, stressing their role in public health improvement, for which they are largely an untapped source.

Case studies are provided at the end of the majority of chapters which we hope will help put the subject matter into a useful practical context to assist pharmacists and other health professionals to whom the public present with symptoms.

Also, for those who wish to find more details about herbal remedies, we recommend *Herbal Medicines* by Barnes, Anderson and Phillipson, published by The Pharmaceutical Press, London.

Clive Edwards
Paul Stillman
2006

Acknowledgements

We would like to thank various past members of staff of *The Pharmaceutical Journal*, who gave us the encouragement to write a series under the title 'Minor Illness or Major Disease?' and provided the medium in which to publish it. In particular, we are indebted to Robert Blyth, who was editor of *The Journal* when the first series was published between 1978 and 1981, and to his successor, Douglas Simpson, who published the second series. On both occasions these two editors were ably assisted by Joanna Lumb, senior assistant editor, who steered us through the basic text which has formed the core of all the published editions of the book.

Our thanks go also to the staff of the Pharmaceutical Press over the years, and especially to Louise McIndoe for her help with this edition.

Along the way we have formed many friendships through the book, and in particular we would like to record that made with Bernard Hardisty, who did much to promote the role of the pharmacist in responding to symptoms, through the medium of his employer, a manufacturer of OTC medicines.

Our thanks also go to various colleagues who have given us the benefit of their wisdom, both in past editions and in the present one.

We are indebted to the following for photographs: Science Photo Library; GlaxoWellcome; Wellcome Trust Medical Photographic Library; the Newcastle Dental School; and the Department of Dermatology, Royal Victoria Infirmary, Newcastle upon Tyne.

About the authors

Clive Edwards studied pharmacy at the School of Pharmacy, London University, and obtained a PhD in pharmacology from the University of Sheffield. He has worked in the pharmaceutical industry and community, hospital and academic pharmacy. From 1978 until 1997 he held lectureships and senior lectureships in clinical pharmacy at respectively the Universities of Aston in Birmingham and Newcastle. He has a wide experience in clinical therapeutics in hospitals and still works as an occasional locum in community pharmacy. He is currently a prescribing adviser for a primary care organisation.

Paul Stillman studied medicine at the University of Bristol, and after vocational training became a principal in general practice in Sussex, where he has remained for 30 years and is now senior partner. He has long had an interest in medical education and is a course organiser and trainer for general practice. He is also involved in the public awareness of health and illness and has worked to promote this through television, radio and the press.

Clive and Paul met in 1977, when Clive was working for a pharmaceutical company in West Sussex and Paul was a GP. They have worked together since that date to promote the role of the pharmacist as an adviser to the public on self-care.

Part A

Responding to symptoms

1

Introduction

Self-care

Self-care is the action taken by an individual to optimise their health and wellbeing, both physical and mental. The term embraces both the prevention of illness and the self-treatment of minor ailments, as well as long-term conditions that have been diagnosed by a doctor.

Society is changing: people want more information, choice and control over their health. Self-care can lead to improved health and quality of life and a reduction in visits to general medical practitioners (GPs) and hospitals.

The promotion of good health and the prevention of ill health includes measures such as treating symptoms and preventing disease by reducing cigarette smoking, encouraging exercise, reducing alcohol intake and healthy eating. Pharmacists can take the opportunity to advise on all of these during consultations with the public based on the topics included in this book.

This 'extra-dispensary' activity complements the advice and education pharmacists already give to those patients for whom they dispense medicines.

Skills and support required

Members of the public can turn to various health professionals, including pharmacists, for advice on self-care. In most cases they will rely on the skills of the pharmacist in addressing a current problem, but part of the treatment the pharmacist provides should, where possible, include education to deal with or prevent problems and symptoms in the future. This is where some simplified explanation of the background of the condition, the mode of action of any recommended medicine and any monitoring required is useful to the sufferer. Also, if referral is appropriate, an explanation of what the doctor might do next or what possible diagnoses need to be excluded is also important.

The NHS Plan (2000) states: 'the frontline in healthcare is in the home'. Arguably the backup or second line is in the pharmacy.

Partnership with medical practitioners

A good working relationship between community pharmacists and local medical practices is to be encouraged, so that local protocols and guidelines, where they exist, are observed. Where such protocols do not already exist, then the two professions should work together to produce new ones. The skills of pharmacists and doctors are complementary and, used appropriately, will enhance the care of individual members of the public. If the two do not gel, or there is conflict in the professional relationship, or even if no relationship exists, then this should be rectified as soon as possible.

The use of over-the-counter (OTC) medicines

A commonly quoted statistic tells us that up to 40 per cent of a GP's time is taken up by consultations with patients who present with minor, self-remitting illnesses. GPs are increasingly recommending self-care to patients. In some cases in the UK this is unacceptable to patients, because about 80 per cent of prescriptions are obtained free of charge and many patients will object to having to pay for OTC treatments. Increasingly, self-care or minor ailment schemes operate in which OTC drugs for defined minor ailments can be obtained free of charge by those patients who fulfil the conditions to obtain free prescription medicines. These schemes operate in the UK and allow pharmacists to be reimbursed for the cost of the drugs provided. Thus the payment barrier is overcome, and it has been shown that such schemes do reduce the workload of the GP.

Self-medication empowers the individual to take care of his or her health and saves in financial public expenditure for prescription drugs as well as releasing valuable doctor time.

In terms of consumer choice, cost and convenience are probably the main factors that determine whether a person obtains a drug over the counter or on prescription. Advertising has a major influence on the purchase of particular OTC brand medicines. Patients have the right to choose what they want, and thanks to increasing consumer demand and limited resources it has been necessary to use the skills and expertise of all health professionals. For pharmacy, this potential in supporting self-care has been outlined in various documents, such as the NHS Plan (July 2000) and *Pharmacy in the Future* (September 2000).

The maxim 'do no harm' is a prerequisite for care given by any health professional and is one of which pharmacists should be mindful. However, the pharmacist is in an ideal position to advise on self-medication, particularly in at-risk groups such as the elderly, who may be taking many prescription drugs and will need advice to avoid drug interactions and duplication of medications.

The motivation for self-care

With so many people eligible for free prescriptions it is often argued that there is little motivation for self-care. This gives no credit to the wealth of OTC medications available in the pharmacy, but not on prescription. It may be that doctors' knowledge of compound OTC medicines is limited, and that they therefore cannot recommend them with confidence for particular symptom complexes. Recent studies also suggest that the traditional medicalisation of presenting symptoms, with closed questions leading the enquirer to a conclusion, leaves the patient still feeling unable to contribute. More patient-centred approaches have helped, sharing ideas and expectations and moving towards an agreed strategy, but the promotion of self-care needs to take this still further. Many people will have thought about their symptoms before presenting them to a professional, and it may be useful to elicit their previous experiences in some detail. What have they done both in this episode and in similar ones in the past? Has it helped, and what were the expectations that prompted it? Then, for example, reassurance that their actions are appropriate but need a little more time may offer them more support than reaffirming that the diagnosis is not serious.

For most, the obstructions to self-care go beyond the financial. Many people will spend money on medication if they feel confident and in control of minor illness. Our task is to support the decision-making process as well as to reassure, and to simplify the complexities of the pharmacology available.

The switch of prescription-only medicines (POM) to OTC status

The availability of drugs over the counter varies from country to country, and indeed in the USA it even varies from state to state. In the UK the variance in control of OTC products ranges from those whose sale must be supervised by a pharmacist (pharmacy-only, or P medicines) to those whose sale is unrestricted and can occur in retail outlets other than pharmacies (general sales list, or GSL medicines)

Generally drugs will be accorded OTC status if they fulfil various criteria:

- The condition for which they are used can be reliably self-diagnosed. However, there are exceptions to this, as for example the sale of antifungal agents for vaginal candidiasis, which are only licensed for use after an initial diagnosis has been made by a doctor. There are some more remote exceptions, such as theophylline (for asthma), glyceryl trinitrate and isosorbide (for angina), which are available legally over the counter.

- Where there is no evidence of irreversible or serious adverse reactions, even in high doses.
- In the UK drugs should have had a long use as a prescription-only medicine before being deregulated to OTC status, to ensure safety. However, some OTC medicines may not be innocuous and side effects may not become obvious until later (e.g. phenylpropanolamine in cold remedies, and herbal medicines such as St John's Wort).
- Where the delay in obtaining a prescription for a drug may cause harm. Examples of such cases are levonorgestrel for emergency contraception.
- Where their use does not require medical supervision or monitoring by a doctor.

There may be other hidden criteria, often of a political or marketing nature.

There have been several high-profile switches of medicines from the POM category to OTC status in the UK, including omeprazole and simvastatin. Simvastatin represents a milestone in the deregulation of drugs to OTC status, in that it is the first drug licensed to prevent serious chronic illness. It is for this reason that the new edition of this book has been extended to include chapters on disease prevention as well as symptom treatment.

Evidence-based medicine

Evidence-based medicine (EBM) should be used to inform clinical decisions, but it should be considered with all the available information about an individual patient before making a decision. Thus pharmacists may recommend products with no evidence base while acknowledging the expectation of the individual member of the public standing before them.

In recent years it has become apparent that many OTC medicines do not have evidence-based effectiveness. However, this should not be interpreted to mean that pharmacists (who have a scientific training) should deny particular

treatments to their 'patients'. Increasingly, with the medical revolution of the last half-century we are in a culture where the public believes that there is 'a pill for every ill'. The placebo effect is huge, and often people come into a pharmacy with a desire or expectation that they will be given a remedy, as well as pertinent advice, to relieve their symptoms.

A parallel situation often occurs in the doctor's consulting room. In the first place it should be remembered that even prescription medicines are not effective to the same extent in every patient. The term 'numbers needed to treat' (NNT) is well known to health professionals and is in effect an admission of this fact. Secondly, patients' expectations, whether real or perceived, often influence the outcome of a consultation, not least the writing of a prescription. Doctors often make clinically inappropriate, non-evidence-based decisions for the sake of maintaining a good patient relationship. Examples are the prescribing of antibiotics for trivial infections and ordering investigations that are not clinically required.

Complementary and alternative medicine

Complementary medicine is very popular with the public. Although in many cases remedies are not supported by placebo-controlled randomised clinical trials, individual choice and experience is important here, just as with more orthodox medicines. Not all patients respond, and it may be that responders are those in whom we are seeing a large placebo effect or who have high expectations. Again, medicine is not a perfect science and patients often respond in an unexpected or inconsistent manner to all kinds of remedies.

There is much to be said for a holistic approach, and pharmacists must make an effort to empathise with individuals who ask for their advice. A sympathetic reaction, a caring attitude and a genuine interest in an individual's problems will contribute to a significant placebo effect, regardless of whatever medicine may be recommended.

Herbal medicines

Herbal medicines are becoming increasingly popular. There are two major issues to be borne in mind: efficacy and safety. Herbal products which are available from a variety of commercial sources will vary in composition. It is therefore difficult to confirm the efficacy of all products, as the amount of active ingredient will vary, often widely, from product to product. Added to this, the identity of the active ingredient may be in doubt. An example of this is St John's Wort, where there is conflict as to whether the anti-depressant activity is due to the hypericins or to hyperforin, and which ingredient causes liver enzyme induction.

Like conventional medicines, herbal medicines often have a controversial evidence base. St John's Wort, for example, has been the subject of many clinical trials and analyses, often with conflicting conclusions.

There is a myth among the public that herbal medicines are safe. Increasingly this is being found not to be the case, as for example in the case of St John's Wort, which is a liver enzyme inducer and can cause many interactions with prescription drugs. There have been other reports, such as tea tree oil being a severe skin irritant, cranberry juice potentiating the anti-coagulant effects of warfarin, and kava causing liver reactions.

Conflicting reports and evidence may be caused by the variation in composition between commercial brands, as referred to above.

The ability of the pharmacist to respond to the public

Pharmacists need to be trained in the differential diagnosis of common minor ailments. They should not be distracted or feel pressured by other elements of their work, such as dispensing, when consulting with a member of the public about a health issue. An effective consultation demands time, empathy and privacy, regardless of what else remains to be done in the pharmacy.

Because of their open availability, pharmacists have been the subject of various covert research activities, particularly by consumer associations over the years, with regard to the advice they give to the public. The publication of such investigations has inevitably highlighted the shortcomings of pharmacists' ability to ask the right questions and give the correct advice. Undoubtedly such research among other professions would produce a range of competencies from practice to practice. The methodology of such research studies is difficult and therefore sometimes of dubious value, but the studies do serve to highlight the fact that care is always necessary in taking a history from an individual who presents with symptoms in the pharmacy.

History taking at this level is an important but not difficult skill to learn, and with experience and practice, pharmacists should quickly become proficient.

A reference sheet or list of questions to ask and when to refer should be available in the desk of the consulting room so that the pharmacist can check that a thorough history has been taken. Pharmacists might also benefit from taking notes of the questions they ask, both as a means of later analysing their efficiency in history taking, as well as with a view to the future when, like doctors, they may be challenged about what they have said.

Diagnosis and history taking

Pharmacists have advised members of the public about the treatment of minor illnesses for as long as the profession has existed. Before embarking on any form of advice or treatment, some initial diagnosis is necessary to exclude any potentially serious cause that may require a medical consultation. This diagnosis of exclusion is one pharmacists should be able to make in the vast majority of cases that they see every day. It may be thought of as a screening or sieving process, which can be achieved by careful, intelligent questioning of the patient. It is a process many patients perform themselves before self-medicating, and generally they are very competent at it. It is also commonly the modus operandi for GPs when a patient presents with symptoms for the first time.

Clearly, this sort of diagnosis can take on various degrees of sophistication, and there is a suitable level at which the pharmacist can participate in the process. At this level it is not difficult, and with a structured approach to questioning, which closely follows that taught to doctors, pharmacists can make valuable judgments as to whether to refer a patient to a doctor or to recommend self-treatment. The suggested format that follows is one approach that can be used to elicit a comprehensive history.

General rules

Almost too obvious to mention, but crucially important, is the question of who is the patient. Is it the person relating the story, or are they a representative of the patient? It is difficult to obtain a satisfactory history from a third party. If the patient is not present, it is useful to establish whether the reason for their absence is the severity of symptoms. Parents of young children will give good histories of a child's illness; if the child is present, the severity of the illness and other signs can be observed. In the absence of the patient, pharmacists should reassure themselves that they are in no doubt as to the severity and nature of the disease. If there is any uncertainty, it is unwise to recommend self-treatment.

The patient should first be allowed to explain the illness in their own words as a response to a general question such as 'What is the problem?' or 'How do you feel?' This allows the patient to relax and encourages them to talk and provide clues that can be followed up by more specific questions later. During this phase of the interview the pharmacist can observe the demeanour or the attitude of the patient so that he or she can consider the question 'Does the patient look ill?' Some patients can articulate the severity of their illness adequately, but in others non-verbal signs (such as body language) must be observed to distinguish a very sick person from a relatively healthy one. This is particularly relevant in babies, who can indicate their discomfort by refusing to eat, by crying or screaming (even after being picked up), or by being irritable or behaving in some abnormal fashion.

Table 1.1 A reminder of questions to ask about symptoms

S	Site or location
I	Intensity or severity
T	Type or nature
D	Duration
O	Onset
W	With (other symptoms)
N	aNnoyed or aggravated by
S	Spread or radiation
I	Incidence or frequency pattern
R	Relieved by

The patient should be asked about current or recent medicines that have been taken, both prescribed (and therefore often for other conditions) and OTC (both for this illness and for other problems). This is helpful for eliciting any drug-induced symptoms, as well as for establishing whether the patient has already tried a remedy for the present complaint. At some point in the questioning, perhaps later in the more specific questions, any relevant past history can be inquired after, such as personal or family history, together with occupation and social habits, for example smoking, drinking and exercise.

The description of the illness can be expanded by asking more specific and structured questions, which can be prompted by a mnemonic (Table 1.1).

Questions to ask

Site or location

This question can be helpful in diagnosis in some instances, for example where pain is the main symptom. For instance, a pain in the abdomen could be caused by appendicitis (central pain, moving to the right iliac fossa), renal colic (pain in right or left loin or iliac fossa), peptic ulcer (central or epigastric) or biliary colic (right hypochondrium). Similarly, headaches can be unilateral (migraine), frontal (migraine, sinusitis or tension) or occipital (tension, muscle spasm or subarachnoid haemorrhage). The site of a skin rash can distinguish a localised reaction, for example to a watchstrap, from the allergy to an antibiotic in which the whole body may be involved.

Intensity or severity

The intensity or severity of a symptom, such as pain, a skin rash or bleeding from a wound, gives information not only about the likely diagnosis but also about the urgency of a situation. This is essential when considering whether to temporise and monitor the course of a symptom or illness for a little longer, to give an OTC medicine or to recommend referral to the patient's GP.

Type or nature

Further description of a symptom can help to differentiate certain conditions. For example, an abdominal pain which is cramp-like or colicky indicates the involvement of a hollow organ, such as the bowel or ureter, which contracts as a result of spasm of smooth muscle in the organ wall. On the other hand, patients often describe the pain of a peptic ulcer as 'gnawing'. Similarly, the appearance of a rash as flat or raised, single or multiple, or blistering or dry lesions can help to differentiate various skin conditions.

Duration

The duration of any symptom must always be established. This information can be helpful to distinguish, say, the headache of migraine (which usually lasts no more than a few hours) from a tension headache (which may persist for several days or weeks). The duration will also help the pharmacist to decide whether to refer in certain situations. For example, a baby who has suffered from diarrhoea for three days requires referral for a medical assessment, whereas a baby with diarrhoea of only a few hours' duration may respond adequately to hydration with a simple electrolyte mixture.

Onset

The history of onset of a symptom or illness can provide clues to its likely cause. Thus, abdominal pain and diarrhoea which starts soon after overindulgence in a restaurant, or headache which occurs on awakening after an alcoholic binge, are likely to require little more than reassurance, sympathy and simple OTC measures.

Accompanying symptoms

Concomitant symptoms may not always be volunteered by the patient, especially if they feel that they are not important or not related to the main symptom about which they are complaining. Such information is, however, crucial to differentiate many disorders. For example, someone who complains of a productive cough or of diarrhoea should be asked whether there is blood in the sputum or motions, to distinguish between potentially serious disease or more trivial illness. Someone with a red eye that is itching and watery may have a simple allergy, whereas a red eye that is painful or accompanied by some disturbance of vision will require immediate medical attention.

Thus, any symptom should be submitted to a systematic review, inquiring first about other symptomatology within the same body system and then, either by direct questioning or by more general open questions (depending on the problem), about any symptoms in other systems.

Factors that aggravate the condition

Although not always relevant, there are some conditions for which inquiry about any factors that worsen the symptom can be valuable. The pain of a peptic ulcer, for example, can be worsened by a heavy meal, or alternatively by fasting, whereas that caused by gallstones will be particularly exacerbated by a fatty meal.

Headaches associated with a raised intracranial pressure will be worse after lying down and hence worse in the mornings, whereas tension headaches may be better in the mornings but worsen as the day goes on.

Spread or radiation

There are several examples of where a sensation – usually pain – spreads characteristically and almost predictably to another part of the body.

In the case of pain, this is known as referred pain. The diagnosis of appendicitis is classically made by the patient describing a pain that starts in the central region of the abdomen and then spreads to the right iliac fossa. The pain of angina often radiates to the arm or jaw, and biliary colic occurs as pain in the upper abdomen that is referred to the back and felt between the shoulder blades. Some skin conditions begin as single discrete lesions in one part of the body before spreading elsewhere, whereas others present in a more generalised way.

Incidence or frequency

If a symptom recurs, then in some circumstances the pattern of recurrence or relapse is characteristic. For example, classic migraine will rarely occur twice in the same week, whereas another form of migraine, known as cluster headache, occurs every day at the same time of day for several weeks. The hayfever syndrome may often be difficult to distinguish from symptoms of the common cold, except that it is notable for its appearance in particular months of the year.

Factors that relieve the condition

Just as some conditions are made worse by particular factors, there are some that can be characterised by factors that relieve them. The pain of peptic ulcer, for instance, is often relieved by small snacks (as opposed to large meals, which tend to aggravate it), and a migraine attack may be terminated by the patient vomiting.

Medicines are often useful to relieve and at the same time diagnose a condition. Thus, an anginal attack may be relieved by glyceryl trinitrate, and reflux dyspepsia alleviated by a large dose of antacid, but not vice versa.

Other factors

The intelligent use of a standard format such as the one we have suggested for asking questions will ensure that the most important areas are covered and that an acceptable standard of interrogation is used. The format we have used here will be applied as appropriate in the topics to be covered in this book, but as all practitioners will

be aware, every question is not always applicable to every circumstance, and the answer to one question often obviates the need for another. With practice, pharmacists will be able to use a standard line of questioning quickly and efficiently, knowing that as long as they have picked out the relevant questions for the symptom under consideration they will have acted in the best possible faith and with acceptable professional competency. They will thus have been able to distinguish between minor illness and major disease. In many cases the cause of a symptom will be obvious, whereas in others a precise diagnosis, at least prospectively, will be impossible, and then the pharmacist will depend on the exclusion of serious pathology.

To complete the skill of diagnosis, even at this level, the pharmacist needs to rely on two further attributes. First, to have in mind a list of the serious diagnoses when considering the symptoms that are presented. Secondly, but no less importantly, to be alert to that unpleasant feeling which develops in a diagnostician's mind when no satisfactory explanation can be reached. This is a developed skill that many call experience. If any of the serious diagnoses cannot be reasonably excluded, the pharmacist should have no hesitation in directing the patient to more suitable assistance, e.g. referring to the GP for a medical opinion.

It is important that pharmacists do not inadvertently raise fears in the minds of patients, especially when recommending referral to a doctor. Obviously it is both educative and consoling to be able to explain to a patient exactly why they should seek a medical opinion, and there is no doubt that patients appreciate a sympathetic ear and a comprehensible explanation of both symptoms and their management. At the same time, when a pharmacist cannot eliminate the possibility of serious pathology it is essential that he or she delivers the message appropriately, depending on the demeanour of the patient. Patients will often have selective hearing and overreact to emotive words such as 'cancer' or 'tumour', perhaps in such a way that they will then avoid seeing the doctor in case the diagnosis is confirmed. It is necessary to avoid the use of such words, and to remember that statistically only a very small number of patients who seek help about their symptoms from a pharmacist will prove to have a serious disease, and an even smaller proportion of symptoms will be due to malignancy. However, there will always be a few instances where there is a degree of uncertainty, or where patients fall into a certain category, in which case it is good professional practice to advise them to see their GP. The same process occurs daily in the doctor's consulting room, where he or she will refer a patient for specialist opinion for similar reasons, to either confirm or exclude a specific diagnosis.

Format of this book

Each chapter in this book contains the main text, in which there is a description of commonly presenting signs and symptoms and their association with various diseases and conditions, together with advice to assist the pharmacist in interpreting them. Potential diagnoses and signals for referral are included, as well as the principles of management with OTC medicines.

A summary of the most common conditions producing the described signs and symptoms is provided, as well as a précis of the warning signals for referral.

A short section called 'Second opinion' gives a brief insight into the actions of the GP when confronted with a patient with similar symptoms to those that may be presented to the pharmacist.

Finally, a number of case histories are provided for illustration.

Bibliography

Department of Health (2000). *The NHS Plan.* London: Department of Health.

Department of Health (2000). *Pharmacy in the Future: Implementing the NHS Plan.* London: Department of Health.

National Prescribing Centre (2004). Community pharmacy minor ailments schemes. MeReC Briefing 27: 1–8.

2

Headache

Most people suffer from headaches from time to time and in the majority of cases they resolve within a short period.

Headache is often no more than a physiological response to circumstances, but it can lead to much anxiety, both for sufferers and for those who aim to unravel its cause. There are two major problems in attempting to discover the origin of a headache. First, there are some potentially very serious diagnoses, which, although rare, may be in the minds of both parties, and secondly, it can be a notoriously difficult condition to explain. There are few definitive signs or tests available to either general practitioners (GPs) or pharmacists that will confirm the diagnosis, yet headache is a common complaint that will bring many people to the pharmacy to purchase analgesics.

Fortunately, in most cases the headache will disappear spontaneously or respond to simple analgesics, proving – albeit retrospectively – to be no more than one of the transient self-limiting episodes to which most people are susceptible at some time or another. However, to distinguish the minority of cases in which serious pathology may be a possibility, it is helpful to understand the mechanisms by which headaches occur, and to arrive at some guidelines to differentiate those types that may relate to an underlying problem from those which are of no lasting significance and can be treated symptomatically by the pharmacist.

Types

Tension headache

Tension is the most common cause of headache. It is sometimes referred to as psychogenic

headache or muscle contraction headache. It can be caused by various emotional stresses, such as tension, anxiety or fatigue. Classically it is thought to result from muscle spasm in the neck and scalp (Figure 2.1).

Chronic daily headache

One accepted definition of this type of headache is one that occurs on at least 15 days of the

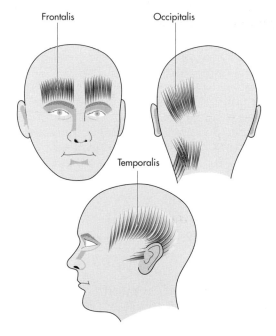

Figure 2.1 Location of the muscles of the scalp that are involved in muscular spasm in tension headache. When the muscles contract, there may be a tightness or band-like feeling around the head. Pain may be due in part to the tension in the muscles as well as a resulting constriction of capillaries within them, reducing their blood supply and causing a lack of oxygen.

month for at least 4 hours. The pain often appears to be there from morning until night and never seems to go away. It can vary in nature from an ache to a dull throb. The most common cause of this type of headache is analgesic overuse. This so-called 'medication overuse headache' is thought to be caused by an increase in the number of pain receptors that are switched on, first by the pain itself and then by increased sensitisation of the receptors when analgesics are used that are not sufficient to remove the pain. Instead, there is an exaggerated response of the receptors that more frequent or more potent analgesia fails to stop, and a vicious cycle between medication and pain begins. Patients with this type of headache will typically be taking simple or combination analgesics on more than three days a week.

Vascular headache

Dilatation or constriction of blood vessels in and around the brain will produce pain. Vascular headaches are the second most common type, as they are associated with any febrile illness (which causes vasodilatation).

Hypertension rarely causes headache (although it is often believed to do so by patients with high blood pressure), except very rarely in severe or so-called malignant hypertension. The headache of migraine may be related to dilatation of blood vessels within or around the skull. More serious cases of headache can be caused by rupture of a blood vessel, as in subarachnoid and subdural haemorrhages.

Traction headache

The brain itself has no sensory receptors within its fabric. A lesion within the substance of the brain will therefore not produce pain until it impinges upon adjacent structures, although if the lesion is severe enough to interfere with cerebral function it may cause other symptoms, such as vomiting, confusion, drowsiness, or disturbances of balance or of intellectual function. Thus, even a lesion as severe as a stroke will not usually be accompanied by headache.

Traction headaches are caused by inflammation (e.g. meningitis), tumours or haematomas (haemorrhages). They are classified as traction headaches because the underlying pathology causes irritation and stretching of the meninges (the protective membranes that envelop the brain and spinal cord). These membranes are richly endowed with sensory pain receptors which, when stimulated, will cause headache.

Tumours and cerebral abscesses are examples of space-occupying lesions, which cause headaches by compressing normal brain tissue against the skull, resulting in a raised intracranial pressure. Head injury can cause a haematoma, leading to a raised intracranial pressure. Infection and inflammation of the membranes surrounding the brain and lining the skull (e.g. meningitis) will cause headache, as will inflammation of the brain tissue itself (e.g. encephalitis) when other structures are involved or the intracranial pressure rises.

Other causes

Headache can be caused by spasm or fatigue of the ciliary and periorbital muscles of the eye, as in eye strain, astigmatism and other refractive disorders. Glaucoma can cause headache. Pain may be referred from the jaw in dental pain, and from the sinuses in sinusitis.

Muscle strain or pulled ligaments in the neck or upper back are a common cause of headache. Shingles affecting the scalp or eyes can cause pain in the face and head. Temporal arteritis is a rare but severe inflammation of the temporal artery and may occur in the elderly, producing pain and tenderness.

Assessing symptoms

Location of pain

Often headache cannot be described as pertaining to one part of the head, but if it is specific the following pointers are useful.

- Frontal pain may indicate idiopathic headache (i.e. of no specific known cause), sinusitis or nasal congestion.

- Occipital pain (back of the head) may suggest tension or anxiety, especially if the pain radiates over the top and sides of the head.
- Tension headache is described as a tight band around the head, often spreading over the top of the head. It is usually bilateral and may be described by the patient as a generalised ache or pain, with no specific focus, felt all over the cranium.
- Hemicranial (unilateral) headache, i.e. headache on one side of the head, is typical of migraine or sinusitis. It often spreads to both sides later. The pain of shingles (herpes zoster) usually starts as a severe localised pain felt in the skin on one side of the scalp, either a day or so before the rash appears or at the same time as the rash develops. Pain on one side of the face may indicate trigeminal neuralgia.
- Pain from within the eye itself may be due to glaucoma or other serious eye diseases, but pain behind or around the eyes is often described in sinusitis, migraine or shingles.
- Pain in the temple area (at the sides of the head) may indicate temporal arteritis in patients over 50, especially if there is sensitivity to touch in this area of the scalp. This requires urgent referral to avoid more general inflammation of the arteries, which could lead to blindness if the blood supply to the optic nerve is compromised.

Radiation

As mentioned above, unilateral headaches such as migraine often subsequently spread to both sides of the head. It is important to remember to ask about the exact site and radiation of pain, as transformation to a generalised headache might obscure the original pattern and location.

Onset, duration and intensity

It is useful to ask the patient to assess the degree of pain by asking 'How severe is the pain?' and then prompting the answer with 'Is it mild and annoying, or is it severe and debilitating?' Another guide to severity is whether the patient is able to carry on with their daily routine.

It is helpful to know if the patient has suffered similar episodes before, as a new pain of some severity should be taken more seriously than recurrence of a headache which has been successfully dealt with in the past. Another useful question is: 'Is this the worst pain you have ever had?' or 'Did this pain stop you in your tracks?' If the answer to either of these is yes, serious consideration should be given to referring the patient to their GP.

If a headache has become progressively more severe over a period of days (or in the case of a child, a few hours) and is not responding to treatment, referral should be considered. In the absence of any other significant factors a headache that is becoming less painful can reasonably be treated with simple analgesics.

A headache that has lasted only a few minutes can be regarded as trivial unless it has occurred suddenly and is described as devastating and the worst pain the patient has ever had. Such a headache might indicate bleeding from a ruptured blood vessel under the membrane covering the brain (subarachnoid haemorrhage), and is a medical emergency. Often under such circumstances the patient collapses and becomes unconscious. A migrainous headache can occur reasonably rapidly, but usually develops over a longer period than a subarachnoid haemorrhage, which may be described as being like a blow to the back of the head.

If a headache is recent in onset but has gradually become worse over a few days, inquiry should be made about recent head trauma, as bleeding may occur slowly, giving progressive worsening of symptoms.

Migraine attacks classically last only a few hours, but in some people they can persist for 72 hours.

The frequency as well as the duration of recurrent headaches should be noted, and may reveal particular patterns. Classic and common migraine usually occur every few weeks and rarely more than once a week, whereas cluster headaches occur for 1 or 2 hours at the same time of day, every day, for several weeks.

Generally, a headache that does not disappear or improve over 1–2 weeks should be considered for referral, with one or two exceptions, such as tension headache (which may occur every day for several weeks in some cases) and cluster headaches.

Headache that is present on awakening can represent a serious cause, such as a space-occupying lesion, but migraines often awaken people, and people can wake up with tension headaches or chronic daily headache. Further history is therefore needed to distinguish between the causes.

Nature of the symptoms

A description of the pain can give valuable pointers to a possible cause of the headache. For example:

- **A sudden pain**, which feels like a blow to the head or an explosion in the head and which stops the patient in their tracks with no warning whatsoever suggests a haemorrhage (see above) and requires immediate referral, to a hospital if necessary, if the patient is in obvious distress.
- **Throbbing or pounding** indicates a vascular cause, e.g. the vasodilatation caused by fever or migraine.
- **Constant or nagging pain** is most probably due to a tension headache, but if it progressively worsens the possibility of something more serious should be borne in mind.
- The pain of migraine is more severe than that of tension headache, but the most easily discriminating factors are the duration and the other associations, such as nausea, vomiting or visual disturbances. Table 2.1 lists signs that differentiate tension headache from migraine.

If the patient complains of vague generalised pain, pressure on top or around the head or short stabbing pain, but does not have any other warning signs, a trial of over-the-counter (OTC) analgesics is reasonable.

Onset of pain/trigger factors

Establishing a pattern to the onset of headaches, especially recurrent episodes, can help not only

Table 2.1   Differentiation between migraine and tension headache

Migraine	Tension headache
Moderate to severe pain	Mild to moderate pain
Usually unilateral	Bilateral
Pulsating	Non-pulsating
Aggravated by normal activities, such that the patient has to stop	Not aggravated by normal activities
Often accompanied by sensitivity to light, nausea and/or vomiting	These symptoms are not usually present

in seeking a possible cause but also in removing trigger factors. When appropriate, inquiries based on the list shown in Table 2.2 will be helpful.

Relieving factors

The avoidance of trigger factors can help in diagnosing the cause of a headache as well as in relieving it. Migraine headaches are classically relieved by sleep or by vomiting.

Premenstrual syndrome, which may present with a headache and other symptoms (see below), classically improves or disappears when menstrual bleeding starts.

Accompanying symptoms

Inquiries about concurrent symptoms can help in differentiating between some types of headache.

Fever

A fever in adults with headache, especially with aching muscles (myalgia), aching joints and/or general malaise, is common in viral infections, sometimes accompanied by other symptoms of upper respiratory tract infection. Fever may also accompany the headache of sinusitis, along with nasal congestion or recent symptoms of the

Table 2.2   Trigger factors for headache

Trigger factors or onset pattern	Possible underlying cause
Food, e.g. cheese, chocolate, caffeine, specific alcoholic drinks	Migraine
Exercise	Migraine, space-occupying lesion
Light	Migraine, meningitis
Hunger	Migraine
Neck movement	Tension, neck injury, meningitis, arthritis or fibrositis of the neck, vascular pathology
Cyclical pattern in women	Side effect of oral contraceptive, premenstrual tension, migraine, depression, tension
Present on awakening or wakes patient at night	Tension, neck muscle spasm, sinusitis, space-occupying lesion causing increased intracranial pressure
Bending down	Space-occupying lesion, sinusitis
Straining, coughing, sneezing	Space-occupying lesion
Sudden and severe with rapid onset	Subarachnoid haemorrhage
Travel	Tension, migraine
Drugs	Various, including oral contraceptives, indometacin, vasodilators (e.g. nitrates, calcium antagonists). Check BNF monographs for individual drugs
Ice cream, cold food	Usually no organic cause

common cold and tenderness of the sinus areas to light finger pressure (Figure 2.2). Fever may occasionally accompany the pain at the side of the head associated with temporal arteritis. In children, fever is one of the distinguishing factors in meningitis.

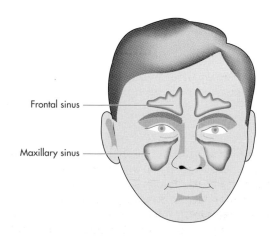

Frontal sinus

Maxillary sinus

Figure 2.2   Position of the frontal and maxillary sinuses.

Tender temples

Elderly patients can develop temporal arteritis, a condition in which either one or both of the temporal arteries is inflamed and may be seen as a red, congested vessel in the temple area, running vertically up the side of the head just in front of the ear. The patient will find that pressure applied to the skin over the artery is very painful. The patient with temporal arteritis may, rarely, have pain or an ache in the jaw, particularly after eating. This is due to obstruction of the blood supply from the cranial artery. If temporal arteritis is suspected the patient requires same-day referral for a medical opinion, as vision can sometimes be affected.

Insomnia

If a headache is severe enough to interfere with sleep the patient should seek a medical opinion, but more commonly patients will complain of early-morning wakening or an inability to fall asleep on retiring, unrelated to the headache, and this may indicate depression and anxiety, respectively. Symptoms of tiredness, poor appetite and mood changes will point to the possibility of a tension headache.

Visual disturbances

Failing vision requires referral, but visual phenomena are a common feature of classic migraine or migraine with aura, and constitute part of the aura that precedes the headache. Common migraine or migraine without aura describe migraine in which no such features are present. The visual symptoms of the aura of classic migraine can take the form of blurred vision, blind spots (scotomas), flashing lights and zigzagging. They disappear within an hour and are followed by severe headache. Nausea also frequently occurs. Restriction of the visual field, or the appearance of haloes around lights, especially in one eye only, suggest glaucoma or the optic neuritis of multiple sclerosis, and same-day referral is required. Visual loss or double vision may occur in temporal arteritis. Any disturbance of vision, unless attributable to migraine, requires urgent referral.

It is noteworthy that only 10–20 per cent of migraineurs have an aura of any description, and therefore other causes of visual disturbance resembling the descriptions associated with migraine should be borne in mind and referral made if there is any uncertainty, or if the duration is longer than 1 hour. Such causes may be acute vascular or neurological deficits such as stroke, retinal occlusion or other intraocular pathology.

Neck stiffness

Neck stiffness in an adult with headache may be related to a neck strain or injury, but it could be a sign of a traction headache. Difficulty in placing the chin on the chest is a signal to refer urgently, particularly in children and young adults, as it raises the possibility of meningitis.

Nausea and vomiting

Nausea, with or without vomiting, is present in patients with migraine, glaucoma, space-occupying lesions and meningitis. Migraine sufferers often find that vomiting occurs towards the end of an attack, and is seen as a relief and a sign that the pain is about to subside. However, effortless vomiting in the morning, associated with a headache, could suggest a potentially serious problem.

Nasal congestion and rhinitis

Nasal congestion accompanies the headache of sinusitis and is also seen in some patients with cluster headaches, together with rhinitis and facial flushing.

Central nervous system symptoms

Patients reporting signs and symptoms of central nervous system involvement require special consideration for referral. Symptoms may reflect general disturbances, such as loss of coordination and balance, drowsiness, irritability, personality changes and even fits. Sometimes the symptoms will reflect more localised lesions, for example slurred speech, muscle weakness in a limb, and disturbances of the senses of smell and hearing. Such problems may accompany the headache of space-occupying lesions, such as tumours, and also subarachnoid haemorrhage and subdural haemorrhage (as in head injuries). Paraesthesiae (pins and needles or numbness), usually in the arm, may occur as part of the aura of classic migraine, but this should disappear within a short time.

Any persistent unusual sensations require investigation, as they may be a sign of a space-occupying lesion.

All of these conditions, with the exception of migraine, are rare, particularly in terms of presentation in the pharmacy. Nevertheless, they are potentially devastating diagnoses and must constantly be borne in mind.

Rash

In children or young adults with headache the appearance of a rash anywhere on the body is a reason to refer immediately for a medical opinion to exclude meningitis. The meningococcal rash is classically purpuric, i.e. it is formed by haemorrhages from small blood vessels and leaves purple marks on the skin which do not blanch when pressed. However, in the early stages the presentation can be confusing.

Weight loss

Although the presentation in the pharmacy of weight loss (over a period of weeks or months) associated with headache will be unusual, it should always be regarded as a potentially serious sign requiring referral. It may occur in cranial arteritis and systemic disease, as well as in patients with malignancy.

Other symptoms

Premenstrual syndrome in women, which may present as a monthly cyclical headache, can also occur in a variety of symptomatic presentations, including irritability, anxiety and depression, abdominal bloating, breast tenderness, and swelling of the hands, ankles or feet.

The aura of migraine can sometimes take the form of food cravings, yawning, mood changes or paraesthesiae (sensation of pins and needles) in the arms or face.

Aggravating factors

Some of the trigger factors mentioned in Table 2.2 will aggravate a migraine attack. These explain the instinct of sufferers who like to lie down in a quiet, darkened room during an attack.

Frequency

Headaches that occur daily are rarely migraine. They are most likely to be due to tension or analgesic overuse.

Special considerations in children

As with all illnesses it is difficult to obtain an exact history from a child, and young children who feel ill may well describe their malaise as a headache without head pain being a feature at all.

Special attention should be paid to the possibility of a head injury, as young children receive more than their fair share of knocks.

Neck stiffness, which could be a sign of meningitis, should immediately alert the pharmacist to refer the patient, but this symptom may be hard to elicit in young children. Meningitis is often notoriously difficult to diagnose, even by doctors, and it is essential that pharmacists should take the time to find out whether a child looks ill or behaves oddly, appears drowsy or irritable, or is vomiting or failing to feed.

The popular conception of meningitis is that of a sudden severe illness which is fatal if not immediately treated. This is true of the rare epidemic meningococcal forms. Rash is a danger signal, but the symptoms do not all develop together and the 'warning' signs often occur relatively late on. The time from the first appearance of symptoms to a stage when the chance of survival is severely compromised can be as short as a few hours. However, viral meningitis often has a more insidious onset and could easily present – particularly in its early stages – in the pharmacy. Great caution is therefore advised in children with headaches. Where any doubts exist, same-day or more urgent referral (depending on the duration and severity) is mandatory.

Children can suffer from migraine, which can start below the age of 10 years, but its onset is more common between the ages of 11 and 15, often around the time of puberty. The symptoms are similar to those experienced by adults, but are usually shorter lasting. Abdominal pain tends to be more prevalent than in adults, and an aura is often present.

Management

Removal of the underlying cause

Once serious pathology has been eliminated, consideration should be given to removing any possible predisposing factors or triggers. It should be emphasised that exercise-induced headache, such as migraine, should be alleviated not by avoiding exercise, but by carefully increasing personal fitness so that the exercise threshold that causes the headache can be raised.

Patients should be encouraged to persist for a week or so with any newly prescribed drugs suspected of causing the headache, as often an adjustment period is necessary, but this will depend on the severity of the headache. In most cases, alternative drugs will be available.

Non-drug methods

The treatment of chronic or repeated headaches, such as tension headache and migraine, lends itself to many types of non-drug therapy, such as massage, acupuncture, osteopathy and hypnotherapy.

OTC drugs

It is easier to prevent a headache or reduce its duration by acting early, rather than trying to treat one that has already developed. This is particularly true for migraine.

Tension headaches should be treated with simple analgesics for a limited period of about 14 days before considering referral.

Anyone suspected of having medication overuse headache should be encouraged to stop taking analgesics even when they are suffering the pain. This is to allow washout of the analgesic from the body. Support from family and friends is very important at this stage.

The response of individual patients to simple analgesics is variable for both pharmacological and psychological reasons.

Pain is a subjective, emotional symptom, and the treatment of chronic headache should be holistic rather than restricted to the symptom itself. The placebo effect is a valuable adjuvant to medication under such circumstances, and a sympathetic ear and reassuring counsel will often help to alleviate the anxiety felt by some patients.

Soluble and effervescent formulations of analgesics, especially aspirin, will reduce the likelihood of gastrointestinal adverse effects. No clear correlation exists between the rapid attainment of so-called therapeutic blood levels and the onset of pain relief after the ingestion of soluble tablet formulations, but the powerful placebo effect of effervescent tablets should not be ignored. They are also a rational choice in patients with migraine, as the reduced gut motility associated with this condition is thought to reduce and delay the absorption of drug from standard tablet formulations.

Citric acid, present in some effervescent formulations, can enhance aluminium absorption and produce toxicity in patients with chronic renal failure who are taking aluminium salts as a phosphate binder.

Paracetamol

Paracetamol, aspirin and ibuprofen have similar analgesic activity, but paracetamol lacks the anti-inflammatory effects of the non-steroidal anti-inflammatory drugs (NSAIDs). Paracetamol is a suitable analgesic to recommend when aspirin is contraindicated, and generally enjoys a reputation as a safe drug in therapeutic doses. Interactions with warfarin have been reported, but at present there is not enough evidence to suggest avoiding its use in anticoagulated patients at normal doses.

Paediatric formulations of paracetamol are recommended for children.

Non-steroidal anti-inflammatory agents

Aspirin is one of the oldest OTC drugs and provides adequate analgesia in most situations. It has anti-inflammatory properties and is therefore suitable for musculoskeletal causes of headache. Aspirin is contraindicated in children under 16 years of age because of its association with Reye's syndrome. It should not be recommended for patients with a history of peptic ulcer or dyspepsia. Five per cent of asthmatic patients are hypersensitive to aspirin, and in its most severe form this allergy can manifest as a life-threatening asthmatic attack.

Aspirin has been widely used in pregnancy but may cause problems in late pregnancy, and paracetamol is regarded as the analgesic of choice.

Aspirin should not be recommended for patients who are taking anticoagulants, nor for those already taking other NSAIDs.

NSAIDs such as ibuprofen are effective in most types of headache. The actions and contraindications of ibuprofen are similar to those of aspirin, but it may cause less gastric toxicity.

Combination products

Products that contain aspirin, paracetamol and codeine in various combinations can be seen as a second-line approach for use when single-agent products fail to alleviate symptoms. Although the evidence for increased clinical analgesia with these drug combinations is minimal, particularly with codeine at a dose of 8 mg, there is a tendency for both the public and health professionals to consider them as more powerful than single agents. This is not totally irrational, and no doubt their use is successful in the management of many patients.

Codeine can cause constipation, and continued dosing should be avoided where this might be problematic, such as in the elderly.

Caffeine is often present in analgesic combinations and is claimed to potentiate the activity and the absorption of analgesics. The data to support the clinical significance of these actions are equivocal and, theoretically, caffeine can be harmful, as it can stimulate the secretion of gastric acid (enhancing the irritant effect of aspirin) and cause central excitation (counteracting the desire to obtain relief of headache by rest or sleep in some patients, particularly in migraine).

Feverfew

Feverfew is a herbal remedy that has had variable success in the prophylaxis of migraine in clinical trials. It can be regarded at best to be of modest benefit, but some patients appear to do well on it. It has definite activity on prostaglandin synthesis, which may partly explain its pharmacological action in migraine. Feverfew is contraindicated in pregnancy because of its stimulant effect on uterine muscle.

Special considerations

Migraine

Gastric motility is reduced during a migraine attack and it is thought that this causes impaired absorption of oral analgesics. It is therefore essential that analgesics be taken at the first sign of an attack, preferably in the form of a soluble or effervescent product to expedite absorption. This is an important point to stress to patients in order to maximise the effect of treatment.

Some proprietary products that are recommended specifically for migraine contain antihistamines, such as cyclizine and buclizine, which are included presumably for their antiemetic effect. Also, some antihistamines do have analgesic activity, and their inclusion in migraine products may be logical in this respect.

Dental pain

Dental pain can be partially or temporarily alleviated by simple analgesics, although persistent pain will not be affected and requires referral to a dentist (see Chapter 16). Following dental surgery, however, aspirin should be avoided because of its antiplatelet activity, which may prolong bleeding.

Drug interactions

Major drug interactions between OTC analgesics and prescribed drugs are highlighted in Table 2.3.

Second opinion

Doctors find the symptom of headache as confusing, and at times worrying, as everybody else. It is common, and there are often no readily available investigations to help in diagnosis. Serious causes are rare, but do exist and will always be in mind.

A clear history is essential. Taking time to identify the features of the headache as outlined in this book will often be the most useful guide

Table 2.3   Interactions between OTC analgesics and prescribed drugs

OTC analgesic	Interacting drug	Consequence
Aspirin	Anticoagulants, e.g. warfarin	Extended clotting time, potential haemorrhages
Aspirin Paracetamol Codeine	Prescribed drugs and combination products containing the same individual components, e.g. co-codamol	Additive toxicity
Aspirin	Methotrexate	Renal excretion of methotrexate reduced
Ibuprofen	Lithium	Renal excretion of lithium reduced

to differentiating it. A neurological examination may follow, but is most often normal. Tenderness over the frontal sinuses may indicate congestion or infection, although if mild may be due to muscular tension. Similarly, spasm felt in the muscles of the back of the neck may be due to tension, or to cervical spondylosis. Tenderness over the temporal arteries at either side of the head may indicate an arteritis.

Raised blood pressure can cause headache, although not as often as is usually assumed. It is commonly measured.

Visual disturbance is always significant, and can be crudely checked for using the Snellen chart found in most consulting rooms. The retina provides a view of a small part of the cranial circulation, and raised intracranial pressure may be reflected in changes in the optic disk. In mild but chronic headache the patient may be advised to have an optometrist check their visual acuity formally.

Persistent headaches, or those where the diagnosis remains in doubt, are often investigated. Blood tests, such as a full blood count, and tests of renal and hepatic function may (when normal) offer reassurance that no serious organic pathology exists. Plain skull X-rays are sometimes done, looking for intracranial calcification,

a rare sequela of long-standing lesions, or evidence of distortion of the cerebral contents, such as is discernible in acute ones.

CT (computed tomography) or MRI (magnetic resonance imaging) scans offer the best views of the brain, but can only be used practically on the few people who require a full neurological investigation. Those with acute and serious headaches will be admitted to hospital, where a lumbar puncture, which draws a small quantity of cerebrospinal fluid from the spinal cord, can show the pressure within that space as well as the presence of infection (meningitis, encephalitis), and suggest other lesions, including malignancies. All are, fortunately, rare.

Bibliography

Fontebasso M (2004). Diagnosis and treatment of chronic daily headache. *Prescriber* 5 February: 13–20.

Steiner T (2001). Guide to the current management of migraine. *Prescriber* 5 November: 62–80.

Steiner TJ, Fontebasso M (2002). Headache. *Br Med J* 325: 881–885.

SUMMARY OF CONDITIONS PRODUCING HEADACHE

Chronic daily headache

A descriptive term used for headaches that occur on a near-daily basis. The most common cause is analgesic overuse, when the condition may be termed medicine misuse headache. Medicine misuse headache may develop within a few weeks in some individuals, but in others may take up to a few years to develop. All types of simple analgesic may be implicated, such as paracetamol and NSAIDs, as well as triptans. Headache must be present in the first instance and chronic use of analgesics worsen it over time.

The pain often seems to be present from waking until going to bed at night, and does not respond to analgesics. Chronic use of analgesics results in the sensitisation of more pain receptors, and a vicious cycle develops.

Withdrawal from analgesics for several weeks is necessary to effect a cure.

Dental pain

Dental pain, especially pain emanating from the jaw, can radiate to the head.

Glaucoma

An increase in intraocular pressure can cause headache, pain from within the eye, haloes around lights, defective vision, red eye, dilated pupils and vomiting – **refer.**

Haemorrhage

Subdural haemorrhage may follow a head injury. Symptoms may appear immediately, or at any time for several weeks. They worsen progressively, and as well as headache there may be drowsiness and sometimes numbness on one side of the body – **refer.**

Subarachnoid haemorrhage is not usually associated with head injury. It occurs suddenly, like a devastating blow to the occipital area, often causing collapse. The patient will show obvious signs of confusion and will be severely ill – **refer.**

Meningitis

Most common in children, but also occurs in teenagers and young adults. Symptoms include headache, fever, photophobia, nausea or vomiting, irritability or drowsiness, confusion and neck stiffness. Skin rash (often appears late) presents as bruise-like spots that do not blanch on pressure. The patient may deteriorate over a few hours and become very ill – **refer.**

Migraine

Classic migraine

This is characterised by an aura that lasts for up to 1 hour preceding the headache. The aura consists of mainly visual disturbances, such as blurred vision, blind spots or flashing and zigzag lights. Sometimes there is numbness or paraesthesiae, usually in an arm. After the aura the headache develops, initially on one side, but it may spread quickly to become bilateral. It lasts for several hours and is usually accompanied by nausea and sometimes photophobia. The attack often ends with the patient vomiting. A period of resolution follows, during which the patient may feel tired and lethargic, before recovery is complete. Migraine attacks usually recur at intervals of more than 1 or 2 weeks. Now often known as migraine with aura.

(continued overleaf)

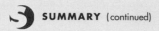 **SUMMARY** (continued)

Common migraine, or migraine without aura
Ninety per cent of migraineurs suffer from common migraine, which resembles the classic type except that there is no aura.

Cluster headaches
These are so called because they occur in clusters, lasting an hour or two, at the same time of day or night, and recur every day for several weeks. The pain is usually around one eye and there is lacrimation and/or a congested or runny nose.

Migraine can often be alleviated by simple analgesics. If unsuccessful, medical referral should be made to consider use of the many drug treatments available on prescription only.

Premenstrual syndrome (premenstrual tension)
A syndrome that presents in women in a variety of forms, often with headache. It is characterised by its regular cyclical appearance, usually commencing 7–10 days before menstruation and disappearing – or at least improving – when bleeding occurs. Other common symptoms include irritability, anxiety and depression, loss of concentration, abdominal bloating, breast tenderness, swelling of the hands, feet or ankles, and weight gain.

Refractive errors
Patients requiring correction of vision or suffering from eyestrain may suffer from headaches.

Shingles (herpes zoster infection)
Infection of nerve tracts in the face or scalp with the herpes zoster virus causes a rash accompanied by shooting pain. Severe pain, often over an eye or one half of the scalp or face, occurs and may persist for several weeks after the rash has healed (postherpetic neuralgia) – **refer.**

Sinusitis
Headache may be unilateral or bilateral, and is often accompanied by a head cold or nasal congestion. There may be a green, purulent nasal discharge. The skin over the sinuses (around the orbit of the eye) is sensitive to pressure applied by the fingers.

Space-occupying lesion (e.g. brain abscess, tumour)
Headache is caused by a raised intracranial pressure owing to the expanding intracerebral mass. The pain may at first respond to simple analgesics, but becomes progressively more severe over several weeks. It is accompanied by other central nervous system disturbances (depending on the part of the brain involved), such as mood change, drowsiness, slurred speech, loss of balance or coordination, vomiting, limb weakness, or strange sensations of taste or smell. The headache is classically worse on awakening and is exacerbated by the raised intracranial pressure produced by coughing, sneezing, straining, bending over etc. – **refer.**

Temporal arteritis
A disease of the elderly, temporal arteritis is an inflammation of the temporal artery, which traverses the side of the head just in front of the ear. The condition is part of a more extensive cranial arteritis, which is an inflammatory process affecting various blood vessels supplying the brain. It is usually seen in patients

→

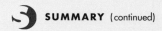

SUMMARY (continued)

who suffer from polymyalgia rheumatica, a collagen vascular disease that presents with morning joint stiffness, pain and weakness, affecting primarily the neck, shoulders, back and thighs. The head pain is usually unilateral and severe, and the temporal artery may be red, prominent and exquisitely tender to the touch. Sometimes there may be jaw pain after eating because of reduced circulation to the jaw muscles. This disease requires same-day referral, as it can lead to blindness if the ophthalmic arteries become affected. The diagnosis can only be confirmed by biopsy of the artery – **refer.**

Tension
Tension headache is the most common type in people aged under 50 years. Causative factors, such as stress, are sometimes easily elicited, but they are not always obvious. Classically, the headache is described as a tight band around the head, spreading over the top of the scalp, but its distribution can also be more vague and generalised, or located at the back of the head or around the eyes. It can persist for several weeks and is notoriously difficult to treat with simple analgesics. It usually resolves spontaneously. It may easily progress to chronic daily headache if the sufferer becomes a habitual analgesic user. Continuous treatment should therefore not be recommended beyond about 2 weeks. Tricyclic antidepressants have been reported to be helpful in some cases.

Trauma
Headache following a head injury may exist as a localised pain in the first few hours but continues as a generalised headache. It may be caused by a subdural haemorrhage (see above), concussion or fracture, and may result in disturbances such as drowsiness, dizziness, slurred speech, nausea and vomiting. The pupils may be unequal in size and may fail to react to light – **refer.**

Trigeminal neuralgia
A rare presentation, trigeminal neuralgia occurs chiefly from middle age onwards. It often takes the form of a sharp, excruciating pain on one side of the face, lasting a few seconds, and is triggered by touching a sensitive area on the face. Sometimes the pain is accompanied by involuntary movements in the distribution of the affected nerve. It is not in itself a danger to life, but it requires treatment with specific drugs such as carbamazepine – **refer.**

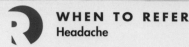

WHEN TO REFER
Headache

Onset/severity
- Sudden, explosive, patient 'stopped in tracks'   Immediate referral
- Occurring some time after a head injury   Immediate referral
- Obvious severity: disabling, patient cannot move,
  interferes with daily routine (and patient has not
  experienced this before), patient appears ill   Same day/immediate*

Frequency and duration
- Unremitting
- Progressively worsening over weeks
- Short duration but worsening over days

Accompanying symptoms
- Nausea/vomiting (unless due to migraine)   Same day/immediate*
- Neurological signs, e.g. paraesthesiae, mood
  change, drowsiness, slurred speech, loss of
  balance, irritability and poor coordination   Same day/immediate*
- Visual disturbance (if migraine has been excluded)   Same day/immediate*
- Pupils unequal in size or not responding to light   Same day/immediate*
- Loss of consciousness   Same day/immediate*
- Jaw pain   Same day
- Tenderness over temples   Same day
- Neck stiffness   Immediate
- Rash
  – on scalp in adult   Same day
  – on skin in child or young adult   Immediate

Pattern
- Worse on awakening

Location of pain
- Temporal area   Same day/immediate*
- Focused above or lateral to eye   Same day/immediate*

*Urgency of referral is a matter of judgement, depending on the signs and symptoms.

CASE STUDIES

Case 1

A middle-aged woman presents with a headache of about 4 weeks' duration. She and her husband are going away on holiday in a month's time. How should the pharmacist respond?

The first priority is to identify the origin of the headache, or exclude serious causes. The phraseology used suggests she may have tried analgesics already, which need to be identified. Her sleep is poor and she is feeling fed up and depressed. She has tried both paracetamol and ibuprofen without success. She feels her holiday will be ruined.

Tension and depression are both a possibility, as are many other diagnoses. Her analgesic use also needs to be quantified.

One problem with headaches is that they are common symptoms of many disorders. This woman has had mounting relationship difficulties with her husband, and is depressed. The forthcoming holiday is, in her view, a 'make or break' chance, which is making her anxious. This in turn has probably contributed to her increasing analgesic use, and the whole episode is spiralling out of control.

None of the above eliminates the possibility, however rare, of serious pathology. This woman's history is of 4 weeks' duration. A recommendation for further analgesia is inappropriate, and she should have been referred to her doctor.

He found no evidence of organic pathology, and a brief prescription for an antidepressant along with relationship counselling removed the need for continuing analgesics.

Case 2

A man aged 70 requests something to relieve pain. Since retiring from the civil service he has enjoyed a peaceful retirement, although recently he has been troubled by headaches. They are vague, nowhere in particular, but becoming progressively worse with time. He is reluctant to consult his GP, believing – or at least hoping – there is nothing serious amiss.

A more detailed and systematic history adds a poor appetite, a gradual loss of weight, and feeling tired and vaguely unwell for more than 6 months. There are few specific symptoms, but he has become increasingly breathless in the last 4–6 weeks.

A definitive diagnosis cannot be deduced from this history, although it is suggestive of a progressive disease. He must be persuaded to see a doctor.

In this case, unfortunately, the underlying cause was a progressive renal failure, for which no remedial cause was found.

Case 3

A woman in her mid-40s reports 'tension headaches'. She has had them before, often premenstrually when she feels stressed. Recently they have become bad enough to need treatment.

The headache is usually left sided. The onset is insidious, but she senses when one is imminent. She often feels nauseated.

The obvious suspicion is of classic migraine, or migraine with aura. The description is not completely typical in that the aura is undefined and the onset is gradual, but is sufficient to warrant a second opinion. On this occasion the woman has requested immediate assistance with pain relief. She has tried paracetamol without effect. An analgesic designed specifically for migraine may help her.

The diagnosis is likely, but not definite. She was given a suitable preparation, which she later reported had helped, but was also encouraged to consult her doctor. The availability of modern prescription-only medicines was offered as possible motivation for her to see her GP, and one was subsequently prescribed.

3

Cough

Cough is a reflex that is stimulated by irritation of the respiratory mucosa in the lungs, the trachea or the pharynx. It is often a reaction to infection or contamination of the respiratory tract and is a protective mechanism to clear the airways of contaminants.

It may sometimes be desirable to encourage a cough, and sometimes to suppress it.

The most frequent cause of a cough in the developed world is an upper respiratory tract infection such as the common cold, but other common causes include allergies and exacerbations of chronic obstructive pulmonary disease.

Types

A cough may be broadly described as either productive – i.e. producing sputum – or non-productive (dry), with no sputum, and questioning along these lines will enable the pharmacist to narrow the list of possible diagnoses. The duration of a cough is also helpful in eliciting the possible cause.

Assessing symptoms

Productive or non-productive

A non-productive cough may be described as dry, tickly or irritating. It produces no sputum, and generally the pharmacist can be reassured that the cause is unlikely to be bacterial infection, although this must be considered along with other symptoms. In some circumstances patients will deny bringing up any sputum, although they will say that they can feel phlegm on their chest. In such cases, the cough is best regarded as productive rather than non-productive.

Non-productive coughs are irritating, not only to the patient, but also to those who live or work with him or her. They occur as a typical response to damage to the upper respiratory tract epithelium caused by viral infection, smoking (active and passive), a dry atmosphere, air pollution (especially in the workplace) or a change in temperature. They may also be a feature of some serious conditions such as asthma or lung cancer, or an adverse reaction to drugs, e.g. ACE inhibitors.

In a patient with a productive cough, the appearance of the sputum can be helpful in eliciting the severity of any underlying cause.

Sputum

Clear or white sputum can generally be considered as being of little significance, unless produced in copious amounts.

Thick yellow, green or brown sputum, or foul-smelling sputum, suggests a lower respiratory (i.e. lung) infection, such as bronchitis, but this is not always the case and sometimes may just represent cell debris being cleared from the airways. Clear, straw-coloured sputum may be seen in disorders of allergic origin, such as some forms of asthma, the yellow tinge being caused by the presence of large quantities of eosinophils from the blood as part of the allergic response.

Blood in the sputum (haemoptysis) may be seen as either copious fresh blood, spots or streaks, and may sometimes colour the sputum brown. It should be regarded with suspicion and referral for further investigation suggested, as it may be a sign of pulmonary embolism, tuberculosis, bronchitis or lung cancer. Check that the blood does appear to be coming from the lung and not from the mouth, throat or nose (caused by trauma, such as nose blowing).

Pink and frothy sputum is sometimes seen in heart failure, where there is congestion of blood in the lungs and some leakage of plasma into the air spaces.

Patients with pneumonia typically produce rust-coloured sputum at first, which may progress to being bloodstained.

Duration and frequency

Coughs may be broadly classified as acute, usually referring to a duration of less than 3 weeks, or chronic, lasting more than 8 weeks. Between 3 and 8 weeks there is a period in which the cough can be described as subacute. Obviously, at first appearance all coughs will be acute, but sufferers will seek advice at different times after onset, and this makes it possible to decide whether self-treatment or referral is more appropriate.

Coughs are usually self-limiting. Viral infections of the upper respiratory tract are the most common cause of acute cough, caused by stimulation of the cough reflex by postnasal drip or clearing of the throat. Any patient with a cough that has lasted more than 2 or 3 weeks without improvement requires referral. A cough that started as a common cold but which has persisted longer than 3 weeks is most likely due to persistent postnasal drip, which is self-limiting, bacterial sinusitis or asthma. Chronic coughs are best referred, as they may be due to chronic lung disease. Recurrent coughs may indicate a serious problem requiring referral. For instance, patients with chronic bronchitis suffer a persistent cough for more than 3 months in the year, and patients with bronchiectasis have recurrent chest infections and require antibiotics. Cigarette smokers often have a recurrent cough, which may be due to chronic bronchitis, and they should be examined by their doctor to exclude infection or lung damage.

A long-standing or recurrent cough, especially in patients over 40, may be a sign of more sinister disease such as lung cancer. Persistent cough may also be an adverse effect of some drugs (see later).

Onset and trigger factors

Coughs may be triggered by various factors, such as a change in ambient temperature, irritants such as cigarette smoke, or simply by taking a deep breath. The onset of a cough may be sudden, acute and devastating, causing collapse or serious illness, as is the case in pneumonia. More often, however, the onset is slower and less dramatic. If it occurs at night and is accompanied by catarrh it may be caused by a postnasal drip (see below). The cough of bronchitis or bronchiectasis is worse on awakening.

Most coughs are worse at night, but special care should be taken to identify a dry night-time cough in children, which could possibly be due to asthma, and night-time cough and breathlessness in adults, which indicate possible pulmonary congestion, as seen in heart failure.

Accompanying symptoms

Nasal congestion, sore throat, fever, myalgia

Cough is commonly associated with or preceded by symptoms of the common cold or influenza-like illnesses. In such cases it is invariably nothing more than a simple viral infection, which may be treated symptomatically with over-the-counter (OTC) drugs.

Shortness of breath, difficulty in breathing (dyspnoea)

These symptoms should alert the pharmacist to refer the patient to the doctor. Such symptoms may be progressive over a number of months or years, indicating chronic bronchitis, emphysema, heart failure or other serious disease, or they may be recurrent, as in asthma, when the characteristic wheeze may be heard. A sudden onset of breathlessness occurs in pneumothorax, pulmonary embolism and pleurisy.

Chest pain

The lung tissue itself has no sensory pain fibres. Pain felt in the chest caused by respiratory disease can arise from the pleura, trachea, bronchi, or the vascular supply. Such pain always requires immediate referral. Pain felt on deep inspiration or coughing may be caused by pleurisy or pulmonary embolism. Intercostal muscle strain following a coughing bout also produces these symptoms and can be difficult to distinguish from pleuritic pain.

Fever

Fever and sweating in a patient with cough suggests infection.

Weight loss

A dramatic loss of weight suggests the possibility of serious disease, such as tuberculosis or lung cancer.

Painful calf

Pain in the calf muscles, possibly associated with swelling in the calf or ankle, may be caused by a deep vein thrombosis; there may also be signs of skin inflammation. The thrombus may break up and be transported by the circulation to the pulmonary artery, where it will lodge as a pulmonary embolus, causing a pulmonary infarct. Chest pain is the predominant feature, along with shortness of breath, but a cough may also be present.

Special considerations: age

In patients over 40, especially if the cough has been present for many years, serious lung disease should be considered. The possibility of chronic bronchitis and some of the consequences of repeated infection and damage to the lung, such as bronchiectasis and emphysema, should alert the pharmacist to refer the patient, especially when other symptoms suggest a serious diagnosis. In patients of this age, especially if they are smokers, the possibility of lung cancer should always be considered.

Children between the ages of about 4 and 8 years may suffer from the catarrhal child syndrome. Such patients experience repeated colds and catarrh, often accompanied by earache. At night, catarrh may run down the back of the throat, irritating the pharyngeal mucosa (post-nasal drip) to produce a cough. Treatment is symptomatic. The child and its parents should be reassured that antibiotics will be of no use and that the episode will be self-limiting, although recurrence is likely until the child grows out of the condition at about 8 years of age. Obviously, any doubts about a child who appears ill or who has had a cough for a number of days should prompt a referral to the doctor.

Young children between the ages of 6 months and 2 years who wake in the middle of the night with a barking or croaking cough may be suffering from croup. Symptoms usually abate the next morning, but may recur the following night. If breathing is noisy (stridor) or there is a wheeze, urgent referral is required. Croup can cause narrowing of the airway because of oedema and so should be taken seriously. The condition can be difficult to differentiate from epiglottitis, in which the child appears ill, has difficulty in breathing and stridor, and attempts to sit or lean forward to breathe. Epiglottitis is a rare condition but is potentially very serious. On inspection of the throat a bright pink lump may sometimes be seen at the back, behind the tongue. If suspected, epiglottitis requires an emergency referral to hospital.

Drug-induced cough or breathlessness

A drug history can sometimes elicit the cause of a cough. For example, ACE inhibitors cause a dry cough in some patients owing to inhibition of the breakdown of bradykinin in the lungs. Clinical trials state the incidence of ACEI-induced cough to be up to 10 or 15 per cent of patients, although many GPs estimate it to be significantly higher. Pharmacists should wait for 4 weeks before referring anyone who is taking an ACEI to the GP to try and differentiate the cause of the cough. Beta-blockers may precipitate heart failure, characterised by breathlessness, with or without a cough.

Management

There is a plethora of proprietary OTC cough medicines and making a suitable choice can present some difficulty to both the pharmacist and the potential consumer. Doubts have been cast on the pharmacological activity of cough medicines, and it seems that it makes little difference to the course of a cough whether such a medicine is taken or not (see Bibliography).

Like any other 'trivial' symptom, a cough with no serious underlying cause will be self-limiting and will disappear spontaneously within a few days. However, public expectations are high, and if someone comes into the pharmacy complaining of a cough then there is a role for a 'cough bottle', even if the evidence suggests that it is little more than a placebo. Clinical studies have shown that some people will find a cough remedy helpful, even if the actual clinical benefit may be questioned. This gives pharmacists the option to recommend that patients try an OTC cough medicine, if they want to. Thus a form of words could be constructed that will acknowledge the pharmacist's awareness of the negative evidence base while not discouraging people who might want to try a cough medicine. This in turn should encourage a dialogue between health professional and patient and allow the patient to retain some choice in managing their symptoms.

It should be borne in mind that many cough preparations do contain drugs with recognised pharmacological activity, even if the clinical significance is unproven. It is pertinent, therefore, that the pharmacist consider some logical rationale when choosing a product containing a mixture of drugs to give symptomatic relief.

The cough mechanism

The cough reflex is a protective mechanism, and in many cases interference with it may delay its disappearance or exacerbate the underlying disturbance that caused it.

The reflex has three nervous components: (a) receptors in the mucosa of the respiratory tract are sensitive to chemical or mechanical stimulation and activate the discharge of afferent impulses along cholinergic (vagus) nerve fibres to (b) the cough centre in the brain stem; (c) efferent impulses from the cough centre are then transmitted along cholinergic nerves to cause contraction of the diaphragm, abdominal and intercostal muscles, resulting in a rapid expulsion of air from the lungs, taking with it mucus and irritating particles on the surface of the respiratory mucosa.

OTC drugs

The active ingredients of cough medicines can be broadly classified into three groups.

Cough suppressants

Cough suppressants can usefully provide symptomatic relief of a dry, irritating or tickly cough that produces little or no sputum. Such a cough may be caused by an irritable mucous membrane in the upper respiratory tract resulting from oedema of the mucosa in the pharynx following a sore throat, or from mucus dripping from the postnasal space, which irritates the pharynx and trachea (postnasal drip).

Non-productive cough is common in tracheitis, in viral infections such as the common cold, and in chronic bronchitis, at times where little sputum is produced. Care should be taken in recommending a cough suppressant to patients with known chronic obstructive pulmonary disease, as the cough reflex is essential to clear the airways of mucus.

Non-productive cough can be distressing and exhausting, preventing sleep at night and irritating other people by day. Cough suppressants may act at different sites in the cough pathway.

Centrally acting cough suppressants Centrally acting cough suppressants act on the cough centre in the brain and reduce the discharge of impulses down the efferent nerves to the muscles that produce coughing. Examples are codeine, pholcodine and dextromethorphan. All are capable of causing sedation (though allegedly less so with dextromethorphan), and long courses will give rise to constipation and may produce dependence. Thus, short courses only should be recommended.

Pholcodine and dextromethorphan reputedly have fewer adverse effects and less abuse potential than codeine, although this is unlikely to be of clinical significance in normal, short-term use.

Antihistamines Antihistamines probably owe their antitussive properties more to their intrinsic anticholinergic activity than to any effect on histamine. They reduce the cholinergic transmission of impulses in the nervous pathway of the cough reflex and thus act as a cough sedative or suppressant. Examples of antihistamines commonly present in cough medicines include diphenhydramine, triprolidine and promethazine.

Antihistamines are not suitable for a productive cough, on pharmacological grounds. Arguments that they are unsuitable for patients with asthma because they may increase the viscosity of bronchial secretions are controversial and may not be of clinical significance. They are particularly helpful when a cough and a head cold coexist, as the antihistamine will also dry the nasal secretions that may cause a postnasal drip and initiate coughing.

Antihistamines used in cough medicines can cause sedation, and because of their anticholinergic properties they should be avoided by patients with narrow-angle glaucoma or an enlarged prostate gland.

Demulcents Demulcents, such as honey, glycerin and syrup, are said to act by coating the pharyngeal mucosa, which may be inflamed, and offer some protection from irritants such as smoke or dust particles. Their efficacy probably relates largely to a soothing placebo effect, but the demulcent effect on the mucosa may be a real one and may also serve to hydrate the delicate mucosal tissues. Where postnasal drip occurs, demulcents may reduce irritation of the pharyngeal mucosa.

Expectorants

Expectorants have traditionally been used to increase bronchial secretions and thus reduce the tenacity of mucus, which can then be coughed up. They have a place in cough therapy, but their efficacy is controversial owing to the lack of strong supportive, objective data, although there is considerable subjective support for their use.

Plugs of mucus and debris in the small airways can cause breathing difficulties and act as sites of infection, and patients who attempt to remove sputum they can 'feel' in their chests may become exhausted by coughing if the mucus is so viscous that it adheres to the mucosal lining of the lungs. There are therefore good reasons for trying to facilitate expectoration.

Hydration of the airways will facilitate adequate production of non-viscous mucus from the glands lining the lungs. This can be simply and effectively achieved by drinking plenty of fluid, so that the tissues remain hydrated, as well as by humidifying the inspired air with steam inhalations.

The addition of substances such as menthol or compound tincture of benzoin (Friar's balsam) to the hot water providing the steam is probably of no extra value except for a psychological effect (which should not be undervalued).

One theory of how expectorants have their effect is by irritating the gastric mucosa, which produces a reflex stimulation of the bronchial tree. The latter responds by secreting more mucus.

Ammonium salts Various ammonium salts have been used over the years and the chloride is still used, albeit less commonly than previously.

Guaifenesin This agent is present in many proprietary cough medicines, although the dosage varies considerably. It would be logical to recommend doses of 100–200 mg for maximum effect.

Ipecacuanha At subemetic doses ipecacuanha stimulates the gastric mucosa and is used as an expectorant.

Other expectorants Citric acid and sodium citrate have expectorant properties, but in the doses used these are probably weak. Squill is an old-established medicine that may be found in some proprietary cough remedies. Liquid extract of liquorice, capsicum, terpin, menthol and eucalyptus oil also appear in proprietary cough medicines.

Bronchodilators

Sympathomimetic agents such as ephedrine and pseudoephedrine are used to relax bronchial smooth muscle. They are also useful as nasal decongestants, and can therefore be recommended when a cough and nasal congestion occur together. Because of their vasoconstrictor effect, sympathomimetics are best avoided by hypertensive patients, those with heart disease, or those taking beta-blocking drugs or MAO inhibitors.

Theophylline is available as a constituent in OTC remedies in the UK. Its exact mode of action is unclear, but it is an effective bronchodilator. The effective and safe dosage is very variable between patients and requires individualisation. The small amounts of theophylline present in proprietary formulations are most likely subtherapeutic for most adults in the doses recommended, but they do at least appear to be safe. However, inquiry should always be made as to whether patients have been prescribed theophylline by their doctor; if this is the case, they should not take any more in OTC medicines because the additive effect of further doses could be toxic.

Combination cough mixtures

Many cough remedies contain mixtures of agents, often from different pharmacological classes. This in itself is perfectly acceptable, provided that individual constituents do not interact in an adverse manner. Unfortunately, this has not been the case with some OTC cough medicines in the past, and some appeared totally illogical from a pharmacological point of view. Fortunately, the number of such irrational combinations has declined in recent years. It might be argued that because there is little clinical evidence to support the efficacy of the individual drugs used, then the selection of one mixture in preference to another will be of no consequence. If, however, we are to have any faith in the preparations on the pharmacy shelves, it is imperative that the pharmacist's product recommendation does have some pharmacological rationale. For example, combinations of expectorants and cough suppressants, or expectorants and antihistamines, are irrational. If a cough is productive and requires an expectorant, then it should not be suppressed at the same time. Similarly, antihistamine drugs will reduce bronchial secretions by an anticholinergic mechanism and this is pharmacologically antagonistic to the effect of an expectorant. Some combinations are entirely logical. For example, a mixture of a bronchodilator and an expectorant, or a bronchodilator and a cough suppressant/antihistamine does not present any obvious pharmacological antagonism (see Tables 3.1 and 3.2).

Special considerations

Children and pregnant women   Because of the self-limiting nature of the majority of coughs and the controversial efficacy of cough medicines, it is advisable to recommend only demulcent syrups to young children and pregnant women. In some instances, where a child has an irritating cough, an antihistamine, such as

Table 3.1   Examples of pharmacologically rational cough mixtures marketed in the UK

Suppressant	Bronchodilator/decongestant	Antihistamine
Dextromethorphan		Triprolidine
Dextromethorphan	Ephedrine	
Dextromethorphan	Pseudoephedrine	Diphenhydramine
Dextromethorphan	Pseudoephedrine	Triprolidine
Codeine	Pseudoephedrine	Diphenhydramine

Table 3.2 Examples of pharmacologically irrational mixtures

Expectorant	Suppressant	Antihistamine
Ammonium chloride		Diphenhydramine
Guaifenesin		Brompheniramine
Guaifenesin	Codeine	
Guaifenesin		Triprolidine

promethazine syrup, will serve the double purpose of suppressant and sedative, to allow the patient (and the parents) to have a good night's sleep.

Patients with diabetes   Except in patients with poor control of their diabetes, short courses of cough medicines containing sugar will have no clinically significant effect in either insulin-dependent or non-insulin-dependent diabetes. If there is any doubt, however, there are a few sugar-free cough medicines that can be recommended. Pharmacists should remember that patients with insulin-dependent diabetes may require more insulin when they have a bacterial or viral infection, even if they have lost their appetite. This is because excess adrenaline and other hormones with an anti-insulin effect are secreted in response to the stress of the infection.

Drug interactions   Major drug interactions between the ingredients of OTC cough medicines and prescribed medicines are shown in Table 3.3.

Second opinion

The symptom of cough is one of the commonest presented to GPs, especially during the winter months. Many patients will consult their pharmacist before or after the GP.

A doctor's initial estimation is based on the history, previous medical history and overall assessment as outlined in this chapter. A physical examination is usual, and often a simple examination of the chest with a stethoscope offers the necessary confirmation. The sounds of both

Table 3.3 Interactions between OTC cough medicines and prescribed drugs

OTC product	Interacting drug	Consequence
Antihistamines	Anxiolytics	Enhancement of sedative and
	Hypnotics	CNS depressant effects
	Sedatives	
	Alcohol	
Antihistamines (because of intrinsic	Phenothiazines	Enhanced anticholinergic effects,
anticholinergic properties)	Tricyclic antidepressants	e.g. blurred vision, dry mouth
Sympathomimetics	Antihypertensive therapy	Reduced antihypertensive effect
	MAOIs	Hypertensive crisis
	Tricyclic antidepressants	Hypertension
Theophylline	Cimetidine	Increased blood levels and risk
	Erythromycin	of theophylline toxicity
	Quinolone antibacterial agents	

inspiration and expiration can be clearly heard, much as they are 'from the outside', and should be the same all over with no added sounds. These may be crepitations, moist crackling noises implying the presence of fluid or exudates in the airway, or rhonchi – whistling, often musical, noises caused by air passing through narrowed airways, and thus common in asthma. Reduced air entry, when breath sounds are diminished or even absent in one part of the lungs, occurs when there is a disease process (e.g. inflammation or obstruction, perhaps by a tumour).

Further confirmation can be sought from auscultation – literally tapping the chest – often with one finger on another. A normally cavernous air-filled space beneath produces a hollow response, a more solid sound a sign of gross inflammation, exudate, or a pleural effusion interrupting the transmission.

The standard investigation is the plain chest X-ray. Air does not reflect X-rays and so provides a contrast against which the heart and major vessels, ribcage and larger airways can be seen. It is most often used to exclude serious pathology in recurrent, persistent or suspicious cases when the development of chronic obstructive airway disease or even carcinoma is feared.

A qualitative assessment of chronic obstructive pulmonary disease (COPD) and of asthma may be assisted by spirometry. In its most basic form the peak flow meter measures the patient's ability to expel air from the lungs, and hence airway resistance. It is used both to diagnose and to monitor asthma.

A spirometer produces a more detailed display, often graphically, of this forced expiratory volume (FEV) against time, and the total forced vital capacity (FVC), basically tells how much air the lungs will hold and how effectively it can be replaced.

The commonest response to a chest infection is the prescription of an antibiotic, usually a short course of a broad spectrum agent. As with upper respiratory infections, the prescriber cannot often be sure that the organism responsible is bacterial, and which antibiotic is going to be effective, but the consequences of allowing the condition to worsen by waiting, and the high probability of primary or secondary bacterial infection, particularly in recurrent cases, is usually sufficient justification.

General practitioners have only a limited number of prescribable linctuses at their disposal in the UK and so they are sparingly used.

Inhaled steroids and a variety of both short- and long-acting bronchodilators are widely used in both asthma and COPD, and short-acting beta-2 agonists may be tried to relieve the bronchospasm associated with acute infections, especially in the young.

Bibliography

Schroeder K, Fahey T (2002). Systematic review of randomised controlled trials of over the counter cough medicines for acute cough in adults. *Br Med J* 324: 329–331.

SUMMARY OF CONDITIONS PRODUCING COUGH

Asthma

Asthma is characterised by wheezing, caused by bronchoconstriction, hypersecretion of mucus and inflammation of the bronchi. There is difficulty in breathing, particularly on expiration, so that patients feel that they cannot remove all the air from the lungs.

Asthma may be caused by allergens (extrinsic asthma) or may show no relation to obvious allergens (intrinsic asthma). It may be triggered by respiratory infection, air pollution, or drugs such as beta-blockers. Acute attacks are sudden in onset, common during the night, and in children may present as a persistent dry cough. Attacks are usually relieved within a couple of hours. The sputum may be straw coloured because of the presence of eosinophils. Note that although wheezing is classically present, asthma can sometimes present solely as a cough, without wheezing – **refer.**

Bronchiectasis

Repeated infections of the lung, such as occur in chronic bronchitis, will eventually lead to irreparable tissue damage. If such damage affects the terminal bronchioles, they become dilated and distorted in shape and their normal mucosal lining is replaced by scar tissue. This scar tissue cannot transport oxygen from the air in the lung to the blood, leading to increased respiratory distress. Cough is persistent and the sputum is purulent, more plentiful in the morning, and occasionally bloodstained. Inflammation and mucus plugs in the small bronchioles predispose to episodes of pneumonia. There is also weight loss – **refer.**

Bronchitis

Acute bronchitis is an infection of the bronchi which is usually bacterial and should be treated with antibiotics.

The bronchial tree is formed of the trachea, main and smaller bronchi, branching into bronchioles and finally to the alveolar tissues. The airways are a succession of passages that decrease in size, and it can be difficult to identify exactly where the infection is, although it is important to do so. The term bronchitis is thus often used to cover several conditions. Tracheitis is common in adults and as it involves the largest airway is rarely serious. The same may be true in children, although the smaller lumen of the corresponding airway must always imply caution, as significant narrowing and obstruction are more likely.

Bronchiolitis is common in children, and, inflaming the terminal and narrowest airways, produces a harsh persistent cough and can be associated with respiratory distress. The overall illness of the child makes medical referral mandatory, and may be urgent.

Acute bronchitis may occur secondarily to upper respiratory viral infections, such as the common cold and influenza, or as an exacerbation of chronic bronchitis. Cough and chest soreness are present and the sputum is purulent. Patients will have chest tightness, wheezing or difficulty in breathing. Often fever is present and occasionally the sputum may be bloodstained – **refer.**

Chronic bronchitis results from repeated trauma to the lower respiratory tract and is often the result of recurrent attacks of acute bronchitis. As well as infection, it may be caused by irritants such as tobacco smoke, atmospheric pollution, dust and irritants in the working environment. Social factors, such as overcrowding in the home, damp, or poor air conditioning, may predispose to chronic bronchitis. It is characteristically seen in middle age and beyond, and is more common in men than women. The patient will have had acute attacks of bronchitis that have increased in duration and severity over the years. Gradually the cough fails to disappear between acute attacks and becomes persistent, often referred to by the patient as a smoker's cough.

(continued overleaf)

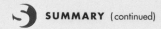 **SUMMARY** (continued)

The classic definition of chronic bronchitis is the production of sputum on most days over at least 3 months for 2 consecutive years. Damage to the lungs occurs and the patient has permanent symptoms, such as breathing difficulties, wheeze and shortness of breath. The disease may progress and cause death, or it may become clinically static – **refer.**

Cancer of the lung
Cough, weight loss and dyspnoea are common symptoms of lung cancer. It is more common in men than in women, usually appears between the ages of 50 and 70 years, and is seen more often in cigarette smokers. Cough may have been present for some time in smokers, but any change in its character is a signal to refer. Blood in the sputum is commonly seen – **refer.**

Chronic obstructive pulmonary disease (COPD)
This collection of conditions includes chronic bronchitis, bronchiectasis and emphysema.

Croup
The term 'croup' is used loosely by both medical and non-medical people to encompass a variety of symptoms associated with an irritant cough in children. Properly used, the term describes an infection (usually viral) of the larynx and trachea which leads to oedema and narrowing of the airway. There is a severe and violent cough, which is often paroxysmal (occurring in bouts). The child often has difficulty in breathing between bouts, and stridor (noisy inspiration) is often present. The condition requires urgent medical appraisal – **refer.**

Emphysema
The recurrent trauma of infection and inflammation, as occurs in chronic bronchitis, can cause hyperinflation of the alveoli, leaving balloon-like processes called bullae which are unable to transfer oxygen efficiently across the lung wall. The bullae disintegrate progressively. Dyspnoea occurs, first on exertion and ultimately at rest, with other symptoms such as wheezing and a productive cough. If the bullae are ruptured at the surface of the lung into the pleural space, a pneumothorax may ensue – **refer.**

Gastro-oesophageal reflux disease (GORD)
This is an uncommon cause of chronic cough and may present with a cough either alone or together with heartburn, oesophageal reflux and oral regurgitation. It is usually diagnosed by various tests and a trial with antacid therapy such as a proton pump inhibitor.

Pneumonia
Pneumonia is usually caused by bacterial infection, producing inflammatory changes (consolidation) in the lung tissue. It has a sudden onset, with a high temperature and cough, and the patient rapidly becomes ill. Chest pain will develop because of inflammation spreading to the pleural membranes that line the lung and chest wall. This pain, characteristic of pleuritic pain, is worse on deep inspiration and on coughing. The cough is initially unproductive, but as the disease progresses, purulent rust-coloured and, later, bloodstained sputum is produced. Viral pneumonia, which often follows an upper respiratory infection, is more insidious in both onset and course; it should be thought of when a cough or other respiratory symptoms persist – **refer.**

→

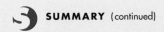 **SUMMARY** (continued)

Pneumothorax

The lung is normally held against the thoracic wall by a negative pressure in the pleural space that 'sucks' it out to assume the shape of the thoracic cavity. If the pleural envelope is ruptured, air enters into the pleural cavity, neutralising the negative pressure, and as a result the lung collapses. This is a pneumothorax. It occurs without warning and for no apparent reason, particularly in healthy young men, as well as in bronchitis or emphysema. It gives rise to a severe, unilateral chest pain which may be either constant or pleuritic in nature, and there may be some dyspnoea. The pain may be felt over the shoulder or sternum and may resemble that of angina or myocardial infarction – **refer.**

Pulmonary embolism

Pulmonary embolism is caused by a thrombus that has formed elsewhere and has detached itself from its primary site (e.g. a deep vein in the calf of the leg) and has been carried by the circulation to the lung, where it lodges in the pulmonary artery. The arterial lumen is blocked, causing lung tissue supplied by the artery to die (pulmonary infarct). The clinical picture is one of sudden onset chest pain and some dyspnoea; there may be blood in the sputum. Cough is a minor feature – **refer.**

Tuberculosis

Tuberculosis is a disease of slow onset and in its early stages the symptoms are often mild. The tubercle bacillus is spread by inhalation of airborne droplets from an infected person. Tuberculosis is common in developing countries but does also occur in the UK. It is often overlooked in the elderly because of its insidious onset and its resemblance to bronchitis and congestive heart failure. Symptoms include a persistent cough, blood in the sputum (not always), fever or night sweats and weight loss. People at risk include the elderly, those who have contact with known cases, immigrants (especially from India) and alcoholics – **refer.**

Upper respiratory tract infection

Cough is a common accompaniment to viral infections, such as the common cold and flu-like illnesses. Irritation of the larynx and trachea by upper respiratory infection or a postnasal drip can cause a cough. The condition is generally self-limiting.

Whooping cough

Although now rare because of immunisation programmes, whooping cough does still occur in children, usually those under 5 years of age. The condition may present initially as a cold, and after a few days a cough develops, occurring at around hourly intervals. After about a week a whoop is heard on inspiration following a spasm of explosive coughing. The cough produces a plug of thick sputum, and is accompanied sometimes by vomiting. The patient will be frightened and distressed. The whoop may last for several weeks or months – **refer.**

Miscellaneous

Various relatively rare lung diseases are worth mentioning to highlight some of the possible causes that pharmacists should be alert to.

Fibrosing alveolitis is a chronic disease that causes reduced lung function, dyspnoea and cough. It is often autoimmune in origin. Rarely it may be due to drugs, the most commonly implicated being amiodarone. Nitrofurantoin and cytotoxic drugs have also been reported to cause the condition – **refer.**

(continued overleaf)

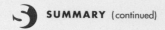

SUMMARY (continued)

Bird fancier's lung and farmer's lung are allergic conditions caused by inhalation of a protein in bird droppings (e.g. from racing pigeons) or of spores of a mould found in stored hay. Again, the picture is one of reduced lung function and cough – **refer.**

WHEN TO REFER
Cough

- Wheezing
- Dry night-time cough in children
- Difficulty in breathing, shortness of breath, breathlessness
- Any concurrent illness or history where infection may be a risk, depending on the severity of symptoms, e.g. chronic respiratory conditions, heart failure or immunosuppression
- Recurrent cough or constant smoker's cough, except where the doctor has given the patient specific guidance for action at a previous consultation
- Chest pain, either uni- or bilateral, particularly if exacerbated on coughing or deep inspiration
- Sputum is purulent, i.e. unusual colour (green, brown) or foul smelling*
- Sputum is bloodstained
- Concurrent medication includes ACE inhibitors
- Weight loss, particularly in patients over 40
- Painful or red, inflamed calf
- General malaise, feeling systemically unwell, persisting sweats or fever
- No improvement of symptoms after 14–21 days, depending on severity, or a deterioration in the condition with time

*Note that green sputum is commonly present in viral infections and may sometimes not justify referral, provided there are no other referable signs or symptoms. Purulent postnasal drip may also be mistaken for sputum, which would not normally require referral.

CASE STUDIES

Case 1

A man in his mid-50s is known to the pharmacist through his visits for two or three prescriptions of antibiotics a year for chest infections, usually during the winter months. He has also spoken about nicotine replacement therapy in the past. He has a heavy industrial occupation in a dusty factory, which probably does nothing to improve his health.

On this occasion he visits about 2 weeks after being prescribed an antibiotic for another chest infection, and says he is much improved but still coughing. The cough is no longer productive but sounds moist and 'rattly', and he feels there is still 'something down there'. He asks for a bottle of cough linctus.

We need to know more about this man's history.

Was there a cough before this infection started?

Does it really appear to be resolved, or might a short course of treatment be inadequate and a relapse occur?

Has he been able to comply with the treatment fully?

Are there any other symptoms, e.g. pain or haemoptysis, that might raise suspicion?

This man went to his GP initially; now he is consulting a pharmacist. Most usually, this is an appropriate understanding of the role of the pharmacist and the range of products available.

As far as possible, other fears must be discovered.

A long-term smoker with recurrent 'winter bronchitis' is always at risk of developing more sinister pathology, and of delay in diagnosis due to the familiarity of his symptoms. Any change, deterioration or unexpected lack of resolution should be referred.

This might also present a good opportunity to enquire as to his current smoking status. Health advice is always most effective when relevant to an immediate problem, and at a time such as this a friendly discussion about smoking cessation might be productive. (See chapter 17 'Smoking cessation')

Case 2

A woman in her late 70s is receiving a regular prescription for digoxin and warfarin. She now has 'a chest cold', and asks for a linctus to help her sleep.

Modern clinical practice is to anticoagulate people with atrial fibrillation. This has undoubtedly prevented many cerebrovascular events, but carries with it certain hazards and the need for careful monitoring.

Although this woman is well enough to visit the pharmacy, more information is needed before suggesting an appropriate course of action, including the duration and severity of symptoms, and in particular any effect on her already compromised cardiovascular system. It would be worth exploring exactly what is disrupting her sleep.

If possible, the stability of her anticoagulation should be considered. Febrile illness and infection can sometimes affect warfarin control, although the effects are of short duration. Unless she coincidentally already has an appointment within the next few days for an INR or can easily arrange a blood test within the next day or two, there is probably little point in making this investigation.

This woman may very well have exactly what she believes, and a pharmacy recommendation for a simple cough medicine can safely be made. The pharmacist needs to be sure she does not have a chest infection requiring medical assessment, and is aware of this possibility in the future.

It is also important to consider her symptoms separately from her own 'diagnosis'. A cough, and perhaps breathlessness on lying in bed, could suggest the infection has precipitated a degree of heart failure which, knowing her prescribed medication, could be a distinct possibility.

(continued overleaf)

CASE STUDIES (continued)

Case 3

A fit 25-year-old man comes into the pharmacy. 'Nothing serious', he explains, 'certainly nothing to keep me off work'. He thinks he has hay fever, the season being appropriate, and the symptoms are of rhinitis, a little wheeze on exertion and a fever, but he feels that it is nothing to worry his doctor about. Although he has a sedentary job, he plays a lot of sport, works out in the gym and prides himself on his health.

What else do we need to know?

A history of this illness should be taken, including its duration and progression, and other features. In this case the man does not look well and is in some discomfort. During conversation it transpires that he has in fact been febrile for 2 days, with an upper respiratory infection at first but now an increasingly painful dry cough, with pain on inspiration and movement, and breathlessness on minimal exertion. He has not seen his doctor, nor is particularly eager to do so. His level of physical fitness and attention to his own health come in part from a belief that illness can be avoided or at least self-managed, and a visit to the doctor is seen almost as a defeat.

A cough that is painful is suspicious. It commonly arises from repeatedly straining the intercostal muscles, and although more significant causes such as pleurisy are rare, they need to be excluded.

Doctors often enquire as to the colour of expectorated sputum. It is a crude judgement, white or yellow possibly suggesting catarrh, green or 'dirty' colours bacterial infection, and a dark colour more serious still. There is little evidence and many exceptions to these associations, although any detective avails himself of all the clues presented. The presence of blood is, however, more significant.

This man must be persuaded to see his doctor, for not only is it impossible to eliminate a serious chest infection, it seems very likely that he has one. He returned later that day from his doctor's walk-in clinic with a prescription for a potent antibiotic, a certificate for work for 2 weeks, and an appointment for follow-up the next morning. On examination the GP found widespread crepitations, crackling noises superimposed over the normal breath sounds, and diagnosed an acute bronchitis, which could have resulted in hospital admission had he not contacted his doctor and started treatment promptly.

4

Sore throats and colds

Conventionally, although somewhat arbitrarily, the respiratory system is divided into an upper and a lower part. For practical purposes, the lower respiratory system can be considered as comprising the lungs, the bronchial tree and associated tissues, and the upper respiratory system comprises the larynx and all tissues above it. Thus, a cough is essentially a lower respiratory problem, whereas head colds and sore throats are upper respiratory disorders.

Colds and sore throats, which often occur together, are common and are usually caused by viral infections. The major symptoms under consideration are sore throat, nasal congestion, catarrh, sneezing and rhinorrhoea (runny nose). Table 4.1 shows the range of common conditions affecting the upper respiratory tract.

Assessing symptoms

Sore throat

A sore throat is generally a self-limiting condition.

Examining the back of the throat by asking the patient to open the mouth as wide as possible and then stick out the tongue will reveal on each

Table 4.1 Differential diagnosis

Sore throat				Rhinitis		
		Examples				Examples
Infection	Viral	'Cold'		Infection	Viral	'Cold'
		Influenza				Influenza
		'Glandular fever'				Sinusitis
		Tonsillitis				
		Pharyngitis				
	Bacterial	Tonsillitis			Bacterial	Sinusitis
		Peritonsillar abscess				
		Pharyngitis				
	Fungal/yeast	Diabetes				
		Inhaled steroid				
	Other	'Vincent's angina'				
				Allergy	Seasonal	'Hay fever'
					Perennial	
					Specific	Animal, food, etc.
					Obstructive	Polyp
						Foreign body
Irritant		Smoking				
		Overuse of voice				

side of the throat the anterior and posterior pillars of the fauces, between which the tonsils are situated (Figure 4.1). It is not possible to distinguish between the appearance of a viral infection and a bacterial infection, although it is thought that at least 70 per cent of sore throats are caused by viruses and are therefore not suitable for treatment with antibiotics.

Thus in the majority of cases, pharmacists have an important role in educating the public, thereby reducing the number of inappropriate visits to the GP. However, there is still an important role in checking the need for referral when certain warning signs or symptoms are present, as described below.

It is worth pointing out that antibiotics were introduced into general practice between the two world wars at a time when severe conditions such as quinsy (peritonsillar abscess), mastoiditis (infection of the mastoid air cells in the middle ear) and rheumatic fever were all common. Widespread antibiotic use, and public health measures, caused the incidence of these three conditions to decline to the state of extreme rarity seen today. Thus, severe sequelae to sore throats are now so rare that the value of antibiotics is questionable, especially as in most cases the cause is viral. Without a throat swab to confirm whether the cause is viral or bacterial, prescribing decisions are made on subjective criteria, which will vary from one doctor to another. The medical profession is being urged to reduce the prescribing of antibiotics for upper respiratory tract infections. The severity of the discomfort, duration of the present condition and of past episodes, systemic upset and appearance of the pharynx may all be influential both for the doctor in prescribing and for the pharmacist in referring.

Severity

If the soft palate, fauces and tonsils are very red or swollen and there are white spots of pus on the tonsils (Figure 4.2) or fauces, the patient should be referred. The pus spots may be a sign of streptococcal infection, which could respond to antibiotic therapy.

The appearance of large, tender lymph nodes in the neck (Figure 4.3) also requires a referral for the doctor to make a decision about the need for antibiotics.

Difficulty in swallowing food or drink requires referral (see Accompanying symptoms).

Duration and frequency

Sore throats caused by either viral or bacterial infections will usually disappear spontaneously within a few days, and as such they are not serious. A sore throat persisting for more than 1 week requires consideration for referral, and if persistent for 2 weeks, the patient should be referred. In teenagers and young adults a persistent or recurrent sore throat requires referral to exclude glandular fever.

Recurrent sore throats should alert the pharmacist to various possible, but rare, causes such

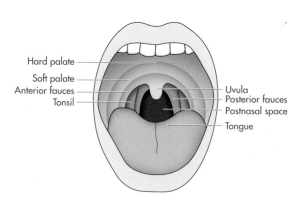

Figure 4.1   Diagram showing the position of the tonsils.

Hard palate
Soft palate
Anterior fauces
Tonsil
Uvula
Posterior fauces
Postnasal space
Tongue

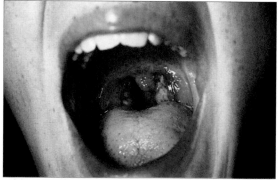

Figure 4.2   White spots of pus on enlarged tonsils.
(Reproduced with permission from Dr P. Marazzi/Science Photo Library.)

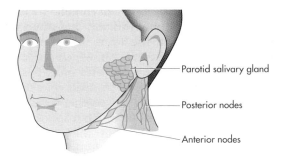

Parotid salivary gland

Posterior nodes

Anterior nodes

Figure 4.3   Main group of lymph nodes in the neck.

as immunosuppression caused by steroids (oral or inhaled) or by AIDS. Sore throat caused by drug deposition during inhalation of steroids can be reduced by advising the patient to rinse the mouth and gargle with water after inhaling.

Patients with undiagnosed or poorly controlled diabetes are susceptible to throat infections, especially those caused by fungi and yeasts, such as *Candida* (thrush). Oral thrush may be recognised by the appearance of white spots on the buccal mucosa and soft palate.

Patients should also be asked if they are taking any drugs, as some can cause bone marrow suppression, resulting in a deficiency of white blood cells and repeated infections of the throat and other organs. These drugs include carbimazole, cytotoxics, gold salts, tolbutamide, chlorpropamide, phenothiazines, antimalarials and some antibiotics. Patients taking these drugs should be referred urgently as the consequences of a lowered white cell count can be extremely serious.

Accompanying symptoms

Common cold   If symptoms of a cold are either already present or developing, it is likely that the sore throat is part of the cold syndrome, caused by a viral infection. For assessment of these symptoms, see below.

Difficulty in swallowing (dysphagia)   Anyone with a sore throat will find it less easy than normal to swallow, but if there is more than the expected degree of difficulty then a referral should be considered. In children and teenagers with throat infections, especially tonsillitis, a sensation may develop of the throat 'closing

over'. This is usually more apparent than real, but if drinking becomes very difficult or saliva cannot be swallowed, referral is advised. In extreme cases, such as quinsy, where there is an abscess on the tonsils, inflammation at the back of the throat may be so severe as potentially to restrict breathing. In very rare cases, dysphagia may be related to an obstruction in the throat or a tumour pressing on the oesophagus. It should be remembered that the reason for asking patients about difficulty in swallowing is to exclude those rare, severe cases where either the pharynx is dangerously inflamed or there is additional pathology causing obstruction that requires a medical opinion. It is often difficult to distinguish between a genuine difficulty in swallowing (dysphagia) and pain on swallowing. The latter can be expected with a sore throat and will be commonly complained of. Dysphagia, however, will be rarely encountered, and apart from indicating a problem in the pharynx could also suggest a possible obstruction in the oesophagus caused, for instance, by a tumour. A pertinent question to ask is whether the patient can swallow liquids. If the answer is negative, then a referral should definitely be made.

Painful and swollen lymph glands   Severe sore throats may be accompanied by swollen lymph glands in the neck (see Figure 4.3). Referral is appropriate if the glands are extraordinarily painful or are not improving after 5–7 days.

Sore throats are often described by the sufferer as painful, and therefore pain alone is not always a cause for referral unless it is persistent and accompanied by painful swollen glands or other symptoms that justify referral.

Earache   Infection in the pharynx can easily spread to the ear via the eustachian tube. Earache should be referred if it has not improved after 48 hours or there is a discharge, as it is not only unpleasant for the patient but may be caused by bacterial infection, which could be assessed for suitability for treatment with antibiotics.

Fever   A raised temperature may be a common accompaniment to a viral or bacterial throat infection and as such is of no great significance.

the different phytochemical compositions of the various preparations that are used. At least three different species of echinacea are used medicinally, and biological variation and the various methods of extraction used can all contribute to the difficulties in standardising and reproducing the same material for scientific study.

Garlic

Garlic has traditionally been used to treat coughs and colds and is reputed to have some immunostimulant properties, but there is little evidence of its effectiveness.

Allergic rhinitis

Some relief of allergic rhinitis can be obtained by allergen avoidance, provided the allergen is known. The measures that can be taken are no more than common sense, but are worth pointing out to sufferers, who may be too focused on hoping that a medicine is going to provide total relief. Examples are show in Case Study 4. The effects of various nasal preparations in relieving allergic rhinitis are shown in Table 4.4.

Oral antihistamines

The first-generation antihistamines such as chlorphenamine, diphenhydramine and promethazine are well known for their sedative and anticholinergic effects, but have been largely superseded by the second-generation drugs such as loratadine, cetirizine and acrivastine, which are less likely to cause sedation. The second-generation antihistamines are more effective in relieving sneezing, itching and rhinorrhoea than nasal congestion.

Topical antihistamines

Nasal sprays and eye drops are available containing azelastine and levocabastine. They have a rapid onset of action compared to oral antihistamines (15 minutes, compared to 1–3 hours). The nasal sprays are effective in relieving nasal itchiness, runny nose and sneezing, but not so effective for nasal congestion. This is because they have some anticholinergic activity and dry up secretions. Nasal decongestants or intranasal steroids can be used with the antihistamine if necessary to relieve congestion.

The antihistamine antazoline is available in combination with the sympathomimetic xylometazoline as eye drops for the relief of itchy, allergic conjunctivitis. Patients should be warned that antihistamine eye drops can cause temporary local irritation.

Intranasal steroids

Nasal sprays containing steroids, such as beclometasone (twice a day) and fluticasone (once a day), are effective in alleviating rhinorrhoea, itchiness and sneezing as well as nasal congestion in allergic rhinitis via a local anti-inflammatory effect. They may take several days to exert maximum effect and should be used regularly as a prophylactic measure. They can be used as combination therapy with an oral or topical antihistamine – the latter used for intermittent flare-ups and the steroid spray for the persistent symptoms.

Cromoglicate

Sodium cromoglicate eye drops are available for the relief of the symptoms of allergic conjunctivitis, such as itchy and runny eyes.

Table 4.4   Effect of types of nasal preparations in relieving nasal symptoms of allergic rhinitis

	Rhinorrhoea	Sneezing	Itchiness	Congestion
Oral antihistamines	++	++	+++	+
Intranasal antihistamines	++	++	++	+
Intranasal steroids	+++	+++	++	+++
Intranasal decongestants	0	0	0	+++

Diet

Dietary interventions are of unproven value in relieving allergic rhinitis, but there is no harm in an individual trial, such as eliminating dairy products.

Second opinion

The medical management of sore throats is in most instances unscientific. Without being able to swiftly determine the causative agent, current medical opinion is that antibiotics are rarely indicated and that symptomatic relief is the aim. However, a small proportion of infections will be bacterial and occasionally potentially serious, and a common rule of thumb is to treat when on clinical grounds they appear to be significant. Thus a high fever, the discovery of exudates on the tonsils or fauces, or palpable cervical glands, although not entirely evidence based, may encourage the doctor to prescribe antibiotics. If the symptoms are of short duration the prescription may be given, to be used only if they persist or worsen. Understandably, different doctors will have their own thresholds for intervention.

Of course, if there are signs of complications at the consultation, such as a major restriction in swallowing or the visualisation of a potential abscess, a medical emergency may result and the patient be admitted to hospital for intravenous antibiotics and possible surgical drainage. Fortunately, such instances are rare.

Simple colds go largely untreated, in any real sense. Where reassurance is insufficient analgesia may be advised, as may be vasoconstrictor nose drops or antihistamines – the last in an attempt to help the catarrh, or at least to offer the patient something. Fifty years ago the psychologist Michael Balint described 'the doctor as a drug', and the power of the placebo remains.

The doctor's main role is therefore to satisfy himself that a cold is the only diagnosis and that there is no sign of a lower respiratory infection or extension to the ear, sinuses or elsewhere that would need separate evaluation. In the very young, where a history is unobtainable and examination difficult, treatment may occasionally be required prophylactically.

Bibliography

Barrett BP, Brown RL, Locken K *et al* (2002). Treatment of the common cold with unrefined Echinacea. A randomized, double-blind, placebo-controlled trial. *Ann Intern Med* 137: 939–946.

Brust JCM (2003). Editorial comment: Over the counter cold remedies and stroke. *Stroke* 34: 1673.

Cantu C, Arauz A, Murillo-Bonilla LM *et al* (2003). Stroke associated with sympathomimetics contained in over-the-counter cough and cold drugs. *Stroke* 34: 1667–1673.

Del Mar C, Glasziou P (2003). Upper respiratory tract infection. *Clin Evidence* 9: 1701–1711.

Watson N, Nimmo WS, Christian J *et al* (2000). Relief of sore throat with the anti-inflammatory throat lozenge flurbiprofen 8.75 mg: a randomized, double-blind, placebo-controlled study of efficacy and safety. *Int J Clin Pract* 54: 490–496.

Yale SH, Liu K (2004). *Echinacea purpurea* therapy for the treatment of the common cold: a randomized, double-blind, placebo-controlled clinical trial. *Arch Intern Med* 164: 1237–1241.

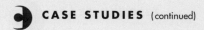

The diagnosis of hay fever has been made by the patient and it seems reasonable to accept this from the history. If she has not used any medication in the past, some education is appropriate.

The girl reveals that she is 16 years old. This means that intranasal steroids cannot be recommended as they are only licensed for over-the-counter use in adults over 18. The pharmacist recommends her to try a non-sedative oral antihistamine for 1 week to judge how it suits her in terms of effectiveness and tolerability. With examinations coming up, it is important to relieve her symptoms and also to avoid any drowsiness.

It is important to discuss ways in which she can avoid exposure to the suspected allergens.

Some empathy with the student at examination time and sensible advice about reducing the exposure to allergens will be helpful. Although they may not be evidence-based measures, they will appear to be sensible and will give her a psychological lift at a time when she may be feeling utterly miserable.

Avoidance measures can be advised, such as staying in the house when the pollen count is high, keeping windows closed, avoiding parks and fields and obvious areas where pollen, especially after grass cutting, will be abundant. When she does go outside, the use of sunglasses should be encouraged and she should wash her hands and face on returning home. If there is a pet in the house, its fur should be wiped down after it has been outside.

A trial with a filter mask that covers the nose and mouth, though not highly fashionable, can be effective, especially if someone's activities cannot be confined indoors. Although not of particular relevance in this case, it is a useful tip for outside tasks in the garden such as grass cutting. For females the use of a scarf to cover the mouth and nose will be more cosmetically acceptable.

5

Eye disorders

Because of the emotive overtones surrounding eye disease, some pharmacists may consider it inappropriate to treat any condition affecting the eye. However, by following the normal protocol to establish the history of the disorder and applying some common sense, it is relatively easy to decide whether a medical referral is necessary (see Table 5.1).

Types

Generally, eye conditions presenting to pharmacists will be disorders either of the eyeball itself or of the eyelids. These can be broadly classified as:

- The painless red eye
- Inflammation of the eyelids
- Disorders of tear formation or drainage
- The painful eye
- Eye disorders which are a manifestation of a more generalised disease.

Foreign bodies in the eye requiring first-aid treatment will not be considered here.

The first three categories are relatively easy to recognise, usually present no immediate danger to the patient, and in most cases can be treated symptomatically in the first instance. The painful eye requires referral and patients will generally need to see a doctor reasonably urgently, according to severity. Diseases in the fifth category will usually manifest themselves with unusual signs or symptoms, so that it will be obvious to an intelligent observer that something serious is wrong. Proptosis (exophthalmos), which is the bulging of the eyes from the sockets, is common in patients with an overactive thyroid gland. Bulging of one eye, however, raises the possibility of some local pathology behind the eye and requires investigation.

Blurred or double vision may be a sign of early demyelinating disease, such as multiple sclerosis, or of a tumour in the brain. Nystagmus, which describes the continuous movement of the eye in a horizontal or vertical direction, may indicate some brain disorder. Nystagmus is also a sign of

Table 5.1 Differential diagnosis of red eye

	Symptoms	Discharge	Vision	Redness	Cornea	Pupils
Conjunctivitis	Gritty, itchy, sore	Purulent (bacterial) or clear (allergic or viral)	Normal	Bilateral	Normal	Normal
More serious pathology	Pain or photophobia	Usually watery	Reduced	May be one or both eyes	Dull or cloudy	May be normal, but can be either small or dilated

phenytoin toxicity, when serum levels of the drug exceed the therapeutic range. These types of more serious disease will be seen relatively rarely in the pharmacy. This chapter will show how to differentiate major and minor disease in the first four categories listed above.

A diagrammatic representation of the eye is shown in Figure 5.1.

Assessing symptoms

Site and type

Conjunctiva

Inflammation of the anterior eye (Figure 5.2) occurs in conjunctivitis, which is the most common cause of red eye. The conjunctiva is a thin vascular membrane that covers the anterior surface of the eyeball and folds back on itself to form the lining of the eyelid. In both allergic and infective conjunctivitis the white (sclera) of the eye is red, and this redness extends to the inner surface of the eyelids (Figure 5.3). Pulling down the lower lid will reveal a very red conjunctiva covering its inner surface, compared with the pale pink seen in a normal eye.

If both eyes are affected, and in the absence of any warning signs or symptoms, the conjunctivitis will probably have either an allergic or an infective cause.

In allergic conjunctivitis there will be no pus, but there is usually a watery discharge, which distinguishes it from that caused by bacteria. (see Accompanying symptoms). The commonest cause of allergic conjunctivitis is hay fever.

Allergic conjunctivitis is often seen in young people, in whom any allergic predispositions are more evident. The patient is commonly female, and the cause is often eye cosmetics, although soaps, cleansers and powders applied to the face can also provoke a reaction.

Hypoallergenic preparations will still affect some people and the condition will only clear after total avoidance of cosmetics around the eyes.

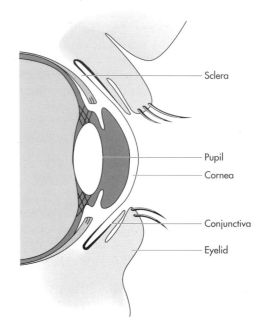

Figure 5.2   Horizontal cross-section of the anterior eye.

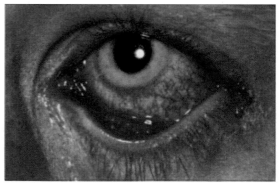

Figure 5.3   Conjunctivitis. (Reproduced with permission from St Bartholomew's Hospital/Science Photo Library.)

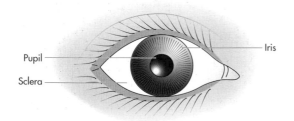

Figure 5.1   Anterior view of the eye.

Conjunctivitis commonly affects both eyes, although one may be affected more than the other. A unilateral red eye is more likely to be related to a condition within the eye, such as iritis (inflammation of the iris) or glaucoma. In such cases the redness typically occurs more around the centre of the eye, close to the iris, and is largely absent from inside the lids, compared to the more peripheral redness of an allergy or infection. However, it is often difficult to distinguish the conditions on this basis.

In wearers of contact lenses conjunctivitis can be caused by a scratched cornea, a reaction to a lens solution, a poorly fitting lens or corneal drying.

A subconjunctival haemorrhage, caused by a burst blood vessel, appears as a red spot or may cover the white of the eye (Figure 5.4). Although it can provoke much anxiety in the sufferer, it is harmless and will heal spontaneously without treatment, provided that no accompanying symptoms are present.

Patients who complain of dry eyes may require artificial tears (as eye drops). This condition is seen as a complication of certain disorders, such as rheumatoid arthritis (Sjögren's syndrome), and in oestrogen deficiency, as occurs in menopausal women. It is wise to refer patients with dry eyes to eliminate corneal ulceration or any other pathology.

A diagnosis of conjunctivitis can only be made after associated pain and vision disturbance have been eliminated (see Accompanying symptoms).

Eyelids

Inflammation of the margin of one eyelid is likely to be caused by a small abscess or stye (an infection of a hair follicle gland at the base of an eyelash; Figure 5.5). The inflammation will be localised at first but may spread to involve the rest of the eyelid, which will become tender and painful. After 1 or 2 days the stye will usually come to a head and may burst, or may simply shrink and resolve. Those that do not resolve may require surgical excision.

Redness and irritation of the eyelid margins (affecting one or both eyes), often with scales adhering to the base of eyelashes, occurs in blepharitis (Figure 5.6). This is commonly associated with seborrhoeic dermatitis or dandruff, or it may be allergic, in which case concurrent conjunctivitis may also be noticed. More rarely, it

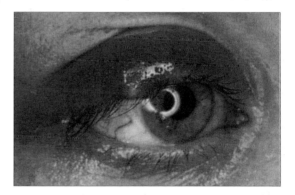

Figure 5.5   Stye on the upper eyelid. (Reproduced with permission from Western Ophthalmic Hospital/Science Photo Library.)

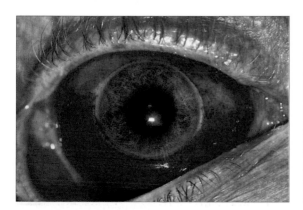

Figure 5.4   Subconjunctival haemorrhage. (Reproduced with permission from Science Photo Library.)

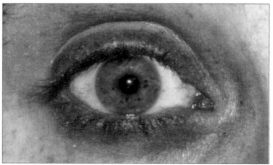

Figure 5.6   Blepharitis, inflammation of the eyelid. (Reproduced with permission of Cosine Graphics/Science Photo Library.)

may be caused by infection. Some eyelashes may be either absent or distorted, sometimes pointing inwards and irritating the surface of the eye. If the cause is infective, pus may be seen discharging from the base of the lashes.

Displacement of the eyelids may be seen, particularly in the elderly. In such cases, the margins of the eyelids do not come together when the eyes are closed. Spasm or atony of the orbital muscles causes the lids either to invert (entropion; see Figure 5.10) or to evert (ectropion; see Figure 5.11). In the former the lid margins and lashes point inwards and irritate the eye, whereas in the latter the lower lid falls away from the eye, offering it insufficient protection and lubrication. In ectropion, the drainage of the tear film is deranged and tears roll down the face.

A hard pea-like lump appearing under the skin of the lid, most commonly the upper lid, away from the margin, will probably be a meibomian cyst (chalazion). They may also be found in the lower lid, and can be visualised by pulling down the lower lid to reveal a small lump resembling an internal stye under the conjunctiva (Figure 5.7). This is an infection of one of the meibomian glands, which are located deep in the cartilaginous tissue on the underside of the lids and secrete fluid on to the conjunctiva. Infection of the outlet of a gland results in blockage and inflammation in the same way that a stye forms. The cyst will normally resolve spontaneously without incident, but may recur from time to time in some patients. A persistent cyst may require surgery.

A drooping upper eyelid (ptosis; Figure 5.8) is often a sign of systemic disease, such as myasthenia gravis, and referral is essential. In babies, special measures are needed to rectify the droop to avoid reduced visual input to the brain and blindness. Ptosis is also a sign of Horner's syndrome, which is caused by a lesion in the cervical sympathetic nerve, often due to trauma, tumours or bleeds.

Retraction of the eyelids may be a sign of a bulging eyeball, which is seen in patients with an overactive thyroid gland. In a mild form it is difficult for the untrained observer to detect, but a gap of white sclera between the iris and the affected lid will be seen if the patient's eye is compared with a normal eye. The accompanying

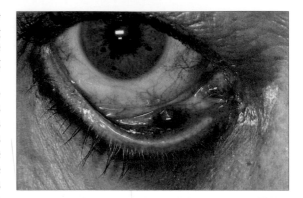

Figure 5.7 Meibomian cyst (chalazion). (Reproduced with permission from Dr P. Marazzi/Science Photo Library.)

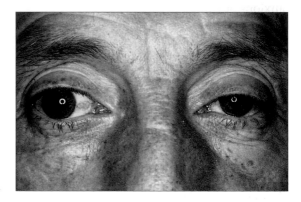

Figure 5.8 Ptosis. (Reproduced with permission from the Wellcome Trust Medical Photographic Library.)

symptoms of thyrotoxicosis (see below) will alert the observer to the condition.

Intensity

It should be relatively easy to distinguish a superficial itching or irritation of the conjunctiva on the eye surface from a more intense pain caused by pathology within the eye itself. Any such pain, which may be accompanied by the other symptoms or signs described below, requires a medical opinion. If severe, referral should be made urgently.

Duration

Styes and bacterial conjunctivitis will normally resolve spontaneously within a few days and can be helped by over-the-counter (OTC) medicines.

Viral conjunctivitis may last for 1–2 weeks. There is no specific treatment and it will eventually resolve spontaneously. Patients should be told to report any worsening of symptoms or the appearance of pain or deterioration of vision, as these may indicate a rare involvement of the cornea.

Meibomian cysts and subconjunctival haemorrhages may take a few weeks to disappear, but will do so without the need for treatment. Entropion and ectropion will usually have been present for a long time when brought to the attention of the pharmacist and will require no urgent treatment, although referral for a medical opinion may be appropriate if the patient is anxious or worried.

Blepharitis that has not responded to appropriate OTC remedies within 7 days should be referred for treatment with antibiotic eye ointment, as a delay may result in the condition becoming chronic.

Any pain within the eye or any visual disturbance requires same-day referral to a GP or hospital emergency department to exclude serious disease.

Accompanying symptoms

Pain

Itchiness, grittiness and soreness on the surface of the eye are common symptoms of minor superficial conditions, such as conjunctivitis. These symptoms should be distinguished from a deep-seated pain arising from within the eye, which indicates possible serious pathology, such as a raised intraocular pressure (glaucoma) or iritis, and requires urgent referral. Similarly, trauma such as flash burns (in welders working with oxyacetylene burners) and corneal injury will cause severe pain.

A feeling of grittiness on the surface of one eye will frequently be caused by a foreign body.

Nasal symptoms

Conjunctivitis accompanied by nasal symptoms, such as congestion, sneezing and rhinorrhoea, suggests an allergic component to the condition. A sore throat, symptoms of a cold or general malaise may be associated with a viral conjunctivitis, which is usually caused by an adenovirus.

Visual disturbance

Loss of vision is a medical emergency. Disturbance of vision may be due to the visual component of migraine, in which case it is likely to be recurrent and recognised by the patient. In conjunctivitis, vision is not significantly affected because the conjunctiva does not cover the cornea and the underlying pupil, and thus light enters and penetrates the eye in the normal manner. Vision may temporarily be affected if the cornea is obscured by fluid or pus. Loss of visual acuity is often accompanied by pain within the eye, but there are exceptions, such as vascular blockage or haemorrhages in the eye, optic nerve damage, temporal arteritis (see Chapter 2) or retinal detachment, which will not be painful.

Double vision accompanied by ptosis and a headache of sudden onset suggests the possibility of an intracranial bleed and requires urgent medical attention.

Bizarre patterns in the field of vision, with haloes seen around bright lights (particularly noticed when coming out of a dark into a lit area, e.g. when leaving a cinema, or driving at night), require referral, as this is seen in glaucoma and multiple sclerosis (known as optic neuritis in the latter case). The patient should be advised to seek advice with the suspicion of multiple sclerosis left unstated, as the diagnosis may prove to be different and in any case requires careful handling by a clinician. The visual disturbances that accompany classic migraine are easily distinguishable from those described here (see Chapter 2).

Tired eyes

Complaints of tired and sore eyes may be associated with conjunctivitis; in the absence of this condition, a referral to the optometrist may be in order to check for eye strain and any defects in visual acuity.

Lacrimation

Lacrimation is associated with interrupted drainage of the tear film and in babies requires referral so that the condition can be rectified. In elderly patients it will be seen in ectropion.

Discharge

A discharge of pus that collects in the inner corner of the eye or which prevents easy opening of the eyelids on awakening is a sign of bacterial conjunctivitis. This may be unilateral, but usually affects both eyes. A clear watery discharge occurs in allergic and viral conjunctivitis.

Pupils

It is wise to carry out a simple physical examination of the eyes, especially if a serious condition is suspected. The pupils should be round and equal in size. They should react equally and oppositely to light, such that each will constrict when a light is directed at it. The pupil should remain circular as it constricts; irregularity suggests adhesions due to iritis. (This may be a previously diagnosed condition, and the patient should be questioned before assuming it is recent.) Any inequality or abnormality of size, shape or reaction will suggest serious pathology within the eye and the need for immediate referral.

A hazy or cloudy appearance to the iris or pupil may be caused by inflammatory exudate in the anterior chamber (as in iritis) or corneal oedema (as in glaucoma), and therefore requires medical referral.

Bulging eye

A rare presentation of a bulging eye (proptosis) or of retracted eyelids (upper, lower or both) may be accompanied by symptoms of an overactive thyroid, such as sweating, hot skin, flushing, tremor of the hands or fingers, weight loss despite an increasing appetite, a fast heart rate and a state of physical overactivity.

Headache

Headaches accompanying eye symptoms can occur in glaucoma, migraine and temporal arteritis. The nature of the headache will assist in differentiating these conditions.

Other symptoms

Although it is likely to be a rare presentation in a pharmacy, Case Study 2 shows that an open question enquiring about any other symptoms not related to the eye can potentially alert the pharmacist and doctor to more unusual causes of conjunctivitis. A question about whether the sufferer feels systemically unwell or has any other, apparently unrelated, symptoms is worthwhile, as is an enquiry about recent long-haul travel, whereby unusual viral and other causes may be responsible for eye infections.

Aggravating factors

Irritation by light (photophobia) may occur in many eye conditions, including conjunctivitis, corneal ulcers and iritis. Although not very helpful in differentiating eye conditions, its presence should be borne in mind as it is a feature of conditions such as meningitis and migraine.

Conjunctivitis may be aggravated by smoke, dust, pollen or cosmetics, and in some instances these irritants will be the causative factors. Contact lenses may cause conjunctivitis, which will usually respond to cleaning of the lenses or to treatment as an allergy, but in some cases where these measures are unsuccessful, referral to an optometrist is approproriate to investigate whether the symptoms are caused by lens intolerance. In any case, it is thought to be a wise precaution to refer any contact lens wearer to a doctor or optometrist to check that the lens has not caused some superficial infection or a more serious one owing, for example, to abrasion or ulceration of the cornea.

Special considerations

Age

All babies under two months old should be referred. Babies with eyes that discharge pus may have specific infections acquired during birth that require appropriate diagnosis and prescription of antibiotics to prevent serious consequences.

Older babies commonly acquire infective conjunctivitis. In their mild forms these infections are of no consequence and can be treated symptomatically by simple measures, such as bathing the eyelid margins with clean water.

Ptosis in babies requires medical attention to keep the lid open. Failure to do so will result in a lack of visual stimulation to the retina and eventual blindness.

A squint in children requires correction to prevent a 'lazy eye', which after the age of about five years cannot be rectified.

Some eye conditions are more common in the elderly and should be borne in mind when assessing an older patient. In temporal arteritis the visual loss, which will be permanent, is preceded by headaches and temporal tenderness (see Chapter 2). Glaucoma has a greater incidence in the middle-aged and elderly population.

The lens of the eye gradually becomes more opaque with age, which can cause cataracts and visual loss in elderly patients. The cornea covering the pupil and iris becomes cloudy. Although cataracts do not require urgent medical attention, referral is necessary if there is any visual loss.

Subconjunctival haemorrhages, dry eyes, ectropion and entropion are all more common in the elderly.

Contact lens wearers

Care should be taken to ensure that lens wearers are not presenting with a condition caused either by irritation due to the lens itself (see below: 'Management: Antibacterial eye drops and ointments') or to preservatives in sterilising solutions.

Management

If an eye condition does not respond to appropriate simple self-medication within 7 days, patients should usually be advised to seek medical advice. This is because some conditions may become chronic, for example blepharitis, and some may need antibiotics, for example severe infective conjunctivitis.

Antibacterial eye drops and ointments

Pharmacists will not be able to distinguish between viral and bacterial conjunctivitis, but even in viral infections antibacterial eye drops will give symptomatic relief because the eyes can feel very uncomfortable. They will also prevent secondary bacterial infection.

The agent of choice for infective conjunctivitis is chloramphenicol. It is active against the bacteria commonly implicated in eye infections, such as staphylococci, streptococci and *Haemophilus influenzae*, and should improve symptoms within 48 hours and completely resolve simple infections within 5 days.

Propamidine is also active *in vitro* against the organisms that are commonly implicated in bacterial conjunctivitis.

Care should be taken in contact lens wearers that infection has not been caused by the lens itself, as in the case of corneal abrasion or dendritic ulcer, and some may consider it wise to refer such people to the doctor or optometrist before attempting to treat such cases.

In any case, lenses must be removed for the whole treatment period with antibacterial drops, because they can cause keratitis (infection of the cornea) to develop as a serious complication. Soft lenses also cause accumulation of preservatives, with resulting irritation, and should not be worn until 24 hours after treatment has finished.

The efficacy of eye drops can probably be maximised in the treatment of conjunctivitis by 2-hourly instillation, at least for the first 2 days of treatment.

Eye ointment containing dibromopropamidine can be used overnight to treat conjunctivitis. It is also suitable as a once- or twice-daily application to the eyelid margins in infective blepharitis and styes. Styes, however, usually resolve spontaneously without the application of antibacterial preparations. Failure to reduce symptoms within 7 days requires referral to the doctor for assessment.

SUMMARY OF CONDITIONS

Blepharitis

Blepharitis is an inflammation of the glands of the margin of the eyelid, most noticeably the eyelash roots. It may be allergic in origin and a long-standing allergic reaction can often produce blepharoconjunctivitis, which is treated in the same way as allergic conjunctivitis. Blepharitis is also sometimes caused by infection. It can also be associated with seborrhoea of the scalp or face.

Cataract

A cataract is an opacity of the lens, most commonly seen in the elderly as a result of degenerative changes with age (Figure 5.9). It presents with some kind of visual impairment and usually occurs in both eyes. Surgery is the treatment of choice – **refer.**

Conjunctivitis

Conjunctivitis is an inflammation of the conjunctiva (the membrane covering the eye, except for the cornea, and the inner surface of the eyelids). It may be allergic in origin, or infective. About 50 per cent of infections are viral, the rest bacterial. The most common bacterial cause is *Staphylococcus aureus*. Most GPs find it clinically difficult to distinguish bacterial from viral conjunctivitis, for although the symptoms and signs are described differently in textbooks there is often confusion clinically. The conjunctiva is inflamed, red and oedematous (see Figure 5.3), and the patient complains of itchiness or grittiness on the surface of the eye. In infective conjunctivitis there is usually a discharge, which may be purulent. When allergy is responsible the discharge is clear or watery. There should be no pain or visual disturbance other than the transient effect of any discharge.

Infective conjunctivitis is self-limiting and there is only limited evidence of the effectiveness of topical antibiotics. Significant complications following conjunctivitis are rare.

What the doctor would do

Doctors will examine the eye mostly to attempt to distinguish between allergic and infective causes, to direct their choice of treatment. They will also need to confirm that any inflammation is confined to the conjunctiva and does not extend to the sclera, and particularly that there is no sign of deeper inflammation in the anterior chamber of the iris.

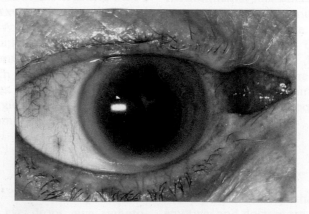

Figure 5.9   Cataract. (Reproduced with permission from
Dr P. Marazzi/Science Photo Library.)

→

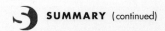 **SUMMARY** (continued)

Topical antibiotics probably do not significantly shorten the course of a self-limiting disorder, and, given the difficulty of distinguishing bacterial infections, are hard to justify with current clinical evidence. Even so, conjunctivitis may cause anxiety in the sufferer or their family, and the expectation is to treat it. Choramphenicol is still commonly prescribed, the unwanted effects being potentially serious but extremely rare, with fusidic acid and other agents used somewhat less frequently. Swabs to culture the causative agent are not often taken, except in resistant or recurrent episodes.

Corneal ulcer
Ulceration of the cornea may be caused by infection or injury and is characterised by pain (though this is not invariably present), photophobia, and either dryness or lacrimation. In severe cases there may be visual impairment. The ulcers may be visible, particularly if illuminated from an oblique side angle, when the catchlight reflects their shape – **refer.**

Dacryocystitis
Dacryocystitis is an inflammation of the lacrimal sac, which drains tears into the nasolacrimal duct, from where they are drained into the nasal cavity. An obstruction of the nasolacrimal duct or, in children, a failure of the duct to open, also results in dacrocystitis – **refer** if gentle massage of the corner of the eye does not relieve obstruction.

Dry eye
Dry eye is a chronic disorder often associated with some underlying systemic disease. The conjunctiva, sclera and cornea can be affected, causing superficial irritation and sometimes photophobia. If untreated it may lead to corneal ulceration – **refer.**

Ectropion and entropion
Occasionally, and usually in the elderly, the eyelids may become displaced. They may invert (entropion; Figure 5.10) so that the lid margins and eyelashes abrade and irritate the surface of the eye, or evert (ectropion; Figure 5.11), so that the lids, particularly the lower one, fall away from the eye, offering it insufficient protection and lubrication. In both conditions there is an overflow of tears. In ectropion the

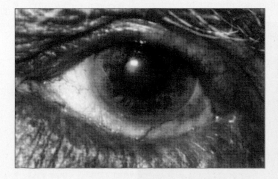

Figure 5.10   Entropion: the lower eyelid is inverted. (Reproduced with permission from the Science Photo Library.)

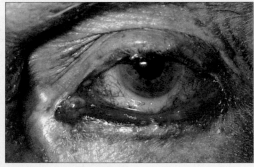

Figure 5.11   Ectropion of the lower eyelid, where the eyelid falls away from the eye. (Reproduced with permission from Dr P. Marazzi/Science Photo Library.)

(continued overleaf)

Table 6.1   Drugs causing constipation

Aluminium (e.g. antacids)
Anticholinergics
Antidiarrhoeal drugs (imprudent use)
Antihistamines (instrinsic anticholinergic activity)
Antitussives (e.g. codeine, pholcodine)
Diuretics (if dehydration occurs)
Iron
L-dopa
Opioid analgesics
Phenothiazines (intrinsic anticholinergic acitivity)
Tricyclic antidepressants
Verapamil

changes to the body, as occur in old age and in pregnancy, cause constipation.

Sometimes, constipation-dominant irritable bowel syndrome starts after a gastrointestinal illness.

Accompanying symptoms

General malaise

If the patient feels ill or unable to work while having constipation this should be regarded as unusual and a referral to the doctor made to exclude any underlying organic cause. The same applies to any fever or night sweats the patient may mention.

Blood in the stool

In the vast majority of cases blood noticed on defecation will have a perfectly innocent explanation. Blood noticed as specks or as a light smear on the toilet paper after a bowel movement is most likely to be due to haemorrhoids or a fissure in the anal canal or the skin surrounding it. Straining at stool can cause or exacerbate haemorrhoids. Fresh blood present only on the surface of the stool has most likely come from the anus or the most distal part of the colon. Blood that is mixed with the faeces, giving a dark colour, often described as tarry, may have a more serious cause, such as diverticulosis, a bleeding peptic ulcer or, rarely, a carcinoma.

Patients taking iron tablets often have a darkened stool, which is of no consequence.

Unless a previous diagnosis of haemorrhoids or a similar condition has been made by a doctor, and there has been no change in the severity of bleeding, it is wise to recommend all patients with rectal bleeding to visit their GP for assessment. If small amounts of blood are seen, as described above, which fit a known diagnosis, then the constipation may be treated by the pharmacist in the normal way for a few days.

Pain

Continuous or severe abdominal pain accompanying constipation, which has been present for 2 days or more, requires a medical opinion. In particular, the pharmacist should be alert to the possibility of obstruction in the bowel (possibly caused by a tumour). In such cases colicky pain, abdominal distension and vomiting may be present, in addition to constipation that is total, i.e. neither stool nor gas is passed.

Nausea or vomiting

The presence of nausea or vomiting with constipation should be regarded as an unusual sign and the patient referred for a medical opinion to eliminate the possibility of intestinal obstruction.

Weight loss

In common with many other disease areas, sudden weight loss for no obvious reason is a suspicious sign that requires referral for the doctor to exclude malignancy.

Diarrhoea

In young adults, alternating bouts of diarrhoea and constipation, together with abdominal pain, are typical of the irritable bowel syndrome. In elderly patients such symptoms are suggestive of spurious (overflow) diarrhoea. If irritable bowel syndrome has been previously diagnosed by the doctor, bulk-forming laxatives are useful when constipation is the predominant symptom. Failure to control symptoms in this way requires referral. Suspicion of spurious diarrhoea in the elderly requires investigation and treatment by the doctor.

Concurrent disease

Hypothyroidism can manifest as constipation, together with lethargy and slowness of movement and mental activity. Depression has been said to cause constipation, although in some cases this may be related to treatment with tricyclic antidepressants (Table 6.1).

Patients who have angina or have recently suffered a myocardial infarction may require laxatives if straining at stool causes chest pain.

Aggravating factors

Various food intolerances have been shown to cause symptoms in some patients with irritable bowel syndrome. These include wheat, dairy products, coffee, potatoes and onions.

Recurrence

Constipation that recurs without obvious cause or with increasing frequency, in the absence of any association with prescribed drugs, may reflect some underlying pathological cause, which should be investigated by a doctor.

Special considerations

Pregnancy

During the second and third trimesters of pregnancy an increased amount of circulating progesterone causes relaxation of the smooth muscle of the bowel. This, together with physical compression of the bowel by the growing uterus and the effects of iron therapy, often results in constipation. Other changes in lifestyle in pregnancy, such as reduced exercise and eating fads, increase the tendency to develop constipation. Patients can be reassured that the symptom is a natural response of the bowel to pregnancy. If dietary management is not successful, treatment is necessary with OTC laxatives, such as bulking

agents or senna, because haemorrhoids may develop if constipation is allowed to persist. Although the risk of inducing uterine contraction is theoretical, stimulant laxatives are often avoided in the late stages of pregnancy.

Age

Babies who are being breastfed normally produce fewer stools than bottle-fed babies. This is perfectly normal and does not require any intervention. Constipation in a bottle-fed baby may be caused by insufficient water being added to the milk powder. Babies or older children who become irritable, feverish or drowsy, or who scream, have pain, feed or eat less or vomit, should be referred.

As in adults, the frequency of bowel movement in children varies, but the majority pass stools at least once per day.

Most children with constipation have ways of withholding the passage of stools. Attempts to defecate are frequently accompanied by pain, causing screaming. The stools become hard, leading to straining and painful defecation, which leads to retention of stools. Common causes in children often relate to unsuitable toilet facilities at school or on holiday, or to teasing by classmates.

Older children may develop phobias about toileting, or may refuse to respond to the call to defecate in order to attract attention. This has the subconscious but desired effect of producing anxiety in the parent, who may become obsessive about the child's bowel habit.

Constipation that is more than transient should be viewed with suspicion the older the patient is, as bowel cancer becomes increasingly more common above the age of about 50.

With increasing age, muscle tone in the bowel is reduced and faecal stasis can occur. In elderly patients regularity of the bowel habit can be an obsession, and they will use laxatives not only to restore the habit to normal but also as a prophylaxis against any future possibility of constipation. This can lead to chronic laxative abuse, causing further reduction in bowel muscle tone and chronic constipation.

Constipation in the elderly should be taken seriously, as it may reflect a state of dehydration

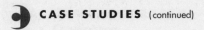 **CASE STUDIES** (continued)

Case 3

A rather nervous young man requests a medication for 'piles'.

What else do we need to know?

However embarrassing, a full history will need to be taken in private. As with all problems rarely discussed in public, the meaning of the terminology used varies. Direct and closed questioning is often needed to establish a clinical picture and diagnosis.

The history is of perianal pain during and after defecation, with a tender lump at the anal margin noticed intermittently and bleeding on a few occasions, although this has been only a smear of bright blood discovered on the paper.

The diagnosis is indeed external haemorrhoids. The presence of a lump and even minor degrees of bleeding is often the source of considerable anxiety and may need both explanation and reassurance.

This man is in his mid-20s, so the risk of malignancy is negligible.

Both haemorrhoids and anal fissures are common in the young, and a suitable topical product may safely be recommended. However, it is always worth inquiring into possible associations that could aggravate or even cause these conditions, constipation being the commonest and a frequent cause of treatment failure.

Like many, this man works long hours in an office, where he eats in the canteen; the menu is fast food, prepared well in advance, and very different from what he was served when living at home. It would be expected that appropriate topical medication would relieve his symptoms and allow healing, but only if his concurrent and long-standing constipation can be addressed. Laxatives of any sort should only be recommended for limited periods, dietary change and fluid intake being a longer-term solution, but important to improve this man's health and future wellbeing.

7

Diarrhoea

Diarrhoea is a symptom that requires a clear, quantitative description by the sufferer, as its definition will vary considerably between patients. A general definition would be a change in normal bowel habit resulting in increased frequency of bowel movements and the passage of soft or watery motions. It is often – but not always – accompanied by colicky pain. Thus, at one end of the spectrum diarrhoea may present as frequent, formed, small stools and at the other as frequent, voluminous watery motions. The difference may sometimes be useful in assessing the severity of a patient's condition.

The commonest type of diarrhoea presenting in the pharmacy is acute, and the most likely causes are dietary insults or bacterial or viral infection. The vast majority of these cases will resolve spontaneously in 2 or 3 days without any specific treatment.

Chronic diarrhoea that lasts for weeks rather than days may indicate a pathological cause. It may represent the recurrence or flare-up of a previously diagnosed disorder, such as irritable bowel syndrome, or a problem that requires medical referral for investigation and diagnosis.

About 10 litres of fluid each day pass through the lumen of the intestines of a healthy adult. Some 2–3 litres of this are ingested orally, and the rest is secreted into the lumen along the course of the alimentary tract; 8 or 9 litres of this are reabsorbed from the small intestine, so that about 1 or 2 litres reach the colon. Absorption from the colon or large bowel results in about 200 ml remaining, and this is excreted in the stool. Both the small and large intestines have spare absorptive capacity to cope with more fluid, but it can be appreciated that, with such huge volumes involved, small changes in either the absorptive or the secretory function of the gut can result in a major loss of fluid. This piece of physiology may be educative for a person who is suffering from diarrhoea and will help them to understand how the condition should be managed.

The causes of diarrhoea are listed in Tables 7.1 and 7.2.

Assessing symptoms

Severity and type

The severity of diarrhoea may be graded arbitrarily in terms of frequency, volume, duration, and the presence of particular accompanying symptoms.

Any patient who suffers severe malaise or pain with diarrhoea for more than 1 or 2 days, without any sign of improvement, should be referred.

Duration

The common acute types of diarrhoea caused by viruses or bacteria (the latter usually from contaminated food or water) generally resolve spontaneously in 2–3 days, but may take up to 5 days. A simple 'stomach upset' – the result of ingestion of toxins but without living organisms – may resolve in only 12–24 hours. It is therefore reasonable to wait to see whether improvement occurs before making any decision to refer, unless concomitant symptoms dictate otherwise.

Persistent night-time diarrhoea requires medical appraisal for the presence of inflammatory bowel disease, such as Crohn's disease or ulcerative colitis.

Table 7.1 Some causes of diarrhoea

Infections
Bacteria: *E. coli, Shigella, Salmonella and Campylobacter* are common causes of diarrhoea in the UK, due to food poisoning, and often acquired during holidays abroad
Viruses: Rotavirus is the most common cause of acute diarrhoea in young children; Norwalk virus is often the cause when large groups are affected, e.g. in restaurants or on cruise ships
Protozoa: *Giardia, Cryptosporidium* and *Entamoeba* are infections usually acquired abroad

Non-infective causes
Alcohol (excess)
Colorectal carcinoma
Dietary changes, spicy foods
Diverticular disease
Endocrine disease (e.g. diabetic neuropathy, thyrotoxicosis)
Inflammatory bowel disease (Crohn's disease, ulcerative colitis)
Irritable bowel syndrome
Malabsorption syndromes (e.g. coeliac disease)

Drugs
See Table 7.2

Table 7.2 Drugs that may cause diarrhoea

Acarbose
Antibiotics
Anticancer drugs
Colchicine
Digoxin (usually with excessive doses)
Iron
Laxatives (overuse or abuse)
L-Thyroxine
Magnesium salts in antacids
Metformin
Metoclopramide
Misoprostil
NSAIDs, especially mefenamic acid and indometacin
Orlistat
Proton pump inhibitors
SSRIs
Statins

In young children with diarrhoea the timescale for referral should be shorter than for older children or adults (see Special considerations).

Chronic diarrhoea, i.e. lasting for weeks or longer, or recurrent episodes usually indicate major pathology, requiring referral. However, in many instances the patient will have a known diagnosis, such as irritable bowel syndrome, inflammatory bowel disease, diverticular disease or some malabsorption syndrome, and they will have been advised how to treat the symptoms by their doctor.

Onset

The patient should be questioned to establish whether the onset of symptoms was associated with any particular event. Symptoms occurring within 72 hours of eating food, particularly dairy products, poultry or meat, especially if others who ate the same food have the same symptoms, suggest a bacterial cause. Onset within 6 hours of eating those foods, together with vomiting, and again, if the symptoms are shared with others who ate the same food, suggests infection with preformed toxins from bacteria.

Association with drug therapy (see Table 7.2) or particular foods should be inquired about. It may be possible to identify an intolerance or allergy to particular food items, such as mushrooms, milk or alcohol (usually beer in large amounts).

Recent travel to tropical or subtropical countries may indicate diarrhoea related to contamination of food or water (so called travellers' diarrhoea). This is usually of short duration. Persistent symptoms might signify more serious infection, such as bacterial or protozoal dysentery, cholera (bacterial) or giardiasis (protozoal).

Accompanying symptoms

Concurrent disease

In addition to previously diagnosed disorders of the bowel, other conditions may cause secondary diarrhoea. For example, hyperthyroidism and diabetes can cause diarrhoea, the latter as a result of either disease of the autonomic nerves in the bowel in long-standing and poorly controlled diabetes, or the effect of drug treatment.

Abdominal pain

Abdominal discomfort is common in patients with diarrhoea. It may present as a sharp, colicky or griping pain, produced by spasm of the smooth muscles of the gut wall and usually felt in the central region of the abdomen, and is generally of no significance. However, severe abdominal pain that is not resolving requires referral.

Rarely, abdominal pain with diarrhoea may represent irritation of the bowel by an inflamed appendix. In such cases the stools are usually not watery or profuse but merely unformed. Acute appendicitis usually begins with pain in the central abdominal region or right flank and there is right-sided tenderness. The pain is continuous, except when perforation occurs, when the pain suddenly stops for 1 or 2 hours and then starts again. The pain of appendicitis wakes the patient at night.

Left-sided pain or tenderness, accompanied either by diarrhoea alone, or sometimes by alternating episodes of diarrhoea and constipation, may be a sign of diverticular disease.

Vomiting

Vomiting and diarrhoea suggest an infective gastroenteritis caused by a virus or bacteria, the latter often from a food source. When vomiting and diarrhoea occur together there is an increased risk that the sufferer will become dehydrated if the condition does not resolve within a few days. Individual patients require appropriate advice, especially the young and the elderly. Generally babies with vomiting and diarrhoea require same-day referral, and young children and the elderly should be referred if there is no significant improvement after 48 hours.

Early signs of mild dehydration in adults include increased thirst and a dry mouth, which will respond to increased fluid intake. In babies and young children, more serious signs may be a lack of alertness, and limpness. In adults, lethargy, confusion, tachycardia and cold, clammy skin and a loss of skin elasticity or retraction of the orbit of the eye (sunken eyes) will indicate dehydration, which requires same-day referral.

Weight loss

Significant weight loss over a few weeks may be a symptom of a previously diagnosed illness causing chronic diarrhoea. However, in all cases where a diagnosis has not been made, referral is necessary to exclude tumours (particularly in the elderly) or malabsorption syndromes.

Blood and mucus in stool

Blood in the stool is usually a signal to refer the patient, especially if it is persistent. Bloody diarrhoea occurs in inflammatory bowel disease (along with the passage of mucus or pus) and cancer of the colon. A distinction may be drawn between smears of fresh blood on the surface of the stool or noted on cleaning, and blood mixed within the substance of the stool. The former is likely to be associated with a local rectal condition and may be secondary to the diarrhoea; the latter is certainly not.

Mucus in the stool is a sign of acute inflammation of the large bowel lining and may present either when there is serious pathology or when there is an acute episode of a less serious, self-remitting condition. It is thus neither diagnostic nor worrying on its own, but should be considered as a sign for referral if it persists, or if it is accompanied by other worrying symptoms, such as blood in the stool.

Frequency and urgency of micturition

Frequency and urgency of urination are commonly present when there is diarrhoea, which is essentially frequency and urgency of defecation. This is caused by the proximity of the colon and the urinary tract, and the general reflex irritability of smooth muscle in the walls of these hollow organs.

Dyspareunia (painful intercourse)

In women dyspareunia is sometimes complained of by sufferers of irritable bowel syndrome. It may be due to proximity to an inflamed or distended colon, although it can be exacerbated by stress.

Upper respiratory symptoms

Symptoms of the common cold occurring at the same time as diarrhoea suggest a viral infection.

Fever

A fever, with or without malaise, suggests infection. In adults this may be monitored for a few days, unless the patient has recently returned from a tropical or subtropical country, in which case referral is necessary to exclude diagnoses such as dysentery and malaria.

Diarrhoea alternating with constipation

In young adults episodes of diarrhoea alternating with constipation may indicate irritable bowel syndrome. In this syndrome the complaint of constipation can occur when the stool is normal in form but after evacuation the patient feels that it is still there; this is known as 'rectal dissatisfaction'. In the elderly this may be a sign of spurious diarrhoea (see Elderly, p 87). As irritable bowel syndrome is essentially a disorder of function, disturbing the normal motility of the large bowel, a common clinical pattern is one of increasingly difficult episodes of constipation eventually relieved by diarrhoea, although with stasis and distension followed by overflow the pattern is often less obvious.

Other chronic symptoms

As mentioned above, patients with a diagnosed chronic condition will often suffer from other long-term symptoms apart from their chronic diarrhoea, and the majority will be familiar with these and able to cope with them. Such symptoms may include abdominal pain, bloating and abdominal distension, nausea and fatigue. Unless there is a sudden change in the severity of these accompanying symptoms or an otherwise unexpected occurrence, reassurance and, if appropriate, simple symptomatic treatment are all that is required.

Aggravating factors

It is well known that stress or anxiety can induce or exacerbate diarrhoea. Although this is typical of the history of irritable bowel syndrome, which is seen particularly in young adults, it is not exclusive to the condition. Apart from any causative agent involved, diarrhoea may be worsened by dietary changes, such as an increase in fibre or fat content, spices, alcohol, or even an excess of tea or coffee.

Incidence and recurrence

Continuous or recurrent diarrhoea strongly suggests some underlying cause and requires a medical opinion.

Nocturnal diarrhoea, other than that experienced immediately after a digestive insult, should be regarded as unusual. Referral is needed to exclude diagnoses such as inflammatory bowel disease.

Diarrhoea caused by drugs will recur in association with administration of the offending agents. Patients should always be asked about current medications.

The presence of symptoms in other members of the household who share toilet facilities may indicate cross-infection or someone acting as a carrier, both of which can cause transference by the faecal–oral route.

Special considerations

Children

In babies the cause of diarrhoea may be infection, and parents should be advised to take special care when sterilising bottles. Some cases of diarrhoea in bottle-fed babies will be caused by insufficient dilution of the milk, resulting in osmotic diarrhoea. Lactose intolerance can also lead to osmotic diarrhoea.

Very young children are at increased risk of dehydration. Babies under 6 months old with stools that are loose and more frequent than normal should be referred after 24 hours if the condition is not improving.

Children under 2 who have diarrhoea for more than 48 hours should be referred if they seem unwell or are not drinking normally.

Dehydration can be difficult to judge, but a limp, non-alert baby should be referred as soon as possible. The important fact to remember is that diarrhoea causes water and electrolyte loss, which must be checked, particularly in young children, by giving adequate fluids and, if possible, electrolyte mixtures. Traditionally, treatment of children has also involved restricting food until the diarrhoea improves, but a more modern approach is described below (see Management).

Elderly

Elderly patients, like children, are susceptible to the dehydrating effect of diarrhoea, especially those who are taking diuretics and those whose fluid and food intake is poor. It is wise to operate guidelines for referral similar to those described for children under 2.

Faecal impaction in the elderly can give rise to constipation and a so-called spurious or overflow diarrhoea. In this condition hard faeces obstruct most of the diameter of the bowel lumen. However, some fluid faeces can seep past the impacted mass, leading to a loose, unformed stool that is produced in relatively small amounts. It is most common in the immobile, frail elderly. Treating this condition as diarrhoea will only cause more constipation.

The patient should instead be referred for a rectal examination and disimpaction of the faeces.

Management

By the time symptoms occur, the bowel mucosa will have already been damaged by bacteria or toxins. It then becomes inflamed and cannot function normally to absorb fluids and electrolytes. Instead, there is a net secretion of fluids into the gut, and although the inflammation will normally subside within a few days, extra fluids are often needed to counteract the fluid loss. The cornerstone of treatment of acute diarrhoea is therefore to maintain an adequate fluid balance. This is particularly important in young children and the elderly. If the patient complains of thirst, this need should be satisfied so that lost body water can be replaced. In adults, bland sugarless drinks, such as water or tea, should be given.

Fasting is generally not necessary if the patient wants to eat. This is also true for babies and children. Patients will, however, often report that food – even a small amount – goes right through them. Some authorities argue that fasting deprives the infecting bacteria of nutrients in the bowel and thus shortens the illness. More recently, others have argued that it makes no difference to the outcome. It is difficult to give definitive guidelines on this issue.

Breastfed babies should continue to feed, as there is no evidence that this is deleterious. Although there is no evidence to show that fasting in bottle-fed babies is of any benefit, it is traditional to stop milk feeding for 24 hours, during which time a proprietary oral rehydration solution should be given instead. The next day, the milk feed can be diluted to a quarter of the normal concentration with water, followed by a 50 per cent dilution the next day, three-quarter strength the next day, and finally upgrading to full strength. Fluids or diluted milk feeds should be offered at least every 3 hours. This will maintain nutrition and fluids at the desired level.

Oral rehydration solutions

Oral rehydration solutions are particularly suitable for babies and children. However, for the mild degree of dehydration suffered by babies and children who commonly present to pharmacists they are not essential, and water alone will provide the necessary degree of hydration. The solutions contain electrolytes, including sodium and glucose, which are actively absorbed across the intestinal epithelium, taking water and chloride with them. The sachets of powders require mixing with water according to the manufacturer's instructions to prevent overloading. A simple rule of thumb is to give one cupful of solution for every loose stool to babies under 1 year, and two cupfuls for older children. As a general rule, over the course of 1 or 2 days the passage of up to four loose motions per day will not put any child at risk of dehydration. However, if the child is particularly ill, or there are abnormal signs, such as unsatisfied thirst, dry mouth, poor urine output, rapid breathing or drowsiness, referral is necessary.

For adults, increased fluids, including salty soups and fruit juices, will suffice.

Antidiarrhoeal drugs

Some authorities decry the use of antidiarrhoeals on the basis that they do not appear to shorten the duration of illness and any benefit is symptomatic. However, for social reasons patients will often insist that symptomatic treatment is desirable, and antidiarrhoeal medicines have an obvious placebo effect. All the spasmolytic drugs below are useful for the diarrhoeal phase of irritable bowel syndrome. They can relieve the urgency of defecation and help with the sensation of incomplete evacuation of which patients complain.

Loperamide

Over-the-counter (OTC) loperamide is an effective symptomatic treatment suitable for adults and children over 12 years old. It decreases bowel motility through its action on opioid receptors in the gut and increases bowel transit time, thus permitting the absorption of fluid and electrolytes. It does not possess the potential adverse effects of anticholinergic drugs such as hyoscine and dicyclomine (dicycloverine), and because it does not cross the blood–brain barrier it has no central effects. In addition to its anti-motility action, loperamide also exhibits some antisecretory properties.

Like other antidiarrhoeal agents, it is not recommended for patients with inflammatory bowel disease except under medical supervision, as it may cause constipation, obstruction and dilation of the bowel (megacolon).

Mebeverine

Mebeverine is a direct-acting spasmolytic drug that has no anticholinergic activity. It has been used for many years for the symptomatic treatment of irritable bowel syndrome, and as such it appears to be effective in relieving the abdominal cramps and hypermotility of the large bowel, with few adverse effects.

Alverine

Like mebeverine, alverine has no anticholinergic activity, but exerts a direct relaxant effect on the bowel smooth muscle and is also an acceptable treatment for the symptoms of irritable bowel syndrome.

Hyoscine

Hyoscine-N-butylbromide is an anticholinergic drug licensed for intestinal spasm and irritable bowel syndrome.

Morphine

Traditional medicines, such as kaolin and morphine mixture, as well as a number of proprietary products containing morphine, have been popular for the treatment of acute diarrhoea, although there is little objective evidence of their efficacy. However, they can lead to addiction if overused. Kaolin and morphine mixture has been reported to cause hypokalaemia because of the liquorice extract it contains, but this is unlikely unless there is chronic usage of large doses.

Codeine, an opioid, like morphine, is available in low dosage in some OTC products, but, like morphine, its efficacy at such doses is dubious and may be outweighed by its abuse potential.

Adsorbents

Adsorbents, such as kaolin, pectin and charcoal, have a traditional place in the mind of the public for the treatment of diarrhoea. They serve little useful therapeutic purpose, although they may adsorb water in the bowel and add bulk to the stool. This may, however, lull patients into a false sense of security because they could still be losing large quantities of fluid from the bowel, but this will be less readily apparent because of the cosmetic effect of the adsorbent agent.

Bismuth subsalicylate

This agent has been successfully marketed because of its dual site of action in the upper and lower bowel. It is promoted for the treatment of heartburn and nausea as well as diarrhoea. It decreases intestinal motility and permits the absorption of fluids to take place. Because it is converted to salicylate, it should not be given to those with sensitivity to aspirin, nor to children under 16 years.

Bulk-forming agents

Bulking agents are usually used to treat constipation, but they can be useful in conditions that produce chronic diarrhoea by absorbing water in the bowel and creating a formed stool. In irritable bowel syndrome, for instance, small doses of ispaghula or sterculia have been used to treat the diarrhoeal phase, but this should be tried carefully because the effect in some patients may be to worsen the flatus and bloating. There is some evidence that bran, in contrast to other types of fibre, may worsen the symptoms of irritable bowel syndrome, but this is controversial.

Peppermint oil

Formulations of peppermint oil have been designed to release the oil in the distal small bowel to avoid potential irritable effects in the mouth and oesophagus. Dispersion of the oil in the small bowel allows transport to the large bowel, where the active ingredient, menthol, exerts a direct spasmolytic effect. It has been a popular prescribable treatment for irritable bowel syndrome for many years and is an acceptable addition to, or replacement for, other spasmolytic agents.

Advice for travellers abroad

The following pointers will help reduce the incidence of travellers' diarrhoea:

- Drink bottled water or water sterilised with purification tablets
- Avoid ice (unless made personally, using bottled water) and ice cream
- Avoid salads and uncooked vegetables (which may have been washed in contaminated water)
- Avoid fruits that cannot be peeled
- Avoid unpasteurised milk
- Avoid murky swimming pools.

Second opinion

Diarrhoea is a common condition and therefore frequently presented to doctors. Children tend to be brought earlier in the course of the illness than adults, their parents being aware of the possibility of dehydration.

The term means different things to different people, and the doctor's first task is to take an accurate history, including duration and frequency of symptoms, to establish an understanding of the presentation. Associated symptoms will be enquired for, including similar problems in close relatives and contacts, or recent foreign travel, to examine the likelihood of infection requiring specific antimicrobial treatment.

An abdominal examination is often undertaken, when tenderness may be found, helping to localise the site of any obvious inflammation. This is most commonly central, but may be epigastric, particularly when there is a coincidental gastritis (perhaps with nausea or vomiting), or suprapubic. Tenderness over the left side of the abdomen may be from direct palpation of the descending colon, but over the right side and iliac fossa is less usual and raises other diagnostic possibilities, including appendicitis.

There should be no discernible masses in this area, and any discovered suggest a neoplasm or abscess and will be regarded as serious. Finally, the abdomen can be examined with a stethoscope in order to listen to the bowel sounds. Increases in activity are to be expected, but otherwise the sounds are essentially normal; however, high-pitched noises, or even the absence of sounds, suggests an imminent intestinal obstruction.

The early signs of dehydration, especially in children and the elderly, should be considered.

The majority of cases will be self-limiting, and symptomatic treatment while observing the natural progression and resolution will, for the majority, be all that is required. In persistent cases or those where clinical suspicion has been raised, a stool sample may be sent for microscopy and culture. This investigation is unhelpful in simple cases, taking at least a few days for the necessary cultures to incubate, and routinely would also be wasteful.

Finally, in the few patients with unresolved symptoms or other suspicions more sophisticated investigations are required, including endoscopy or barium contrast X-rays, perhaps with blood tests to check on haemoglobin status and renal and hepatic function. These inevitably take time to organise in primary care, and an urgent referral to secondary care is the obvious way of accelerating the process.

Bibliography

Banks M, Farthing M (2003). Acute diarrhoea: guide to acute management. *Prescriber* 19 Oct: 48–59.

British Society of Gastroenterology (2000). *Guidelines for the Management of Irritable Bowel Syndrome.* www.bsg.org.uk/clinical_prac/guidelines.htm

 SUMMARY OF CONDITIONS PRODUCING DIARRHOEA

Colorectal cancer (carcinoma of the large bowel)
A tumour in the large bowel can cause constipation or diarrhoea. Signs to look out for are blood in the stool, mucus in the stool (noticed as slime passed with the motion, often in the mornings), patient middle-aged or older, abdominal pain, swelling in the abdomen and weight loss. Any change in bowel habit in a patient aged over 50, particularly accompanied by weight loss or malaise, should be referred for investigation. Increasingly some surgeries and clinics are offering routine testing for occult blood and even sigmoidoscopy – **refer.**

Diverticular disease
See Chapter 6, p 79.

Inflammatory bowel disease
Inflammatory bowel disease includes Crohn's disease, a disorder characterised by inflammation in any part of the digestive tract, including the large bowel, and ulcerative colitis, a disorder affecting the large bowel only. These conditions usually present in the teenage years and young adulthood. The classic symptoms are bloody diarrhoea, with repeated visits to the toilet that do not abate during the night. The

→

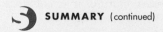 **SUMMARY** (continued)

patient will feel ill and there will be weight loss and anorexia. The conditions are chronic, and are characterised by temporary remissions and flare-ups – **refer.**

Food poisoning
Food poisoning is caused by bacteria such as *Salmonella*, *Campylobacter*, *Shigella*, *Clostridium* and *Staphylococcus*. Common sources of infection are meat, poultry and dairy products. In mild cases the condition is self-limiting over the course of 1–3 days. If symptoms (diarrhoea, vomiting and abdominal pain) are severe, **refer.**

Irritable bowel syndrome
Irritable bowel syndrome is a relatively common condition, affecting about 15 per cent of the population and often commencing in the under-40 age group. It is often a diagnosis of exclusion, as there is no specific disease marker. Symptoms vary among sufferers, but characteristically there is recurrent abdominal pain that is relieved by emptying the bowel, urgency, diarrhoea which sometimes alternates with episodes of constipation, abdominal distension and bloating, a feeling of rectal fullness and incomplete evacuation. The diagnosis is often by exclusion of other conditions after the patient has had thorough tests and investigations. See also Chapter 6.

Malabsorption
Malabsorption syndromes, such as coeliac disease, are rare but should be borne in mind when there is weight loss, fatigue or anaemia, with or without abdominal distension. In children, malabsorption is often associated with lactose intolerance.

Protozoal infection
Visitors to or from some tropical and subtropical countries may become infected with protozoa that cause diseases such as amoebic dysentery and giardiasis. These conditions may resolve spontaneously, but if symptoms persist referral is advisable. In addition to diarrhoea, symptoms can include vomiting, abdominal pain, malaise and fever – **refer.**

Travellers' diarrhoea
Travellers' diarrhoea is an acute diarrhoea that may be caused by a change in diet (e.g. an increase in oily or spicy food), in climate, or in the mineral content of drinking water. It is usually self-limiting but can be disruptive to holidays or business trips. If it persists, it may be due to infection, often with bacterial toxins such as from *Escherichia coli*, *Campylobacter* or *Shigella*. In some cases the infection may be viral. Infection usually occurs in a country where sanitary conditions are poor or drinking water is contaminated. Persistent cases require further investigation and referral.

Viral infections
Viral gastroenteritis is one of the most common types of diarrhoea in the UK in both children and adults. It is usually self-limiting.

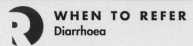

WHEN TO REFER
Diarrhoea

Onset
- Recent travel abroad

Medical opinion on the same day

Severity
- Patient obviously ill, e.g. showing signs of dehydration, such as being delerious or confused, or small child with very dry mouth and lips

Refer urgently

Duration
- Symptoms have changed or worsened and patient not improving after 1 or 2 weeks (depending on severity of original symptoms)

Accompanying symptoms
- Blood in stool
- Nausea (for more than 3–4 days)
- Loss of appetite (for more than 3–4 days)
- Weight loss (over previous 2 weeks)
- Fatigue
- Fever
- Pregnancy or breastfeeding

Same/next day
Same/next day

Incidence
- Diarrhoea wakes patient at night several times for more than 2 or 3 consecutive nights

CASE STUDIES

Case 1

A well-dressed woman in her late 50s requests a confidential consultation with the pharmacist. She and her husband have returned from a perfect Caribbean holiday, marred only on the last 2 days by intermittent abdominal pain and diarrhoea, which have persisted since their return. She is eager to point out that they stayed at a good hotel and were careful to observe the guide's recommendations.

What else should the pharmacist know?

The care this couple took while abroad may be reassuring, but does not eliminate the possibility of an acquired infection.

A standard history reveals that they have both suffered from diarrhoea approximately four to six times a day, preceded by colicky central pain lasting for 4 days now. They feel reasonably well, and are keen to get on with the tasks that commonly await on return from holiday.

After noting the details, the pharmacist advises symptomatic relief in the short term, but stresses the need for further investigations if symptoms persist, and points out that holiday diarrhoea, whatever its cause, does not reflect adversely on either the traveller or the resort.

A week later the woman returns, asking an assistant for more of the same medication.

Two potential alarm signals may be present now. A request for continuing medication beyond the period when resolution might reasonably be expected should always be followed up closely, and the request for someone not personally present also warrants enquiry.

The woman is now completely well but her husband is worse, with more pain and diarrhoea that prevents him leaving the house.

Whatever follows, this woman should be firmly advised that her husband see his GP. A further history adds the more recent symptoms of some bleeding and the passage of mucus. Without these new symptoms or this latest opportunistic visit, the pharmacist could easily have fallen into the trap of assuming either that the original diagnosis remained correct or that no other pathology could have occurred. Fortunately, his alertness prompted him into advising referral for this man.

In this case the diagnosis was a diverticular abscess. The patient was admitted to hospital as an emergency, where the abscess was surgically resected along with a length of diseased colon shortly before it perforated. The diverticular disease would have been present for some time, but can be asymptomatic. It is possible that the enteritis acquired abroad seeded the abscess in a pre-existing diverticulum, and that the conscientious attention of the pharmacist had an important part in the patient's successful recovery.

Case 2

A woman in her early 20s comes to the pharmacy one Saturday afternoon with her son, who is about 1 year old. He has had diarrhoea for 3 weeks. Everything he eats goes straight through him. The surgery is now closed, the weekend stretches before her and she feels she cannot cope. Her boyfriend and mother agree that something must be done.

What else do we need to know?

The prospect of diarrhoea for a prolonged period in a child of this age is alarming, and would imply a potentially serious disorder, if the child (fortunately present) did not appear so well. Clearly a full history is necessary. This must include an account of all professional and other advice solicited so far, and a description of the presenting complaint.

Slowly it emerges that the diarrhoea is in fact loose stools, but not invariably and not every day. Several times a week he produces voluminous and offensive motions, which spill from his nappy and soil both adjacent clothing and the atmosphere.

(continued overleaf)

CASE STUDIES (continued)

The boy has repeatedly been taken to the doctor, where he has been examined, his mother told that he is fine, and prescribed nothing. In the past she feels he has never eaten well, always picks at food and is frequently at the doctor's with colds and coughs. This is the woman's first baby, and as she is receiving what feels like criticism from all sides she can only conclude that the problem must in some way be her fault.

Whereas in some ways the history, including the medical opinion, is reassuring, this is nevertheless likely to be a difficult problem to resolve. Objectively the patient himself appears to be a well-nourished, contented child, but this perception clearly conflicts with those of his parents and other observers. It is important to be personally confident of the absence of serious pathology, but equally necessary to communicate this in a meaningful way to all concerned with his wellbeing.

It is important to explore the ideas, concerns and expectations not only of the patient when appropriate, but also of his family and carers. Sympathetic listening and encouragement may elicit useful information that forms the basis of useful communication and a shared understanding, not merely a summary of the clinical findings.

Further questioning suggests an erratic diet. With a working mother, childminders and grandparents, his diet is grazing, often unsuitable, and mostly a selection of snacks rather than meals. Anxieties have been raised over a period of time, fuelled by a lack of knowledge and hence confidence, and perhaps shared feelings of guilt.

Reassurance should be positive, including practical advice and continuing support. Goals should be realistic to the individual circumstances and set in a certain timeframe.

A team approach may be useful, especially at first, involving the GP for medical advice and the health visitor for follow-up and reinforcement.

8

Abdominal disorders

One of the most common symptoms presented to the pharmacist is abdominal discomfort or pain. This can encompass a multitude of possible diagnoses relating to the gastrointestinal tract, the genitourinary tract, and sometimes to other body systems from which pain may be referred to the abdomen. This chapter will deal principally with the common disorders of the upper gastrointestinal tract, allowing the pharmacist to recognise gastro-oesophageal reflux disease, non-ulcer dyspepsia and peptic ulcer disease. For conditions affecting the lower gastrointestinal tract (the large bowel) the reader should refer to Chapters 6 and 7.

A reasonably accurate diagnosis can often be made on the basis of a clear history, although sometimes the precise cause will remain a mystery. In such cases it is sufficient to determine the severity of the symptoms and the need for referral.

In this chapter the term 'pain' is used to describe all symptoms ranging from a mild or vague discomfort, such as indigestion, to the more commonly accepted lay definition of pain as a sensation that hurts.

An important part of the history of a patient with abdominal symptoms is the location of the pain. The system used in medicine to describe the site of symptoms is to divide the abdomen into nine areas by mentally drawing across its surface two vertical and two horizontal lines, as shown in Figure 8.1.

Assessing symptoms

Location of pain

The information in Table 8.1 will be helpful in considering the possible cause of abdominal

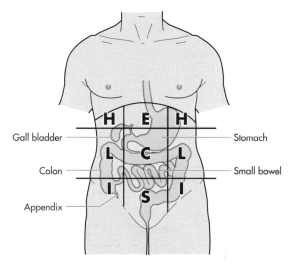

Figure 8.1 The nine areas of the abdomen used to locate symptoms (H, hypochondrium; E, epigastrium; L, loin; C, central; I, iliac fossa; S, suprapubic).

pain. It should be emphasised that this table indicates the sites where pain is typically felt, but there will be variability between patients and the presentation will not always be a classic textbook case. Abdominal pain is often not localised but will be described vaguely as covering all the abdomen. This may represent either a non-specific gastritis or enteritis with no known cause that will resolve spontaneously or, alternatively, the early presentation of a disorder that is not yet sufficiently advanced to show all of its typical features. Thus, the rest of the history must be considered along with questions about the site of pain.

Patients may give a clue to the diagnosis by the manner in which they show the location of their pain. In answer to the question 'Show me

Table 8.1   Differential diagnosis of pain according to site

Chest

(Although anatomically distinct from the abdomen, symptoms felt in the chest may arise from the gastrointestinal tract)

Acid reflux, with or without hiatus hernia
Angina
Muscular strain
Myocardial infarction
Oesophagitis or oesophageal obstruction (difficulty in swallowing, lump in throat)
Peptic ulcer

Epigastric

Angina (atypical presentation)
Biliary colic (atypical presentation)
Gastritis/dyspepsia
Duodenitis
Oesophageal ulcer
Gastro–oesophageal reflux disease
Peptic ulcer (gastric or duodenal) disease
Pancreatitis
Tumour

Central

Abdominal aneurysm
Appendicitis (central pain which spreads after a few hours to the right iliac fossa)
Biliary colic (caused by infection of the gallbladder or common bile duct, or obstruction with gallstone)
Bowel ischaemia
Colitis

Diverticular disease
Gastritis/gastroenteritis
Inflammatory bowel disease
Irritable bowel syndrome
Mesenteric adenitis
Obstruction
Pancreatitis
Peptic ulcer (gastric or duodenal)
Tumour

Suprapubic

Cystitis
Colitis
Diverticular disease
Irritable bowel syndrome
Tumour

Rectal pain

Rectal carcinoma
Haemorrhoids
Spasm of pelvic anal muscles

In women

Ovarian cyst
Salpingitis
Tubal (ectopic) pregnancy
Uterine disorders (e.g. dysmenorrhoea, endometriosis)

Hypochondrium

Either or both sides

Atypical presentation of pneumonia, pleurisy, angina
Muscular or ligamentous pain from the back
Peptic ulcer
Shingles

Left side

Gastritis

Right side

Biliary colic (often radiating to the back and shoulder)
Liver disease

Loin

Either or both sides
Lumbar muscle strain (felt in the lateral and posterior aspects of the loins)
Renal stone/ureteric colic
Shingles

Iliac fossa

Either or both sides

Bowel tumour
Colitis
Diverticular disease

In women

Ovarian cyst
Salpingitis (inflammation of fallopian tubes)
Tubal (ectopic) pregnancy

Right side

Appendicitis

Groin pain

Inguinal ligament strain (groin strain)
Inguinal or femoral hernia

where the pain is', a patient with a peptic ulcer or other distinct lesion may point with a finger to an exact spot on the abdomen, whereas someone with a less specific symptom may place a whole hand over the area where the discomfort is felt. The typical locations of pain in common abdominal disorders are shown in Figure 8.2.

Spread

The pain of myocardial ischaemia, as in angina or infarction, is classically described as spreading from the chest to the jaw, neck, shoulder and arms. This helps to distinguish it from oesophagitis, although the classic radiation of

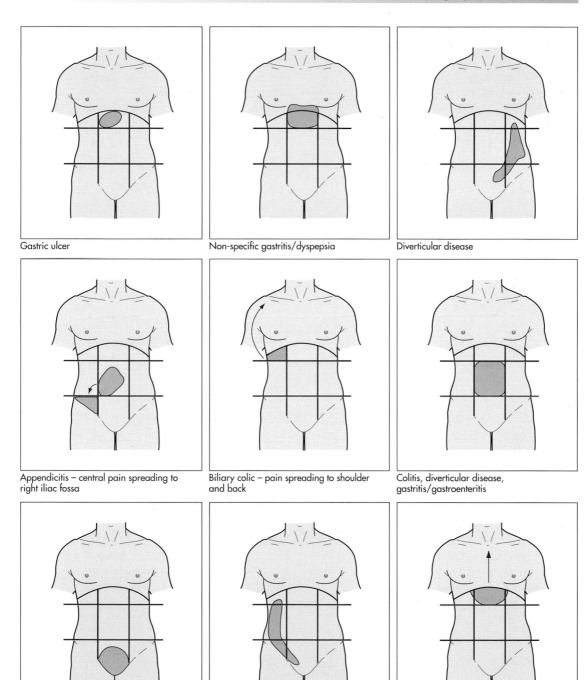

Gastric ulcer

Non-specific gastritis/dyspepsia

Diverticular disease

Appendicitis – central pain spreading to right iliac fossa

Biliary colic – pain spreading to shoulder and back

Colitis, diverticular disease, gastritis/gastroenteritis

Cystitis (infection in the bladder) – pain in the suprapubic area, often spreading to the back

Renal colic – left or right side, pain starts in the back and then spreads as stone moves down urinary tract

Oesophagitis, angina, myocardial infarction – in angina and myocardial infarction, pain can also spread to jaw, neck and arms

Figure 8.2 Typical location of pain in common abdominal disorders.

pain from the chest is not seen in every patient with cardiac ischaemia. The sufferer of cardiac symptoms will often indicate the location of pain with the palm of the hand across the chest, or sometimes by clenching the fist to indicate the sensation of tightness or squeezing felt in the chest.

Appendicitis is often first felt as central pain, which after a few hours radiates to the right iliac fossa; again, this history will not be reported by every patient with appendicitis.

Pain that radiates to the back or shoulders is typical of biliary colic (e.g. due to gallstones), peptic ulcer and, more seriously, pancreatitis. The pain of cystitis may spread from the suprapubic area to the back.

Pain in one loin that moves downwards into the suprapubic region or the testis is typical of renal colic, caused by a stone passing from the kidney, along the ureter to the bladder and then the urethra. This journey may be spread over a long period (days or weeks).

Intensity and duration

Severe pain that is continuous for more than a few hours may indicate serious pathology and possibly a medical emergency. If there is no previous history and the pain is sudden in onset, such severe pain is described clinically as an acute abdomen. It may be caused by conditions such as pancreatitis, peritonitis, an active or perforated peptic ulcer, abdominal aortic aneurysm and gynaecological emergencies. The severity of abdominal pain will govern the decision as to how soon a doctor should be seen.

Milder pain that occurs at some time during every day and persists for 2 weeks despite a course of treatment requires referral if it is troublesome. Obviously, the presence of certain accompanying symptoms (see below) may shorten the period before a doctor should be seen.

Symptoms that do not occur on a daily basis may be left for a little longer – say up to 4 weeks – to assess the effect of symptomatic treatment before referring to the doctor.

Type

Descriptions of the type of pain can be helpful, but they depend on the intelligence and articulacy of the patient.

Colic is a term used to describe waves of severe pain superimposed on a more constant duller pain, and occurs when a hollow muscular organ is in spasm. Thus, a colicky or griping pain is most likely to indicate involvement of the stomach or bowel, the genitourinary system (such as the ureter, bladder, uterus or fallopian tubes) or the bile duct system.

Abdominal pain will sometimes be described as a vague discomfort. This is typical of, but not exclusive to, the common indigestion seen with a non-specific gastritis. The condition is self-limiting, its cause usually being dietary over-indulgence or poor eating habits. Patients may use various words to describe indigestion or dyspepsia: reflux, trapped wind, burping, a bloated feeling or a grumbling stomach.

A sharp burning sensation in the epigastric region or behind the sternum is typical of oesophagitis due to reflux of stomach contents, and is referred to by the lay person as heartburn. This acid reflux occurs in everyone, particularly after or during meals, and is quite normal, although usually asymptomatic. When it causes symptoms, indicating damage to the lower oesophagus, it is referred to as gastro-oesophageal reflux disease (GORD). Such a sensation may also be caused by a peptic ulcer, although sometimes a patient with an ulcer will complain of a more specific gnawing pain that can be pointed to with a finger.

The pain of angina or a myocardial infarction can mimic oesophagitis and other causes of abdominal pain. Although these conditions will be seen relatively rarely in the pharmacy, they should always be borne in mind.

An inflammatory process in any organ in the abdomen may result in a sensation of tenderness over the affected area. It is therefore important to ask not only about pain but also about any tenderness, particularly when light pressure is applied with a finger or when the patient bends or stretches.

Onset

Factors surrounding the onset of abdominal pain can provide some useful clues about the diagnosis.

Pain related to meals generally indicates a lesion in the stomach or bowel and is a classic symptom of a peptic ulcer (as well as non-ulcerative inflammatory conditions of the gastric and bowel mucosa). Epigastric or central pain that occurs a few minutes after a meal is typical of gastric ulcer, and pain that occurs 1–2 hours after a meal is more typical of duodenal ulcer. The pain of a duodenal ulcer is usually worse during the night. Both of these types of pain may respond to antacids, H_2 antagonists or proton pump inhibitors, but pain that persists despite such treatment requires referral.

Pain or other abdominal symptoms following a single incident of overeating or excess alcohol may represent either a non-specific (or non-ulcer) gastritis or indigestion, which will resolve quickly without the need for referral. However, if symptoms become severe or persist, they could represent some underlying pathological cause, such as food poisoning.

Angina or myocardial infarction may be brought on by large meals. If this seems a possibility, it is important to establish whether the patient has a past history of ischaemic heart disease, and also to bear in mind how ill they appear to be. Angina may also be brought on by the cold or by exercise.

Any pain or discomfort that starts immediately on eating could represent oesophagitis or reflux, or even a nervous dyspepsia. If simple over-the-counter (OTC) treatment is not successful, this condition requires attention and it is best to refer the patient for reassurance or investigation.

An acute hernia caused by lifting or straining may be felt as a severe pain in the groin or suprapubic region, whereas a muscle strain in the back may be referred to the lateral aspects of the loins, the hypochondria and the chest.

Severe pain or a throbbing or burning sensation on or after defecation is typical of haemorrhoids, but could also indicate anal fissure, fistula or rectal abscess. This type of pain requires referral.

Any abdominal injury or trauma with symptoms requires referral.

Abdominal symptoms such as pain, diarrhoea or constipation may be related to prescription drugs. Gastrointestinal symptoms can be caused by aspirin and other non-steroidal anti-inflammatory drugs (NSAIDs) and iron, whereas oesophageal symptoms may be caused by bulking agents, potassium salts, NSAIDs, tetracyclines, bisphosphonates and steroids, especially if the patient is lying in bed. Calcium channel blocking drugs are also associated with dyspepsia.

It is important to establish whether the onset of pain relates to the menstrual cycle. Midcycle pain may be caused by an ovulation syndrome, whereas pain around the time of menstruation is likely to be due to some uterine spasm (such as dysmenorrhoea) or endometriosis.

Pain that occurs or is worse when the patient passes urine is likely to indicate cystitis or, less commonly, renal colic caused by a stone.

A sudden onset of abdominal pain, particularly in a previously fit individual, may well represent an acute abdomen, which has already been referred to.

Abdominal symptoms, especially indigestion or epigastric pain, that occur for the first time in a man of middle age or beyond and which do not respond to OTC products require referral, as gastric carcinoma is most common in men in this age group.

A sudden onset of chest symptoms, no matter how reminiscent of oesophagitis, should alert the pharmacist to consider the possibility of ischaemic heart disease and to question the patient further to exclude this possible diagnosis.

Accompanying symptoms

A great many other symptoms may accompany abdominal pain or discomfort. They have been arranged here in approximate decreasing order of importance or severity.

Alarm signals, as defined by the National Institute for Health and Clinical Effectiveness (NICE) in 2004, are shown in Figure 8.3. If they occur, then a referral to the doctor is appropriate.

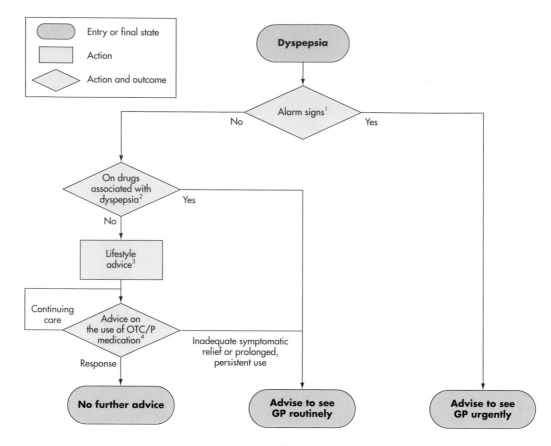

Legend:
- Entry or final state
- Action
- Action and outcome

Dyspepsia

Alarm signs[1] — No / Yes

On drugs associated with dyspepsia[2] — No / Yes

Lifestyle advice[3]

Advice on the use of OTC/P medication[4] — Continuing care / Response

Inadequate symptomatic relief or prolonged, persistent use

No further advice

Advise to see GP routinely

Advise to see GP urgently

1 Alarm signs include dyspepsia with gastrointestinal bleeding, difficulty swallowing, unintentional weight loss, abdominal swelling and persistent vomiting.
2 Ask about current and recent clinical and self care for dyspepsia. Ask about medications that may be the cause of dyspepsia, for example calcium antagonists, nitrates, theophyllines, bisphosphonates, corticosteroids and NSAIDs.
3 Offer lifestyle advice, including advice about healthy eating, weight reduction and smoking cessation.
4 Offer advice about the range of pharmacy-only and over-the-counter medications, reflecting symptoms and previous successful and unsuccessful use. Be aware of the full range of recommendations for the primary care management of adult dyspepsia to work consistently with other healthcare professionals.

Figure 8.3 Flowchart to guide pharmacist management of dyspepsia. (Reproduced with permission from National Institute for Health and Clinical Excellence (2004). *Dyspepsia: Managing Dyspepsia in Adults in Primary Care.* NICE Clinical Guideline no.17. London: National Institute for Clinical Excellence. Available from www.nice.org.uk<outbind://8/www.nice.org.uk>.)

See also the section 'When to refer' at the end of this chapter for a more comprehensive list of symptoms that require referral.

Weight loss

Weight loss is a significant sign in anyone with abdominal symptoms, and becomes more so from middle age onwards. It may be caused by a peptic ulcer, but it could signify a sinister pathology, such as a carcinoma, and should always be referred.

Blood in the stool

Melaena (blood in the stool) is a warning symptom that needs referral for either reassurance or investigation, particularly in the older population. If the patient gives a past history of haemorrhoids, it may be possible to differentiate spotting of blood on toilet tissue due to haemorrhoids from a black tarry stool containing blood from a lesion further up the bowel. However, if the symptoms have changed in a patient with previously diagnosed haemorrhoids, or if there is any doubt whatsoever in the pharmacist's mind, then it is wise to refer the patient for a medical opinion.

Fresh (bright red) blood smearing the stool in a young person, associated with symptoms of haemorrhoids, is probably acceptable in the short term. However, in those over the age of 40 any type of blood in the stool requires investigation.

Anaemia

The commonest cause of anaemia in patients admitted to hospital is a gastrointestinal bleed, and it is therefore necessary to refer any patient with signs of anaemia, with or without abdominal symptoms, to the doctor.

Signs of anaemia are tiredness, facial pallor, pale conjunctiva (seen by everting the lower eyelid and comparing with the red/pink conjunctiva lining the lower lid of a healthy person) and pale palms of the hands (again observed by comparing with the pink palms of a healthy individual). Severe anaemia may cause shortness of breath.

Menstrual disorders

Abdominal symptoms associated with specific times in the menstrual cycle, such as midcycle, premenstrual or perimenstrual pains, suggest that the problem relates to the genital tract. Where involvement of the genital tract is suspected or requires exclusion, any irregularity should be inquired for, such as a missed period, vaginal discharge, abnormal bleeding, and particularly any symptoms associated with early pregnancy, such as nausea, breast changes and nocturia. Patients with pain associated with any of these features will generally require referral to exclude serious conditions such as a tubal pregnancy, salpingitis or endometriosis.

Jaundice

Frank jaundice can be recognised by a yellow discoloration of the skin. More subtle signs can be detected by inspecting the sclera of the eye, which will have a yellow colour or tinge compared to the white of a normal eye. Jaundice suggests liver or biliary involvement and requires referral.

Dysphagia

A genuine difficulty in swallowing food or drink requires referral to exclude oesophageal obstruction.

Patients with GORD may complain of this symptom, which is due to a narrowing of the oesophagus caused by a stricture created by the irritant reflux. This may improve with symptomatic treatment. A feeling of a lump in the throat that does not affect swallowing should also be followed up, although perhaps not as urgently as genuine dysphagia.

Swelling

Localised swelling in the abdomen is associated with hernias. General abdominal distension may be real or imagined, and can occur with relatively benign dyspepsia as well as with more serious diagnoses. However, referral is necessary if there is a real change in the abdominal girth measurement together with abdominal symptoms.

More often the patient will complain of feeling bloated, usually with flatulence. This is a common symptom of many abdominal disorders and is not really helpful in making a differential diagnosis.

Vomiting

Vomiting that persists for more than 1 or 2 days requires a medical opinion. Usually the cause will be food or alcohol intolerance or gastrointestinal infection, but it can occur as a result of severe pain (as in renal or biliary colic and appendicitis), in reflux oesophagitis and in nervous dyspepsia. In the presence of severe abdominal pain vomiting may be a sign of obstruction.

Vomiting can also arise from extra-abdominal causes, such as migraine or a raised intracranial pressure.

In children, vomiting may be caused by fever, unassociated with other abdominal symptoms. This is common in acute systemic viral infections in the young. It is usually of no consequence, unless frequent enough to raise the possibility of dehydration or an alternative cause.

Diarrhoea and constipation

These two symptoms are considered in Chapters 6 and 7. Diarrhoea is often associated with abdominal colic and is common in gastroenteritis, diverticulitis and colitis. It may also occur with pain in appendicitis. In older patients, the pharmacist should be alert to the possibility of sinister causes.

Abdominal pain with constipation may be caused by a temporary impaction of the stool; if simple laxatives are not effective, the patient should be referred for exclusion of other causes of obstruction.

Dysuria/frequency

Pain or a burning sensation on passing urine, frequency and urgency may suggest a urinary tract infection or a renal stone. Inflammation of other organs in the abdomen, such as the bowel or appendix, can also irritate the urinary tract, causing these symptoms.

Rash

Severe pain on one side of the trunk is characteristic of herpes zoster infection (shingles), and often precedes the appearance of a rash. The rash follows the course of sensory nerves and may be seen across the front of the upper abdomen or chest, around the side of the trunk and on the back. The rash looks like that of chickenpox (flat at first, then forming pustules and vesicles). Immediate referral is necessary for the doctor to consider treatment with antiviral drugs, which should be started as early as possible after the diagnosis has been made.

Waterbrash

Waterbrash, the regurgitation of bitter gastric contents, is a common and not very specific symptom that may occur in almost any kind of dyspepsia, but is most often associated with GORD.

Cough

Sometimes patients with acid reflux may have a cough. This is thought to be due to stimulation of the vagus nerve by the reflux of acid into the oesophagus.

Aggravating and relieving factors

Pain from a peptic ulcer is not always aggravated by food: sometimes food acts as a buffer to the acid attacking the damaged mucosa and hence provides some relief. Classically, a gastric ulcer is said to be aggravated by food and a duodenal ulcer relieved by it. Food will trigger heartburn, and patients will often complain of a sensation of obstruction at the gastro-oesophageal junction if a stricture is present.

The pain of oesophagitis or acid reflux may be aggravated by lying down (and is therefore a problem at night) or bending. Sometimes smoking, alcohol, chocolate or coffee can lower the pressure in the oesophageal sphincter and allow reflux to take place.

Antacids, H_2 antagonists and proton pump inhibitors (PPI) usually provide some relief in peptic ulceration and oesophagitis, but do not help in nervous dyspepsia or in biliary colic due to gallstones. Pain in a patient with biliary colic due to gallstones will be exacerbated by fatty foods, and a reduction in the amount of fat eaten will relieve or prevent the pain to some degree. This is not always diagnostic, however, as the pain of peptic ulcer may be affected in the same way.

The colicky pain of colitis or gastroenteritis will often be temporarily relieved by passing a stool, which differentiates these conditions from appendicitis, in which no such relief will usually occur.

Pain caused by non-specific gastritis, peptic ulcer, oesophagitis or hiatus hernia can normally be relieved temporarily by antacids, H_2 antagonists or PPIs. This may be helpful in distinguishing these conditions from angina. The pain of angina usually responds to sublingual glyceryl trinitrate, which may have been prescribed for the patient. Chest pain not responding to either type of drug should be evaluated in terms of the possibility of a myocardial infarction.

Special considerations in children

Abdominal pain in babies from the age of 2 weeks to 4 months may indicate colic. This usually occurs in the evenings. The baby will draw up its knees and cry, despite being picked up. The condition resolves spontaneously by the age of 4 months.

One serious cause of abdominal pain in babies aged between 4 months and 2 years is intussusception. In this condition, two adjacent sections of bowel telescope together, causing obstruction and an acute abdomen. The condition is a medical emergency.

Projectile vomiting in babies at about 6–8 weeks of age is a possible indicator of obstruction, such as pyloric stenosis. Referral is necessary.

Viral conditions can cause enlargement of the mesenteric lymph glands (in the abdomen) in children. This may produce a non-specific abdominal pain, usually associated with fever, which may be confused with other potentially more serious conditions. It usually resolves spontaneously.

Management

Normally, excessive reflux is prevented by tone in the lower oesophageal sphincter and by oesophageal peristalsis. Patients can be advised on lifestyle measures that might help to reduce the symptoms caused by a failure of the former mechanism. Small, regular and frequent meals are better than hurried greasy food binges, and eating late at night should be avoided. Fat in food lowers the tone of the lower oesophageal sphincter, which is undesirable in acid reflux. Sphincter pressure may also be lowered by smoking, alcohol, chocolate, coffee, or even peppermint, which is present in some antacid preparations. Heartburn can often be relieved by raising the head of the bed and by avoiding bending and stooping.

Weight reduction may be helpful in relieving symptoms in patients who are overweight.

Acid suppressants and mucosal protectants

Gastric acid suppression can be achieved by traditional antacids such as aluminium and magnesium salts (see below), by H_2 receptor antagonists such as ranitidine, cimetidine and famotidine, and by PPIs such as omeprazole. Additional agents such as alginates, which form a protective cover over the oesophageal endothelium, can also be used either alone or in combination with acid suppressant therapy. The most appropriate class of agent can be chosen according to the severity or frequency of the symptoms. Traditional antacids are perceived to be the less potent of the three classes, but large doses may be as effective as the H_2 antagonists. Patient choice and convenience and the type of formulation will often determine which to use. Antacids and H_2 antagonists are both relatively fast acting in suppressing symptoms (about 1 hour) and are particularly suitable for isolated episodes of dyspepsia. H_2 antagonists can be taken once a day and if, for example, they are taken at night, they will provide relief over a period of about 12 hours. PPIs such as omeprazole tend to be more potent acid suppressants, but there can be a delay of up to 2 days before maximum symptom relief is felt. They are thus appropriate for treating recurrent symptoms, which may occur several times a week, rather than the isolated episode following a dietary extravagance the night before, although this may be a theoretical strategy rather than a proven practical difference with respect to their use as OTC remedies.

Antacid preparations should be taken either 1 hour before or 1 hour after meals for maximum efficacy. Earlier administration after meals will result in the antacid being ejected from the stomach into the duodenum by gastric emptying, which normally occurs within an hour of eating. Also, food acts as a good buffer against acid attack on the gastric mucosa.

A combination of an acid suppressant with alginate (see below) can also be recommended for symptoms of GORD.

There is an abundance of evidence for the efficacy of all three H_2 antagonists mentioned and of omeprazole as ulcer healing drugs and symptomatic remedies in GORD, peptic ulcer and non-ulcer dyspepsia.

The H_2 antagonists should not be taken continuously for longer than 2 weeks without consulting a doctor, to avoid masking symptoms of serious disease.

The licence for omeprazole in the UK permits its occasional use for longer periods, provided there is symptomatic relief within 2 weeks and that symptoms are controlled by 4 weeks.

Omeprazole interacts with phenytoin, warfarin, azoles, digoxin and tacrolimus.

Cimetidine should be avoided in patients taking phenytoin, theophylline and oral anticoagulants, but ranitidine and famotidine do not interact with these drugs and are suitable for use in these cases.

The most significant drug interactions with antacids are shown in Table 8.2.

Table 8.2 Major drug interactions with antacids

Drug	Effect
Chlorpromazine	Reduced absorption
Ciprofloxacin, norfloxacin	Reduced absorption
Digoxin	Reduced absorption
Enteric-coated tablets	Coating disrupted in stomach
Iron	Reduced absorption
Lithium	Serum levels reduced by sodium (bicarbonate)
Penicillamine	Reduced absorption
Rifampicin	Reduced absorption
Sucralfate	Efficacy reduced as pH increases
Tetracyclines	Reduced absorption
Warfarin and phenindione	Reduced absorption

Traditional antacids

Magnesium salts

Magnesium salts are effective antacids but in doses required to give symptomatic relief they can cause diarrhoea.

Many products, for example magnesium carbonate mixture and magnesium trisilicate mixture, contain a relatively high sodium content, which may be unsuitable for patients with heart failure or hypertension.

Aluminium salts

Antacids containing aluminium are also effective. They are considered by some to be longer acting than magnesium salts because of a slowing effect on gut transit time. This in turn can lead to constipation. For this reason, they may be considered less suitable than magnesium salts for elderly patients.

Many proprietary antacids contain a mixture of aluminium and magnesium.

Calcium salts

Calcium salts have the reputation of being fast acting. They can lead to constipation and, theoretically at least, may cause acid rebound by stimulating the secretion of gastrin, which in turn causes more acid to be secreted by the stomach. The clinical significance of this is unclear.

Bismuth salts

Bismuth is an old established antacid that is effective but which can cause constipation.

Sodium bicarbonate

Sodium bicarbonate is a fast-acting antacid but should be avoided in patients whose sodium intake needs to be limited. It should not be used on a long-term basis, as it is absorbed and may cause metabolic alkalosis.

Other agents

Domperidone

Domperidone is a prokinetic agent that stimulates gastrointestinal peristalsis and is licensed for OTC use for the relief of postprandial symptoms of dyspepsia, heartburn and nausea. It is thus a useful agent to consider when acid suppressants have been tried without success, or when nausea is an accompanying symptom of indigestion.

Dimeticone

Dimeticone reduces the surface tension of the mucus-coated gas bubbles in the stomach and small bowel so that small bubbles coalesce. It is claimed to act as a defoaming agent, allowing gas to be eliminated. It is included in many proprietary antacid mixtures.

Alginate

Alginates are present in some proprietary medicines and are useful for relieving symptoms of GORD. They are said to form a floating viscous gel on top of the stomach contents. This protects the vulnerable mucous membrane of the oesophagus when the gastric contents are forced up into it. Such medicines are suitable for hiatus hernia and other causes of reflux.

A combination of cimetidine and alginate is available for the treatment of heartburn.

Treatment strategy by the doctor

There are various consensus guidelines for the management of ulcer-like dyspepsia and reflux in primary care, and pharmacists should be aware of the strategies of local GPs so as to be able to educate and reassure their patients.

Spasmolytic drugs

Drugs that relax smooth muscle can relieve certain abdominal symptoms. Loperamide is a useful antidiarrhoeal agent and was mentioned in the earlier chapter on diarrhoea (Chapter 7). It will give some relief of intestinal colic associated with diarrhoea.

Dicyclomine (dicycloverine), alverine and hyoscine are antispasmodic drugs and are suitable for the treatment of gastrointestinal colic (the products differ in their recommendations for minimum age of use). Hyoscine is also licensed for use in primary dysmenorrhoea (i.e. dysmenorrhoea that is not secondary to another condition).

Anticholinergics, such as hyoscine and dicyclomine (dicycloverine), may cause dryness of the mouth, some blurring of vision and palpitations. They are contraindicated in patients with glaucoma or prostatitis.

Analgesics and NSAIDs

Paracetamol can be used for the relief of abdominal pain. Aspirin is best avoided because of its irritant effect on the gastrointestinal tract.

Ibuprofen can be useful for the relief of dysmenorrhoea and other pain associated with the genital tract in women.

Second opinion

The symptoms and signs classically described in medical textbooks do not always reflect the reality of individual patients, and this is probably as true in the abdomen as anywhere in the body.

Abdominal pain, nausea and vomiting, or changes in bowel function are common in people of all ages and the possible underlying causes are numerous. A systematic approach is needed, and doctors will rely on as precise a history as can be obtained, with an emphasis on the objective severity and duration of symptoms and the presence of signs. When examining the abdomen they take each of the areas we have indicated, testing for tenderness and the presence of masses. Tenderness is pain on direct pressure, rebound tenderness (a suggestion of involvement of the peritoneal lining of the affected organ) or guarding (a protective muscular rigidity over that site) being more significant. The kidneys can be tested by bimanual palpation at each loin. The rectum and prostate can be palpated digitally.

The abdomen is normally soft, the organs not being individually identified. An enlarged liver may be felt under the right costal margin, or very rarely a spleen in the left hypochondrium. The bladder in urinary retention is usually obvious, as may be the descending colon in severe constipation. Enlarged kidneys may become palpable. A mass can also be found when a tumour arises from within an organ.

Abdominal disorders can be investigated by testing the urine for sugar or protein, microscopic examination for cells or blood, or culture of any infection. The stool can also be examined microscopically and bacteriologically, and can be tested for blood or the malabsorption of nutrients.

Blood tests reveal an insight into the function of the renal and hepatic systems, the prostate and, by measuring hormone levels, the female reproductive tract.

Plain X-rays do not differentiate individual organs well, but can show air and fluid levels in the bowel if obstruction is suspected, or the calcification of some renal calculi. Barium is still used as a contrast medium, in swallows, meals, follow-throughs to the small intestine or in enemas.

Ultrasound scans can identify the gallbladder and stones, and the renal and reproductive tracts. Endoscopy can visualise and allow for biopsy of the upper GI tract as far as the proximal jejunum, and the rectum and latter part of the colon. All of these investigations will be openly available to many GPs, offering a comprehensive system for investigating patients with suspicious or unexplained symptoms and signs.

Referral to specialists, hospital physicians and surgeons will be made urgently in acute conditions or where malignancy is suspected, and more routinely when further investigation such as a CT scan seems appropriate, or when surgical management is indicated.

Bibliography

National Institute for Health and Clinical Excellence (2004). *Dyspepsia: Managing Dyspepsia in Adults in Primary Care*. NICE Clinical Guideline no. 17. London: National Institute for Health and Clinical Excellence.

 SUMMARY OF CONDITIONS PRODUCING ABDOMINAL PAIN

Acute abdomen

Acute abdomen is the term used to describe a potentially life-threatening situation. Because of the severity of the illness, the patient will not present to the pharmacy but a relative may describe the symptoms. The patient will have sudden severe pain of recent onset, be obviously ill, have abdominal tenderness, and will lie still because movement causes more pain. There may be fever, vomiting and abdominal distension. Causes include peritonitis, bowel infarction, bowel obstruction, pancreatitis, abdominal aortic aneurysm and gynaecological emergencies – **refer** urgently.

Abdominal aortic aneurysm

An aneurysm is a localised abnormal dilatation of a blood vessel. In the abdominal aorta this is often due to an atherosclerotic/ageing process. The aneurysm weakens the wall of the aorta, which may rupture. Symptoms are abdominal pain, usually epigastric, radiating to the back, and a pulsating mass may be felt in the abdomen. It is a medical emergency – **refer.**

→

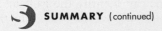 **SUMMARY** (continued)

Appendicitis

An inflamed appendix may occur at any age but is relatively rare in babies. It presents as pain that is central or in the right iliac fossa, often moving from the former to the latter region within a few hours of onset. The pain is continuous and there is right-sided tenderness. The pain may be accompanied by vomiting and either diarrhoea or constipation, related to inflammation of the surrounding bowel – **refer.**

Biliary colic

Spasm of the common bile duct may be caused by obstruction of the duct by gallstones or by infection of the biliary network. It presents as abdominal pain, epigastric or central but often high in the right hypochondrium, and is also felt in the back and in the tips of the shoulders. There is often nausea and vomiting – **refer.**

Carcinoma

Carcinoma of the oesophagus occurs mostly in adults over 50 years old. There is a period of silent growth before the appearance of symptoms (food lodging in the oesophagus, loss of weight, and sometimes pain on swallowing).

Carcinoma of the stomach causes few symptoms until the growth of the tumour is advanced, and the prognosis is usually poor at the time of diagnosis. Although it sometimes occurs in patients with a long history of indigestion, it often arises in those without previous symptoms. The peak incidence is between 40 and 60 years of age and it is more common in men than women. The patient will complain of indigestion at first, and later of pain on a daily basis, with loss of weight and vomiting. Although antiulcer therapy may give some relief for a few weeks, the patient eventually deteriorates.

Cancer of the large bowel or colon is slow growing and potentially curable if diagnosed early. It presents as a change in bowel habit in patients beyond middle age, with abdominal pain, distension, and blood or mucus in the stool.

Cancer of the rectum usually presents as diarrhoea, with blood present, but occasionally it may present as constipation. There is abdominal discomfort and pain in the rectum, with loss of weight. Rectal tumours vary considerably in their rate of growth – **refer.**

Diverticular disease

Diverticulitis produces a colicky pain. This may last from 1 to 3 days and then settle, and is followed by a symptom-free period before recurring. It may be accompanied by diarrhoea and blood in the stool, or by constipation – **refer.** See also Chapter 6.

Dysmenorrhoea

Dysmenorrhoea presents as severe pain around the time of menstruation and is caused by uterine spasm. Primary dysmenorrhoea usually occurs in younger women, whereas secondary dysmenorrhoea, which is associated with an underlying condition, such as fibroids or endometriosis, can occur in older women too. The pain is either colicky or dull, usually in the lower abdomen, and often radiating to the back. It starts either a few days or hours before menstruation and ceases 1 or 2 days after menstruation begins. Mild cases may respond to NSAIDs such as ibuprofen, but if it is persistent or severe, **refer.**

(continued overleaf)

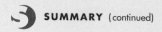 **SUMMARY** (continued)

Endometriosis

Endometriosis is the abnormal presence of endometrial tissue at sites outside the uterus. These are usually located in the abdomen and include the peritoneum, ovary, bladder and intestines. It is a cause of dysmenorrhoea (see above) and can also cause pelvic inflammation and infertility – **refer.**

Gastritis and gastroenteritis

Irritation leading to inflammation of the mucosa of the stomach or small bowel, giving variable and often diffuse abdominal pain or indigestion, is often caused by overindulgence in either food or alcohol. Vomiting may also be present. It is often referred to as non-specific gastritis or non-ulcer dyspepsia (in which the cause is undiagnosed) and resolves spontaneously within 1 or 2 days. In children, non-specific gastritis is associated with fever. Other causes of gastritis or gastroenteritis include bacterial contaminants in food (food poisoning), viruses (gastric flu), and protozoal infections in travellers from abroad. If the condition does not respond to rest, fluids and simple OTC measures within a few days, **refer.**

Gastro-oesophageal reflux disease (GORD)

GORD is the tissue damage caused by a retrograde flow of gastric contents into the oesophagus, producing symptoms of heartburn and acid regurgitation. It is a common condition caused by a loss of tone in the lower oesophageal sphincter and decreased peristalsis. It can result in oesophagitis and stricture, causing obstruction to the passage of food. It can be treated with acid suppressants.

Hernias

Abdominal hernias are caused by a weakening of the muscles and supporting tissue in the abdomen, which allows protrusion (herniation) of the contents. They are common in the lower parts of the abdomen, where structures leave the abdominal cavity. They are often brought on by lifting or straining. The commonest types are inguinal (where the spermatic cord leaves the abdomen) and femoral (where femoral vessels leave the abdomen). The former, seen in males, presents as a swelling in the suprapubic area which eventually pushes into the scrotum. It is felt as an ache in the groin. Femoral hernias occur in both sexes and may be felt as a colicky pain. The swelling is small. Umbilical hernias, with protrusion of the umbilicus, are common in babies. They are usually of no consequence and in most cases resolve as the baby grows – **refer.**

Hiatus hernia

Hiatus hernia is a weakness at the oesophageal hiatus (where the oesophagus penetrates the diaphragm) such that the lower oesophagus and/or part of the stomach is able to slide up through the diaphragm into the chest. The oblique entry of the oesophagus into the stomach disappears and reflux of gastric contents into the oesophagus readily occurs. Hiatus hernia may be congenital, but more usually develops in later life. It also occurs when there is an increase in intra-abdominal pressure, as in obesity or pregnancy. Hiatus hernia is sometimes asymptomatic but generally produces heartburn, which can be treated with antacids. Surgery is occasionally required to rectify the abnormality – **refer.**

Inflammatory bowel disease

See Chapter 7. Abdominal pain is usually mild, the main symptom being bloody diarrhoea. A colicky pain may precede a bowel motion – **refer.**

→

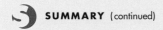 **SUMMARY** (continued)

Irritable bowel syndrome
See Chapter 7.

Nervous dyspepsia
The main symptoms of nervous dyspepsia (functional gastritis) are pain and vomiting. Psychological causes, such as tension or anxiety, are usually easily found.

Non-ulcer (non-specific) gastritis/dyspepsia
In this condition there is inflammation of the gastric mucosa caused by smoking, NSAIDs, alcohol, or no known cause, whereas in gastric ulcer gastritis may follow or precede the development of a crater or ulcer in the gastric wall.

Oesophagitis
Oesophagitis commonly occurs either as a result of a primary inflammatory lesion in the oesophagus or as a result of reflux of gastric contents (see above). Oesophagitis is a common symptom in peptic and oesophageal ulceration and hiatus hernia.

Pancreatitis
See also biliary colic. Pancreatitis is an inflammatory condition of the pancreas, commonly caused by gallstones, alcohol, infection or tumours. It causes sudden acute abdominal pain, as described under biliary colic and acute abdomen – **refer.**

Peptic ulcer disease (PUD)
Peptic ulcers destroy the mucosa and submucosal tissues of the stomach and duodenum. Their first occurrence is most common in males under 35 years of age. The chief symptom is abdominal pain, usually epigastric, but sometimes in the right hypochondrium in duodenal ulcer. Pain is relieved by simple antacids, H_2 antagonists and PPIs. The onset of pain is related to food. It may occur either soon after a meal (gastric ulcer) or 1–2 hours after a meal (duodenal ulcer). Alternatively, food may relieve the pain. The pain of duodenal ulcer is often worse at night and when a meal is delayed or missed. Other symptoms include heartburn, waterbrash, belching and abdominal distension. If untreated, there may be perforation of the ulcer, bleeding and anaemia – **refer.**

Renal colic
Renal colic is usually caused by a renal stone blocking a ureter. There is severe pain in one loin, which may initially start as an ache. The pain then spreads down the flank and into the suprapubic region or, in males, the scrotum. The episode of pain may last several hours and will recur at intervals of days or weeks as the stone passes down the urinary tract. There will often be blood in the urine. Vomiting may occur because of the intense pain – **refer.**

Salpingitis
Salpingitis, an acute form of pelvic inflammatory disease, is a relatively rare condition in which there is inflammation of the fallopian tubes caused by infection. The condition produces lower abdominal pain, tenderness in the iliac fossa, and usually a fever. A pregnancy in the fallopian tube (ectopic pregnancy) may be suspected if there is pain, often with bleeding, following 8–10 weeks of amenorrhoea – **refer.**

(continued overleaf)

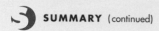 **SUMMARY** (continued)

Urinary tract infection
Pain (usually a burning pain on passing urine), frequency and urgency are symptoms of a urinary tract infection. Infection is most common in the bladder (cystitis). There may be fever and suprapubic pain and tenderness. Recurrences are common, particularly in women. The condition is less common in men and unusual in children, and should be referred. In women, individual mild cases will resolve spontaneously, but if the patient has frequent recurrences, **refer.**

 WHEN TO REFER
Abdominal disorders

• Sudden onset of intense pain that does not abate	Immediate referral
• Symptoms related to medication	
• Pain unrelated to meals	
• Persistent symptoms, not responding to OTC medication	
• Age over 55 with recent onset of dyspepsia and continuous symptoms	
• Blood in stool	
• Weight loss	
• Dysphagia	
• Swelling (not bloating)	
• Vomiting for more than 1–2 days	
• Diarrhoea or constipation for more than 1 week	
• Anaemia	
• Jaundice	Immediate referral
• Dysuria	
• Aggravated by exercise or effort	Immediate referral
• Pain radiates to arm, neck or jaw	Immediate referral
• Pain radiates to back	
• Pain radiates to testis or suprapubic region	Immediate referral
• Pain radiates from central region to right iliac fossa	Immediate referral

CASE STUDIES

Case 1

A man in his 60s requests the purchase of an antacid or preferably 'one of the stronger medicines advertised on the television' for indigestion. He looks well and fit.

What more should be known?

A history of the nature, frequency and severity of symptoms is essential. Even though the man appears well, the absence of alarm signals should be established.

A history given was of infrequent dyspepsia, usually provoked by certain foods, which he felt was not serious but rather annoying. An H_2 antagonist was recommended.

He returned about a week later with his wife, requesting a further supply. Would you consider it safe to continue?

The medicine appears to have been used more quickly than expected, raising concerns about the severity of symptoms. This demands enquiry.

A lack of response to medication, or early relapse afterwards, should be referred.

The presence of this man's wife on this occasion was important. It was she who was the sufferer, with symptoms for over 3 months, often after food or at night, progressively worsening. Her diet was good, she had never smoked, and only drank alcohol occasionally, but she looked unwell and rather pale, and had recently lost weight. She feared both cancer and the surgery she thought must follow, and had persuaded her husband to seek treatment for her in the hope that she was wrong and it would resolve.

The lesson for the pharmacist was never to assume that the customer is the patient, and always to ask the question directly.

The lesson for this woman and her husband is that it is always better to seek advice quickly, whatever might be the diagnosis.

In this case there was a happy ending. A referral to her doctor followed by an urgent appointment with a gastroenterologist resulted in an endoscopy and biopsy. The findings were of non-ulcer dyspepsia, moderate reflux and *Helicobacter* infection. Eradication therapy improved her symptoms considerably and maintenance PPI medication still further.

Case 2

A man and his wife consulted the pharmacist after returning from a holiday in the Far East. They were both very anxious, the man suffering from an upset stomach that had spoiled the later part of their trip. 'It cannot be the holiday' they protested, both having eaten the same food.

What more does the pharmacist need to know?

A full history of the symptoms and their duration is required. The absence of any illness in this man's wife does not eliminate the possibility of an acquired infection in him, although any differences in their eating and drinking should be explored. Other differences, such as the use of bottled rather than tap water, should also be identified.

A discussion between the couple followed, comparing differences in details about the use of tap water to clean teeth, and their consumption of alcohol. The pharmacist was able to elicit a story of several episodes of central abdominal pain and diarrhoea, often following large meals with wine. In between the man was left with a general abdominal discomfort and feeling generally unwell. Prior to the holiday he had suffered episodic abdominal pain and diarrhoea, considered by both of them to be stress induced. 'He has a very busy and important job', the pharmacist learns.

(continued overleaf)

CASE STUDIES (continued)

It is now imperative that he return to work and medication is requested. How should you respond? A medical referral would probably result in a full abdominal examination and possibly a stool culture, which may in turn produce a diagnosis.

Why this couple have chosen the pharmacy rather than the surgery for advice is worth exploring.

A mild gastroenteritis following a holiday abroad is common, and frequently settles with symptomatic treatment and time. These people are anxious, and it would be helpful to know why. This may affect the advice given and the need for a prescriptive course of action.

This couple had seen both their GP and the practice nurse in connection with immunisations before the trip. They had mentioned the abdominal symptoms and the diagnosis of irritable bowel syndrome was suggested, which they both refuted. They were not keen to return to the surgery.

They were reassured, with a suitable medication recommended and the proviso that the problem should be reassessed if resolution did not occur. The man returned only a few days later reporting that his pain was worse. On further questioning he disclosed that on one occasion while away he had got up at night to go to the toilet and found his urine bright pink. This followed a particularly rich dinner, there had been no pain, and in the cold light of day he even doubted the accuracy of his memory. He was referred and investigated, and eventually a renal calculus was removed cystoscopically.

Once a strategy, and particularly an attitude, has been adopted, it can be difficult to undo.

Despite the symptoms and signs described in this book and others, many patients will not follow a classic presentation. The pharmacist here kept an open mind, recognised a possible alarm signal and acted upon it, even though this meant reversing his earlier approach of reassurance.

Case 3

This man in his late 60s was well known to his pharmacist. He visited regularly for his repeat prescription for well-controlled hypertension, and occasionally for self-medication. He was now seeking advice for diarrhoea, mild and of only a few days' duration. What should be recommended?

In the absence of any worrying associated symptoms, it would be reasonable to recommend medication, within a suitable timeframe. This man's age, and a change of bowel habit, reduces the acceptable time before further investigation is warranted.

He has had no previous similar episodes, although a review of recent self-medication showed records of the purchase of an antacid and paracetamol for a headache. As the pharmacist felt uneasy about this man's past and recent history, he was advised to seek medical advice. He attended his GP, although by the time of the appointment the diarrhoea had stopped and clinical examination was normal.

A month later he returned to the pharmacy for a paracetamol and codeine combination analgesic. This was advised by the nurse when he was at the surgery for a blood pressure check to relieve the vague but not severe pain and the occasional looseness in the bowel more effectively.

It is always difficult to contradict colleagues. It is also difficult to ignore what are growing suspicions of serious pathology. An insidious onset can often be overlooked.

With a further request a month later, the pharmacist felt obliged to voice his concerns again. The history was of repeated attacks of vague central abdominal pain, despite feeling well in between attacks. The hypertension remained controlled, and the practice nurse had suggested that the occasional can (or sometimes more) of beer in the evenings most probably explained not only the abdominal symptoms but his moderate obesity as well.

He was referred back to his GP on the premise that an analgesic, if prescribed, would be free of charge, but with instructions that he should advise the doctor of the nature and particularly the duration of his symptoms.

→

CASE STUDIES (continued)

Often suspicions come to nothing. With this man, a series of blood and urine tests, as well as an X-ray, were normal and he was extremely fortunate to have an ultrasound scan. The aneurysm thus discovered was resected and grafted urgently, and it was noted at the time of the operation that a number of minor leaks into and through its wall had already occurred. This diagnosis is often difficult clinically in the presence of even moderate obesity.

It is satisfying to make or suspect a diagnosis, but equally important to respond to the almost subconscious feeling that something is wrong.

9

Perianal and perivulval pruritus

Pruritus in the genitalia and the perianal region is a minor symptom that can be treated with over-the-counter (OTC) medicines, provided that certain criteria are met. The symptom is relatively common, but because patients may be embarrassed to discuss it, some will self-diagnose and medicate without consulting a pharmacist. Many of the common conditions that give rise to pruritus are recurrent, and it is important that patients are educated and advised appropriately. Inappropriate or prolonged medication might exacerbate the condition or mask some underlying pathology.

The most common conditions that cause perivulval itch are cystitis or urethritis and vulvovaginitis. The latter can be caused by infection of the vagina, most commonly with yeasts (candidiasis or thrush), bacteria (bacterial vaginosis) or protozoa (trichomoniasis). Perianal itch may be due to haemorrhoids (piles) or threadworm (pinworm) infestation.

Assessing symptoms

Site or location

Although the symptoms of haemorrhoids and threadworm are easily located to the perianal region, there may be some overlap in the symptoms of vulvovaginal infection and cystitis in women. This is partly because of the close proximity of the vulva and the urethral opening, but also because of irritation of the vulva in cystitis caused by urine dripping from the urethra. It is of course important to locate the site of pruritus to differentiate cystitis from vaginitis. This is sometimes difficult to do.

A rash on the perivulval skin may be caused by sensitisation to toiletries, synthetic underwear, or the use of products containing local anaesthetics.

Type and severity of symptoms

Vaginal candidiasis (thrush) usually presents as vulval soreness, itching, and a burning sensation in the vulval area. There is often redness or swelling of the vulva and a thick, white, odourless discharge. By contrast, the discharge of bacterial or trichomonal infection is smelly and offensive (see Accompanying symptoms for details). Sometimes these conditions may be asymptomatic.

Although less common in men, thrush can cause itching, burning and/or redness at the tip of the penis or under the foreskin. A burning sensation is felt on urinating. A penile discharge is best referred to exclude a sexually transmitted infection (STI).

Patients with cystitis (usually women) will complain of itching at the opening of the urethra. Cystitis in men is much rarer, and should be referred for investigation to exclude conditions such as prostatitis. A burning sensation will be described when passing urine (dysuria). Patients may also complain of urinary frequency and urgency. Rarely, loin pain will be felt. In such cases, the infection may have ascended into the kidney and the patient should be referred. Cystitis can also be an accompanying symptom of all the above causes of vulvovaginitis.

Patients with mild cases of haemorrhoids, or in the early stages of the condition, will complain of itching in the perianal region. More severely affected patients, especially those with external haemorrhoids, may suffer intense pain.

Anal fistulae or fissures in the anal canal are also painful. Any patient complaining of pain should be referred for examination and an accurate diagnosis.

Threadworm causes itching around the anus, particularly at night. This may produce acute pain in some children, particularly when scratching has caused excoriation of the skin in the perianal area.

Onset

Infections of the vagina can be a complication or accompany a course of antibiotics or steroids. Pregnancy predisposes to an overgrowth of *Candida*, and the use of oral contraceptives may alter the vaginal environment and cause candidiasis, but this is controversial and may not be the case with low-dose oestrogen pills. Pregnancy or suspected pregnancy requires referral. Diabetes is another predisposing factor for candidiasis.

In cases of vaginal candidiasis, patients should be asked about their use of local topical applications, such as vaginal deodorants or bath additives, as these can predispose to or exacerbate the condition.

Sexual intercourse can cause trauma, with a resulting urethritis. This gives rise to the well-known condition of 'honeymoon cystitis'.

In men, candidal infection of the penis may be noticed after sexual intercourse.

A change in sexual partner is often associated with the onset of bacterial vaginosis.

Antibiotics can affect the vaginal flora and cause an overgrowth of *Candida*.

Dysuria, frequency, vaginitis, discharge, urethritis and rashes in the genital region are all possible symptoms of an STI and may occur within a few days of sexual intercourse with an infected partner. STIs will not present frequently to pharmacists, but it is important to regard symptoms associated with such a timescale with a high index of suspicion, especially in young adults, the single, those returning from holiday, or whose job involves a lot of travel, and individuals (or their partners) who have been treated previously for STIs. There are frequently concerns about the possibility of HIV infection,

when no symptoms will be evident. These should be handled sensitively, explaining the low probability among heterosexuals, the need for safe sex, and that the antibody blood test will not be accurate until 3 months after exposure. Referral for counselling is recommended.

A patient may relate the onset of haemorrhoids to a cough, sneeze, or episode of physical exertion. They may first appear when straining at stool, or during episodes of constipation.

Symptoms of threadworm infestation have a sudden onset, commonly at night. This is because the eggs are laid by the female worms at night when the environment is warm. Scratching by the patient causes the female worms to rupture, liberating more eggs. The pruritus is associated with some chemical in the eggs.

Duration and frequency

Most patients will seek relief of symptoms promptly. Vaginal candidiasis may be treated with topical OTC imidazoles for 1 week or with an oral azole as a single dose. If there is no obvious improvement after 1 week the patient should be referred to exclude other conditions. Referral should also be made if the patient has suffered from similar symptoms on more than two previous occasions in the past 6 months, so that any underlying predisposing condition, such as diabetes, can be identified and a differential diagnosis made to exclude other diseases.

If the patient is known to have diabetes and has recurrent episodes of candidiasis she should be questioned about the control of her diabetes and referred if appropriate, as high levels of glucose may encourage an overgrowth of *Candida* in the vagina.

Mild cases of cystitis usually resolve spontaneously within a few days. Symptoms that persist beyond 3 days require referral so that antibiotic treatment can be considered. As with candidiasis, frequent recurrence may suggest that the patient has some predisposing condition, such as diabetes, or an anatomical or physiological abnormality in the urinary tract. Changes in the urethral and vaginal epithelium at the menopause may increase the likelihood of infection in some women; in such cases, local application of oestrogen may be helpful. If symptoms are recurrent around the time of menstruation in younger women and do not respond to OTC medicines, the patient should be assessed by a doctor.

Thrush can be a chronic complaint and patients may complain of a discharge for several weeks. A long-standing discharge, however, is unlikely to be vaginitis, and is more often associated with pelvic inflammatory disease (PID), hormonal disturbance or other systemic illness. PID is a complication of bacterial vaginosis and requires referral.

Patients with threadworm will usually seek help within a few days of symptoms occurring. They can be treated at any stage of the disease with OTC anthelmintics, provided there is no reason for referral. Initial treatment may be followed with a repeat dose 14 days later (see Management). Any cases that have not resolved within a few days or which recur after 2 weeks require special consideration for referral or counselling on prophylactic measures.

Mild cases of haemorrhoids may not present to pharmacists or doctors for a long time after the condition first becomes symptomatic. Ideally, any rectal bleeding requires a diagnosis by a doctor, especially in middle-aged and elderly patients, to exclude any serious cause. However, if bleeding is noted just as spotting or streaks on the toilet paper after defecation, and there is only a mild pruritus, OTC medication and advice will usually be appropriate, at least for a short time, if the patient is reticent about seeing a doctor.

Haemorrhoids can often recur. Aggravating factors, such as constipation, can sometimes be identified and it is important that these are dealt with as well as the haemorrhoids themselves.

Accompanying symptoms

Vaginal candidiasis

In this condition there is often (but not always) a characteristic vaginal discharge, which is usually described as thick and white or creamy (resembling cottage cheese) but odourless. However, the discharge can sometimes be thin and watery or yellow in colour; this type of discharge is also typical of some other vaginal infections, which may not respond to topical imidazoles and require referral for investigation.

A thin, watery discharge in a postmenopausal woman may be due to candidal infection. However, if the condition does not respond to OTC azoles referral is necessary, so that atrophic vaginitis and carcinoma can be excluded. Note that the OTC preparations are not licensed for use in women over 60.

The discharge associated with candidiasis is odourless. Any offensive smelly discharge requires referral, as it may represent a trichomonal or bacterial infection. The discharge of bacterial vaginosis has a fishy odour, which is often prominent after intercourse. That of trichomoniasis is often profuse and frothy, and may be white, yellow or green in colour. Similarly, blood in the discharge or any bleeding not associated with menstruation should be referred to exclude a sinister cause. A slight discharge is normal in some women and reassurance is all that is needed, provided the discharge has not changed in any way, such as amount, smell or texture, and is not irritant or bloodstained.

Other symptoms in a patient with vulvovaginitis that should be regarded as unusual and require referral include vaginal blisters, abdominal pain, fever, vomiting and diarrhoea. These may indicate other local pathology or pelvic inflammation. Dyspareunia (painful intercourse) may be caused by candidiasis, but could indicate other pathology. The patient should be referred for a full examination and assessment. If the patient is pregnant, receiving immunosuppressive drugs or is known to have HIV infection, referral is necessary. Referral should also be made if the patient, or their partner, has a known history of STIs so that both can be treated and relapses prevented.

Any patient with symptoms lasting more than 7 days despite treatment should be referred. This is because the differential diagnosis can be difficult, and conditions such as STIs, bacterial infection, trichomoniasis, genital herpes and warts may present with similar (although often more severe) soreness, inflammation and oedema.

Cystitis

If the symptoms of dysuria and frequency are accompanied by pain in the loins, with or without vomiting (suggesting infection or other conditions high in the urinary tract), fever or blood in the urine (indicating more severe infection or inflammation), the patient should be referred.

The urine may be turbid or smell 'fishy' and this may cause no concern on its own, unless persistent. However, if the symptoms of cystitis or urethritis are accompanied by a vaginal discharge, then it is wise to refer the patient.

Pregnant women often present with the symptoms of cystitis. These may represent nothing more than the mechanical effects of pressure from an enlarging uterus and will often resolve spontaneously in a few days. However, if symptoms are either persistent or recurrent, the patient should be referred.

Urinary frequency is a presenting feature of diabetes. If this symptom has lasted for more than a few days, is marked at night and is accompanied by thirst and weight loss, the patient should be referred.

Patients who are known diabetics should present no special problems unless any of the referrable symptoms above are described. However, the patient should be advised to keep a close watch on blood glucose concentrations, as a return of symptoms may indicate hyperglycaemia.

Cystitis is rare in young men. It may be a manifestation of a renal stone, causing damage and infection in the renal tract. In such cases, the patient will complain of episodes of severe colicky loin pain spreading downwards, over days or longer, to the groin and the testicles. It requires a medical appraisal. Referral is also necessary if there is a penile discharge or a known history of STDs.

In older men cystitis is more common, but referral is needed for exclusion of prostatic disease and bladder neoplasms. Blood in the urine, hesitancy on starting urination, a weak flow or dribbling of urine are all signs for referral.

Threadworm

In a child, perianal itching that is worse at night will almost certainly be caused by threadworm.

The diagnosis is confirmed by finding the small white worms, which measure 5–10 mm in length, either in the stool or, very occasionally, on the skin between the buttocks.

Perianal itching in adults, in the absence of a family history of threadworm or visual confirmation of worm infestation, may be due to irritation by deodorants, tight nylon underclothes, or the other causes of perianal and perivulval itch considered in this chapter.

Scratching of the perianal area can cause the skin to become inflamed and sometimes broken. If this is troublesome, the patient should be referred to exclude infection or dermatitis, both of which will be resistant to treatment.

Persistent or particularly heavy cases of threadworm in children can cause loss of appetite, weight loss, insomnia and irritability. Such cases should be referred. Migrating worms have been said to cause inflammation of the vulva and vagina, causing itching and discharge.

Haemorrhoids

Constipation can cause or aggravate haemorrhoids.

Blood in the stool is common in patients with haemorrhoids, and this is well known by most lay people. Because the vast majority of patients will not consult their GP about mild cases of haemorrhoids, it is easy for them to become blasé about this symptom. Although the correct advice is to refer all patients with rectal bleeding who have not received a diagnosis from a doctor, some with mild haemorrhoids will prefer to self-diagnose. Because blood in the stool can signify serious disease, some working guidelines are appropriate. These, of course, depend on the patient being able to give a clear description of their symptoms.

Fresh blood coating the stool is typical of lesions in the descending colon and rectum, and patients with this symptom should be referred to exclude serious pathology. Similarly, any blood that is evident in the flush water in the toilet requires referral. Blood mixed in the stool, giving a dark red or black tarry appearance, suggests that the source is higher in the gastrointestinal tract. This is typical of bleeding gastric or duodenal ulcers, or lesions such as polyps or cancers in the colon. Such cases should be referred.

If blood is present as spots or streaks on the toilet paper, accompanying other symptoms of haemorrhoids, referral for a medical opinion may not be necessary, provided that no severe pain, diarrhoea, loss of appetite, nausea or vomiting have occurred and the pruritus is mild. However, if there is any doubt, referral should be made, especially in middle-aged and elderly patients, in whom colorectal cancer is relatively more common.

Conditions that require referral, and which may be suspected if there is severe pain, include a thrombosed haemorrhoid (when a prolapsing varicocele strangulates and clots) and various infections, such as a perianal abscess or Bartholin's abscess (an infection of a fluid-secreting gland opening into the vagina), or an anal fissure or fistula.

Aggravating factors

Various factors that can initiate or predispose to perivulval and perianal pruritus have been referred to already. Symptoms can be aggravated by the following factors.

Passing urine will cause a burning sensation or other discomfort in cystitis, and also in some cases of vulvovaginitis, such as candidiasis, when urine dribbles on to the sensitive area.

Constipation will aggravate haemorrhoids, and the symptoms of haemorrhoids are usually worse after a bowel motion.

Perfumed soaps, bubble bath, locally applied deodorants and disinfectants may aggravate an already sensitive skin or mucosa caused by any of the conditions described above, producing pruritus and vaginitis.

Tampons and intrauterine contraceptive devices may aggravate vaginal candidiasis, as may menstruation and sexual intercourse.

Tight underclothing made from synthetic material, such as nylon tights, will increase the temperature and humidity of the perianal and perivulval region, thus fostering ideal conditions for the growth of bacteria and candida, as well as encouraging the female threadworm to lay eggs. Nightclothes and bedding will create a similar warm environment.

Hot baths also aggravate the symptom of pruritus.

OTC products advertised for the treatment of 'embarrassing itching' and which contain local anaesthetic agents, such as benzocaine, can sensitise perianal and perivulval skin, thereby aggravating rather than relieving the condition.

Special considerations

Age

Children under 16 years should be referred if they have any of the symptoms described in this chapter, except for threadworm, as such symptoms are rare in this age group. Any suspicion of child abuse or of sexual intercourse under the age of 16 should be handled delicately and diplomatically, but in every case the doctor, health visitor or social worker should be informed. Confidentiality should be respected whenever possible, although the interests of the child at risk are paramount.

Because the incidence of cancer increases with age, OTC treatment should not be recommended in the elderly if there is any doubt about the diagnosis. For instance, vaginal candidiasis is rare in women over 60, and symptoms suggesting such a diagnosis should therefore be referred for confirmation.

Males

In older patients (from middle age onwards) the possibility of prostatitis should be considered if perineal pain with hesitancy and dysuria is present.

In younger men cystitis is relatively uncommon compared with women, and any symptoms suggesting this condition should be referred either to the GP or, in cases where an STI is suspected, to the local genitourinary outpatient clinic.

Patients with suspected STI

Any patient with a history of STI, or with a partner suspected of having an STI, is best advised to consult the local genitourinary outpatient clinic for rapid diagnosis and treatment. Pharmacists should reassure patients that they will be dealt with in a friendly, confidential, anonymous and professional manner.

Management

Threadworm

Treatment of threadworm itself is relatively simple, but compliance with additional hygienic measures is necessary to prevent reinfestation.

Mebendazole and piperazine are both available as single-dose OTC treatments for threadworm. All family members should be treated to obtain the maximal effect, even if they are asymptomatic.

Piperazine is presented as a powder that should be dissolved in water or milk. The initial dose should be followed by a second dose 14 days later to kill the worms that hatched from eggs present at the time the first dose was taken. Piperazine should not be recommended for patients with epilepsy, or in pregnancy. The powder can be used in children over 3 months. Piperazine elixir is taken daily for 7 days and repeated after 1 week if necessary. For children under 2 it should be used on medical advice only.

Mebendazole is suitable for children over 2 years old. It is contraindicated in pregnancy. It is available as a chewable tablet and is effective often without the need to repeat the dose after 14 days, although this is a sensible precaution, as with piperazine. Parents of children with threadworm should be reassured that it is a common condition, is harmless and, despite the stigma once attached to it, does not reflect poor hygiene or diet.

Various measures should be taken to break the cycle of reinfestation, otherwise any recommended medicine may fail to have a lasting effect. Bedlinen and towels should be washed frequently, and underwear and nightclothes changed daily. Hands should be washed and nails scrubbed before eating and after going to the toilet to reduce the transmission of eggs from anus to mouth. Airborne transmission is also possible, and as eggs will be found in dust on floors and furniture, thorough vacuuming may be helpful. A bath or shower taken early in the morning helps to remove eggs laid overnight. Some patients may not obtain instant relief of symptoms after use of an anthelmintic. In such cases crotamiton cream has been suggested to be useful as an adjuvant to treatment.

Cystitis

Symptomatic relief from cystitis is commonly achieved by drinking plenty of fluids and taking sodium bicarbonate (5 g every 3–4 hours), sodium citrate or potassium citrate to alkalinise the urine.

Patient counselling can include advice to empty the bladder as completely as possible after urinating, and to avoid delay in emptying the bladder. Perianal hygiene is important, and patients should be encouraged to wash the area with water and unperfumed soap after a bowel movement, and to wipe from front to back to prevent reinfection.

If symptoms are related to intercourse, the perianal skin should be washed beforehand and the bladder should be emptied before and after intercourse. A lubricant should be used to prevent trauma and soreness.

Care should be taken to avoid tight underclothes made of synthetic material. Detergents should be thoroughly rinsed out after washing underclothes.

Cautions regarding the use of OTC cystitis products are outlined in Table 9.1.

Haemorrhoids

OTC treatments for haemorrhoids are available as suppositories, creams and ointments. Most contain mixtures of astringents (bismuth salts), local anaesthetics, antiseptics, antipruritics, zinc and other miscellaneous substances. However, the most effective preparation is likely to be one that contains hydrocortisone, a proven anti-inflammatory agent. Care should be taken against protracted use, because the perianal skin can become steroid dependent if topical steroids

Table 9.1 Contraindications and need for care in the use of potassium- and sodium-containing preparations

Contraindication	Need for care
Renal disease	Patients may have impaired ability to excrete potassium in potassium citrate
Pregnancy, hypertensive patients	Caution with extra sodium intake with sodium bicarbonate and citrate
Patients taking ACE inhibitors or potassium-sparing diuretics	Potassium citrate may cause hyperkalaemia
Patients taking nitrofurantoin	Nitrofurantoin is inactivated in alkaline urine
Patients taking lithium	Sodium salts can reduce plasma lithium levels

are used for a prolonged period. Preparations containing local anaesthetics should only be used for short periods because of the risk of sensitisation of the skin.

Patients who are constipated should be advised that this will exacerbate the symptoms of haemorrhoids. They should be recommended a laxative for the short term and counselled about adding more roughage (or bran) to the diet and increasing fluid intake. Bulking agents, such as ispaghula and sterculia, are suitable, but if constipation has been present for some time, or is particularly stubborn, a stimulant laxative such as senna may be appropriate to obtain the first motion.

Patients should be advised not to put off the call to defecate and to avoid prolonged straining.

Pregnant women who suffer from haemorrhoids should be advised to increase the fibre content of their diet, as the high progesterone levels in pregnancy have the effect of relaxing the smooth muscle of the bowel.

The cornerstone of relieving the symptoms of haemorrhoids is perianal hygiene. The perianal skin should be washed at least once daily and then patted dry, to prevent irritation by faecal matter in the perianal folds.

Vaginal candidiasis

The decision to treat vaginal candidiasis rests on whether the patient has had the symptoms diagnosed before and whether it is a recurrent problem. If this is the first time the symptoms have appeared, or if the woman has had more than two recurrences in the past 6 months, she should be referred. This is because in the first instance it is crucial that serious diagnoses such as bacterial vaginosis, which can cause serious complications, are excluded. Recurrent cases of candidiasis may suggest an underlying condition such as diabetes causing relapses and reinfection, or the presence of a more resistant species of *Candida*, which is resistant to short-term azole treatment.

OTC antifungals are not licensed for use in patients aged under 16 or over 60.

The most effective treatment for vulvovaginal candidiasis is one of the azole preparations. The choice is between a single-dose oral preparation (such as fluconazole) and topical preparations in the form of creams or pessaries (imidazoles such as clotrimazole). These are recommended for OTC use only for uncomplicated candidiasis in women who have previously suffered from, and are able to recognise, the condition. Patients may prefer a single-dose treatment, either orally or intravaginally.

An intravaginal preparation or oral dose is necessary to treat the infection, which lies high in the vagina. Imidazole creams may be applied night and morning and can give symptomatic relief where there is extensive vulval or labial irritation. If seepage occurs from daytime use of the cream, usage can be restricted to a bedtime dose when the patient is lying flat.

Patients with symptoms that have not resolved within 7 days should be referred.

Patients should be asked what treatment they have already tried. Creams containing local anaesthetics are widely advertised to the public for this condition but can cause sensitisation and irritation of the perivulval skin. Non-drug remedies, such as the local application of yoghurt or of acidifying agents, such as dilute vinegar, should be discouraged for a few days before and after the use of imidazoles, as the latter are less effective in an acid environment.

Male sexual partners may be asymptomatic carriers of *Candida*, but the value of treating them with antifungal creams is unclear. However, symptomatic men can be treated with a single dose of oral fluconazole and an imidazole cream.

Patients should be advised of other measures that can be taken to reduce symptoms. These include avoiding perfumed products, such as soaps and bubble baths, which may exacerbate the skin irritation. Hot baths can cause irritation, as can wearing synthetic underwear, tights and tight-fitting trousers.

Women taking oral contraceptives who are having recurrent candidal infections may benefit from switching to a low-dose oestrogen pill or an injectable progestogen.

After defecation the anus should be wiped from front to back to prevent the transfer of infection from the bowel to the vagina.

Azoles are inhibitors of the hepatic microsomal metabolism of some drugs. Caution is therefore advised in patients taking warfarin, and it is suggested that the prothrombin ratio (INR, measured routinely in such patients) be checked within or at the end of a 7-day treatment period. In theory, the arrhythmogenic potential of the antihistamines known to cause arrhythmias, i.e. terfenadine and astemizole, might be enhanced by both oral and topical imidazoles. Blood concentrations of theophylline, ciclosporin, rifampicin and oral sulphonylureas may be increased by the imidazoles. Except for ciclosporin, these latter interactions are unlikely to be of any clinical significance.

Second opinion

Despite the confidentiality of the consulting room and the frequency of physical examinations, many doctors find it as difficult as other people to discuss intimate problems. Fortunately, the profession now includes many more women than formerly, and patients will have a choice of doctor to confide in.

The history taken will not differ from that available to the pharmacist, and some conditions, such as cystitis, can be investigated or treated without resort to physical examination.

For many, however, this remains a prerequisite to diagnosis and a careful and sensitive examination, with a chaperone if required, is mandatory. Vaginal swabs or cervical smears may be required to investigate gynaecological disorders, a rectal swab to identify colonic and perianal infections. Worm infestations can be identified by the use of clear sticky tape, applied to the skin of the anal margin and then removed, with the organisms trapped and sent for microscopy.

External haemorrhoids or an anal fissure can be visualised, a digital rectal examination used to identify internal haemorrhoids, low rectal lesions or, in males, an assessment of prostatic size and shape. Some GPs will perform sigmoidoscopy in their surgeries to visualise these, although the presence of suspicious symptoms such as unexplained rectal bleeding will need further investigation. This may include barium enema X-ray, or colonoscopy.

Referral to secondary care is required when symptoms such as rectal or vaginal bleeding cannot be explained, or further investigation is required. Suspected sexually transmitted diseases may be better dealt with by the genitourinary medicine clinic, where specimens may be obtained using specialist techniques, often involving rapid microbiological inspection. These clinics are also usually better placed to pursue contact tracing.

The majority of patients attending their GP will bring with them fairly straightforward problems such as cystitis, vaginitis, and minor rectal conditions that can be identified and treated in primary care. More significant problems are rarer, but therefore require a high level of diagnostic suspicion if they are not to be missed.

Bibliography

Anon (2004). An update on vulvovaginal candidiasis (thrush). *MeReC Bulletin* 14: 13–16.

Clinical Effectiveness Group (Association for Genitourinary Medicine and the Medical Society for the Study of Venereal Disease) (2002). *National Guidelines on the Management of Vulvovaginal Candidiasis*. www.mssvd.org.uk

SUMMARY OF CONDITIONS PRODUCING PERIANAL OR PERIVULVAL PRURITUS

Anal fissure

An anal fissure is a tear in the mucosa of the lower anal canal. It is painful and often associated with haemorrhoids – **refer.**

Anal fistula

An anal fistula is a deep communicating sinus or channel connecting the anal canal either to the perineum or to adjacent organs. It causes swelling, pain and pruritus. It is sometimes preceded by an anorectal abscess – **refer.**

Bacterial vaginosis

This is the most common vaginal infection and is caused by a number of organisms, particularly *Gardnerella*, *Mycoplasma* and *Bacteroides*. There may be coinfection with *Chlamydia* and *Trichomonas* spp. The condition commonly relapses after successful treatment of an episode. It usually presents with a vaginal discharge that has a characteristic offensive fishy odour. It usually responds to oral metronidazole or topical clindamycin.

In the doctor's surgery or laboratory bacterial vaginosis can be distinguished from candidiasis by a pH >4.5 and an enhancement of the smell when potassium hydroxide is added to a sample of the discharge fluid.

Chlamydial infection

Chlamydia is a bacterium that causes a sexually transmitted infection of the urogenital tract, predominantly in women. It is often asymptomatic for long periods, but when symptoms occur they include purulent vaginal discharge, postcoital bleeding, intermenstrual bleeding, dyspareunia and abdominal pain. Complications include pelvic inflammatory disease, which can lead to infertility or ectopic pregnancy – **refer** (to either GP or to local genitourinary clinic for follow-ups, contact tracing and advice on prevention of reinfection, e.g. use of condoms)

Carcinoma

Cancer of the colon and rectum (see Chapter 8), or vulva in women – **refer.**

Cystitis

Cystitis presents as itching in the urethra, a frequent and an urgent desire to pass urine, and pain on passing urine. The condition is more common in women than in men. This may be due to organisms being carried from the perianal area to the urethra, which is relatively short in women, thereby facilitating the passage of bacteria to the bladder. In 50 per cent of cases no bacteria can be isolated from the urine. In men complaining of these symptoms referral is necessary to allow investigation, particularly for prostate and renal causes. Predisposing factors for cystitis include diabetes, trauma during sexual intercourse, and an alteration in the skin environment caused by vaginal deodorants, bubble baths etc. Treatment with OTC medicines may be tried for 3 days in women.

Haemorrhoids

Haemorrhoids are divided into two general types: internal and external. Internal haemorrhoids (first-degree haemorrhoids) are abnormally large or symptomatic dilatations of blood vessels engorged with

(continued overleaf)

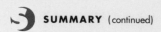

blood that bleed. They require only symptomatic treatment. They are present in the mucosa of the anal canal, but sometimes may become so swollen with blood that they drop down outside the anal sphincter (prolapsed or external haemorrhoids). They may retract and resite themselves spontaneously (second degree) or require manual assistance (third degree). Sometimes they remain permanently prolapsed (fourth-degree haemorrhoids).

Pruritus is a common early symptom of haemorrhoids. There may be bleeding, especially after a bowel movement. With internal haemorrhoids there is usually no pain unless there is a prolapse, when the patient feels a sensation of something moving down the anal canal, followed by acute pain. External haemorrhoids are extremely painful – **refer.**

Polyps

Polyps are benign or malignant tumours that can arise anywhere in the large bowel. They are often asymptomatic, but can bleed, cause pain, or eventually disturb bowel function to the point of subacute obstruction. Recurrence is common. There is a familial tendency to polyps. If there is a history or family history, **refer.**

Sexually transmitted infections (STI)

Those STIs (venereal diseases) that may produce symptoms suggestive of cystitis or candidiasis include the following:

- **Gonorrhoea** Gonorrhoea is characterised by a urethral discharge in males and a vaginal discharge in females, dysuria and frequency. It usually manifests itself within 1 week of intercourse – **refer.**
- **Genital herpes** In genital herpes a vesicular rash affects the tip or shaft of the penis or the labia and vulva. There is local pain, which is aggravated by intercourse, and there may be dysuria – **refer.**
- **Genital warts** There are two forms of genital warts: a frond-like growth, which is almost certainly sexually transmitted, and a flat, common skin wart, which is not. Warts affect the labia, vagina and cervix in women, and the shaft, glans and particularly the foreskin in men. They may be found around the anus, particularly in homosexual men. They are not serious but are difficult to treat and often recur – **refer.**

Threadworm

Enterobius vermicularis (threadworm) is a small thread-like worm between 3 and 10 mm long. Swallowed ova develop in the gut and infect the large bowel. The female lays eggs outside the anus, usually in warm conditions, such as when the patient is in bed. This causes intense pruritus and sometimes pain, with symptoms being worse at night. Children are particularly susceptible, but threadworm spreads in families and at school and all ages can be infested. The condition normally responds to OTC treatment and good hygiene.

Trichomonal vaginitis

Infection by *Trichomonas vaginalis* (trichomoniasis) is rarer than candidal infections. *Trichomonas* is a protozoon. The symptoms of infection with this organism are similar to those of candidiasis but more severe. The vaginal discharge has an offensive odour and is yellow or green – **refer.**

→

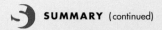 **SUMMARY** (continued)

Vaginal candidiasis (thrush)

Vaginal candidiasis is an infection with *Candida* species, most commonly *C. albicans*. In a small minority of cases *C. glabrata* is the causative organism, which is more resistant to treatment. There is vulvovaginal itching and often an odourless, white vaginal discharge. Sometimes there is a burning sensation in the vulval area and dysuria. The source of the infection is often the alimentary tract, including the mouth. Infection spreads to the vagina from the anus via the perianal skin. Predisposing factors include pregnancy, diabetes, the use of vaginal deodorants etc., antibiotics and steroids.

The importance of a diagnosis of the initial episode by a doctor cannot be overstated.

Sometimes candidiasis and bacterial vaginosis can be concurrent, so that any failure to respond to treatment should be referred to the doctor. Candidiasis may be treated with OTC azole preparations if it has been previously diagnosed by a doctor. If a patient presents with symptoms suggestive of candidiasis for the first time, she should be referred to confirm the diagnosis. Patients with frequent attacks should be referred to identify the presence of any predisposing factors. Women over 60 should also be referred.

WHEN TO REFER
Perianal and perivulval pruritis

Vaginitis
- Not had before
- Had more than twice in the last 6 months
- Foul-smelling discharge
- Bloodstained discharge
- Loin pain   Immediate referral if severe
- Abdominal pain   Immediate referral if severe
- Abominal pain and fever and/or vomiting   Immediate
  and diarrhoea
- Pain (other than just soreness) on urination
- Patient is taking immunosuppressants   Immediate
- Patient is diabetic   Immediate
- Pregnancy   Immediate
- Breastfeeding
- Age over 60
- Age under 16
- Failure to improve significantly within
  7 days of OTC treatment
- Ulcers in genital area   Immediate
- Anyone with a history of STI
  (sexually transmitted infection)

Threadworm
- Recurrent
- Failure to respond to OTC remedy within a
  few days

Haemorrhoids
- Pain in anal area
- Abdominal pain
- Weight loss
- Age over 40 and bleeding noted for first
  time
- Going to toilet more frequently
- Failure to respond to OTC products

Cystitis
First attack, or more than three in 12 months, that fails to respond to short-term symptomatic treatment.

CASE STUDIES

Case 1

A man in his late 60s was collecting his repeat prescription for left ventricular failure and aortic valve disease. He appeared unwell, and reported several epistaxes and some spontaneous bruising over the last week or so. He asks the pharmacist's opinion.

His medical history suggests he may be anticoagulated: this should be enquired for, or checked with his medication list.

Any reason for loss of control, such as poor compliance or failure to have it checked, should be identified.

His warfarin control was normally stable, the dose constant, and the INR had been checked about 2 weeks previously. He was advised to see his practice nurse for a further check immediately, and not to take any further warfarin until advised.

Are there any other considerations that need exploring?

A drug interaction is a further possibility. This man's wife had purchased miconazole cream 2 weeks previously, not remembered by the pharmacy staff. It was intended for her husband, who did not wish to mention a fungal infection in his groin. His INR the same day was >10, but control was rapidly regained after the topical application was stopped.

Case 2

A woman in her late 50s believes she has developed piles and requests medication. How should the pharmacist respond?

A full history is as important here as elsewhere, but the reasons for the enquiry should be explained first. This should be conducted in as much privacy as possible.

After using the toilet the woman had noticed 'something come down' which is irritant and occasionally streaks the paper with a little fresh blood. This had been present for only 10 days, and was accompanied by perineal irritation.

What are the differential diagnoses?

Her diagnosis of haemorrhoids seems likely. An anal fissure could be responsible for irritation, pain on defecation and superficial bleeding, but not the feeling of a lump. Her bowel frequency, especially any constipation, should be noted.

The exact nature and location of the lump should be defined. Occasionally early and minor degrees of uterine prolapse in women can be confused with rectal lesions.

This woman is in the age group where rectal bleeding should not be allowed to persist without investigation.

A topical application was provided, with advice about the need to avoid straining and for review. She was encouraged not to continue the medication, but to see her doctor (a) if the condition did not resolve within a week; (b) if it recurred after treatment; or (c) if the bleeding persisted.

Case 3

A woman in her 30s has requested medication for 'worms' for all of her three children. What should the response be?

The symptoms behind her suspicion need to be identified.

The ages of her children need to be known.

A history of previous infections and any medication is important.

(continued overleaf)

CASE STUDIES (continued)

Any possible sources of the infection also need treating.

On questioning, threadworm seems most likely. Two of the children have perianal itching and one has seen small white worms with her stool. A recommendation for treatment is provided, although the history revealed the family had acquired a puppy some months ago, and that this was their second infection since then. They believe the dog to be to blame. Is this reasonable?

Dogs are frequently affected by worm infestations, which could be transmitted to humans. Infections in domestic animals are easily treated, and can be prevented by regular medication.

Surveys have reported considerable numbers of pets which are rehomed because their owners believe they are the source of illness or allergies in humans. In this instance a review of hygiene practice within the family and other contacts suggested a number of potential human hosts, and no further infection occurred.

10

Ear disorders

Symptoms in the ear are often associated with upper respiratory tract disorders and are common in children. The inner ear is continuous with the upper respiratory tract, being connected by the eustachian tube, which functions to equalise pressure in the ear. Symptomatic relief can be obtained in some cases with over-the-counter (OTC) medicines, but examination by a doctor is necessary if symptoms persist.

Assessing symptoms

Site or location

Disorders of the ear can be conveniently listed in terms of the site of the lesion (Table 10.1). A diagram of the ear is shown in Figure 10.1.

Table 10.1 Disorders of the ear

Outer ear	**Middle ear**
Otitis externa:	Otitis media (infection)
dermatitits (pinna or external ear canal)	Secretory otitis media (glue ear)
infection (external canal)	Trauma and perforation of eardrum
Tumour (pinna)	Otosclerosis
Trauma, e.g. laceration (pinna)	
Excessive wax (external canal)	**Inner ear**
	Vertigo (including Ménière's disease)
Foreign bodies	Eustachian catarrh or barotrauma
Furuncles (boils)	

Severity

The severity of symptoms will determine the need for and the urgency of referral. Any severe pain in the middle ear is distressing to the patient and requires an examination with an otoscope by the doctor. If a lesion causing discomfort in the external ear is visible then the pharmacist must make a judgement based on the severity of the symptoms and the possible diagnoses. Thus, dermatitis on the pinna may be itching and uncomfortable, but may be treated with OTC creams in the first instance without the need for referral. On the other hand, a patient with an isolated blister, ulcer or unusual lesion on the pinna, which is growing in size but causing only minimal itch, should be tactfully but firmly referred so that malignancy can be excluded.

Because of its abundant blood supply, trauma to the pinna can result in profuse bleeding. The ear should be compressed with a clean pad and the patient sent to a hospital Accident and Emergency department.

Duration

Acute otitis media generally lasts for less than 1 week. However, if there is severe pain, referral is necessary before this time so that the ear may be examined to exclude perforation of the eardrum or the development of chronic suppurative otitis media. The latter is more common in adults than in children. Eustachian catarrh, which may accompany the common cold, usually lasts less than 1 week, but occasionally it may continue and develop into a chronic catarrhal state.

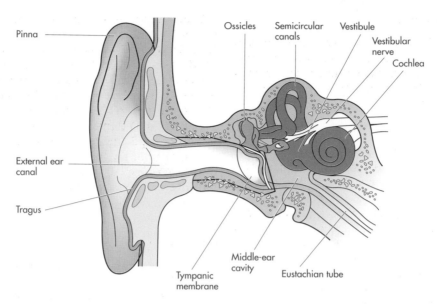

Pinna

Ossicles   Semicircular   Vestibule
            canals

Vestibular
nerve

Cochlea

External ear
canal

Tragus

Middle-ear
cavity

Tympanic
membrane

Eustachian tube

Figure 10.1 Diagram of the ear.

Glue ear (secretory otitis media) may persist for several weeks or months without being recognised because it is often symptomless until the associated deafness becomes apparent.

Vertigo may occur briefly during an ear infection associated with an upper respiratory tract infection. In such cases, the symptom will resolve in a few days. However, the vertigo associated with Ménière's disease will either persist or recur and become more severe. It will often be accompanied by nausea, vomiting and tinnitus.

Onset

Eustachian catarrh and otitis media may develop during a common cold. Both of these disorders can also be caused by swimming, diving and air travel, when pressure differentials between the middle-ear cavity and the outside can suck fluid and microorganisms from the nasopharynx through the eustachian tube.

Accompanying symptoms

Pain

Pain may be associated with a furuncle (boil) in the external ear canal, but otherwise it is not a major feature of otitis externa. Problems caused by ear wax do not generally produce pain, and it is rarely a major feature of glue ear. Earache is complained of by the majority of patients with otitis media – this is the commonest cause of earache in children. It requires referral for a diagnosis.

Earache may or may not be a feature of Eustachian catarrh. It occurs in chronic suppurative otitis media only if the drum perforates. Pain may be experienced during descent in an aircraft (barotrauma), particularly if the sufferer has catarrh.

Earache should generally be regarded as a referrable symptom.

Cold, sore throat

Infection easily passes from the mouth and nasopharynx to the ear via the Eustachian tube, and ear infections may therefore be the result of bacterial or viral invasion.

Swelling and discharge

Redness, swelling and a discharge are common features of a furuncle in the ear canal, but may also reflect an infective dermatitis in the canal. A discharge may be seen in both acute and chronic types of otitis media.

Bleeding and bruising

Bleeding in the pinna is often copious and may not respond to the application of pressure. Patients should therefore be referred. In addition, any trauma to the pinna, with or without external bleeding, may result in large haematomas between the skin and the cartilage. These should be assessed by a doctor to determine whether they require surgical drainage to prevent fibrous scarring, which can result in the familiar 'cauliflower ear'. Any blood discharged into the ear canal requires a medical opinion to exclude perforation of the eardrum if the bleeding does not appear to arise from the canal itself.

Itching

Itching or irritation of the ear canal or pinna usually represents a form of dermatitis, which can be treated with OTC topical preparations. It may sometimes be caused by the presence of a discharge in the canal.

Deafness

Deafness can be caused by obstruction in the external ear canal, inflammation in the middle or inner ear, or a disturbance of the auditory nerve. It is therefore to be expected when the ear canal is blocked by wax, debris or a discharge (as from an infection), and in otitis media (chronic and acute), eustachian catarrh and barotrauma. In glue ear the onset of deafness is insidious and may only be recognised when a child is observed to be failing at school because he or she cannot hear properly. Deafness with no apparent cause in young adults may be due to otosclerosis (see p 136) or may be industrial deafness, a permanent result of long-term unprotected exposure to high levels of noise, mostly from machinery.

Deafness can be tested with a tuning fork to determine whether it is conductive or perceptive. Conductive deafness is caused by failure of conduction of sound waves. Normally, sound waves enter the ear canal and cause the eardrum to vibrate, which then moves the chain of ossicles to transmit the vibrations to the cochlea in the inner ear. Perceptive deafness is failure of the system beyond this point, such as the cochlea failing to transmit the vibrations and stimulate the auditory nerve, or the nerve itself failing to transmit impulses so that the sound can be appreciated in the brain.

Red eardrum

Using an otoscope, many ear conditions can be differentiated by the state of the tympanic membrane (eardrum). It appears normal in otitis externa, Is often normal in glue ear, but is red in otitis media or following trauma. This is important, because the instillation of ear drops is contraindicated when the drum is perforated. Often the drum cannot be seen during examination with an otoscope because of occlusion by a discharge or wax.

Fever and malaise

Otitis externa does not usually produce any signs of systemic disturbance, even in the case of a furuncle in the ear canal, unless the infection is severe. Fever is generally a sign of infection and is common in children with otitis media; it is often accompanied by vomiting. It is also a common sign of teething in babies with earache.

'Something in the ear'

Although patients may describe occlusion of the ear canal and the associated deafness as a feeling of 'something in the ear', it should be remembered that foreign bodies can also be real rather than imaginary. They can cause anxiety and, in the case of live insects, acute pain and appalling irritation as they struggle and flap their wings. Insects can be dealt with in the first instance by the pharmacist (see Management). Foreign bodies may sometimes be removed, depending on what the object is and its accessibility.

Neck stiffness

Neck stiffness associated with symptoms in the ear requires referral to exclude the rare cases of an abscess in the mastoid air cells, or thrombosis of the adjacent cavernous venous sinus, the associated inflammation spreading to involve the meninges or even the brain.

Tinnitus

Tinnitus is the complaint of an extraneous noise arising in the ear or anywhere in the head. It is usually described as ringing, buzzing, hissing or even pulsating. It may be a symptom of any disorder of the ear. It can be an accompaniment of senile deafness, otosclerosis, industrial deafness, Ménière's disease or drug toxicity (e.g. high-dose aspirin, furosemide, gentamicin).

Vertigo

Disturbances of the inner ear may cause vertigo, the most important causes being Ménière's disease, vestibular neuronitis and positional (postural) vertigo. Vertigo is best described as a sensation of the room spinning around the sufferer. It should be distinguished from unsteadiness on the feet (as occurs, for example, in muscle weakness or Parkinson's disease) or lightheadedness (a feeling of dizziness, as in postural hypotension, which may be associated with some drugs, particularly antihypertensive drugs in elderly patients). Vertigo is a referrable symptom if it occurs at some time of the day for more than a few days.

Nausea and vomiting

Nausea and vomiting in association with vertigo, tinnitus and eventual deafness is seen typically in Ménière's disease, but may also reflect other disorders of the internal ear.

Incidence and recurrence

As might be expected, infections of the middle ear (otitis media) are more common in winter because of the association with upper respiratory infections. In the summer, such infections may result from swimming, diving and air travel. Symptoms may not become significant until several days after acquiring the infection, and patients should be questioned about their activities, especially after a holiday.

Glue ear can develop into a chronic condition but it may be difficult to identify until deafness becomes apparent.

Otitis externa can also develop into a chronic condition that is symptomatic from time to time.

Trigger factors

Recurrent episodes of otitis media may be associated with swimming and water sports. In children, frequent upper respiratory infections and attacks of otitis media may be associated with the development of a persistent catarrhal problem. Repeated barotrauma in frequent air travellers can have the same effect.

Patients who have an inflammatory lesion, such as a furuncle in the ear canal, will complain that it is painful when the pinna is pulled upwards and back (as when an observer attempts to examine the ear) or when the tragus is pressed.

Patients with positional vertigo will often have momentary vertigo when getting out of bed.

Management

Problems of the external ear

Dry skin on the pinna can be treated with an emollient such as aqueous cream, emulsifying ointment or a similar proprietary preparation. If the skin of the external ear canal is affected, olive oil may be more convenient to use. If there is a contact dermatitis caused by sensitivity to earrings, patients should be encouraged to wear nickel-free earrings or to use a proprietary clear lacquer to coat the earrings, so that the nickel is not in contact with the skin. Topical hydrocortisone should also be used in such a case of contact dermatitis, provided the pharmacist is confident there is no infection present.

Aluminium acetate solution may be a useful astringent for itching otitis externa and can be used when there is a wet dermatitis either on the pinna or in the ear canal.

If an infection is suspected or the lesion is not showing signs of improvement after 7 days, the patient should be advised to see a doctor to evaluate the need for antibiotics.

Many cases of otitis externa affecting the external ear canal are aggravated by water and by scratching. These factors, and poor cleaning of the ear, will predispose to infection. The patient should be advised either to avoid swimming or at least to use earplugs when doing so, to dry the ears gently but thoroughly, and to perform an aural toilet before instilling drops into the ear canal. The removal of debris from the ear canal and the maintenance of a clean, dry environment will deter invasion by pathogenic organisms. Cleaning should be done with cotton-wool buds, which should be used once and then disposed of. The cotton wool should be gently rotated along the entire length of the canal.

Although it is necessary to keep the canal dry, it should not be occluded with a plug (except when swimming) if there is any exudate, as this will only serve to keep the exudate inside and provoke further irritation. The use of an appropriate proprietary preparation or aluminium acetate solution should assist in drying up excess moisture, and such a preparation can be used prophylactically.

Adults should be told not to poke hard objects, such as hairgrips or matchsticks, down the ear canal as they may scratch the canal and promote infection, and there is also a small risk that the eardrum may become perforated.

Fretful children who writhe are at risk of damage to the ear during cleaning. They are best dealt with by sitting the child sideways on the parent's lap while another person performs the cleaning procedure. One parental arm can be placed around the child's shoulders and the other around its head, holding it against the parent's chest.

Furuncles in the ear canal are difficult to treat, but some relief can be obtained by the application of a hot flannel and oral analgesics.

Cerumenolytics

Water- or oil-based ear drops can be used to dissolve excess wax. They are not always successful and take several days to produce their effect. However, they do facilitate syringing, which may have to be resorted to by the doctor or practice nurse if the drops alone are not effective within 1 week. Problems may arise if drops are instilled into an ear with a perforated drum, as this may cause irritation or pain and perhaps infection of the middle ear.

It is often impossible to visualise the eardrum using an otoscope when there is a large amount of wax in the canal, and the doctor then has to rely on taking a brief history to assess the likelihood of a perforated drum. The pharmacist can do this by asking if the patient has had a recent ear infection, or whether there has been a history of perforation or a chronically discharging ear. Perforation may have occurred recently without being diagnosed by a doctor, and so the patient should be asked about any discomfort or pain, especially after diving or any other water sports or air travel. If any of these questions is answered in the affirmative, the patient should be referred. Similarly, if patients experience pain when instilling ear drops, they should be referred.

Some cerumenolytics will sometimes cause ear wax to swell at first, and patients should be warned that deafness may be worsened initially.

Several proprietary drops contain wetting agents, such as docusate, which may be helpful. On the other hand, some contain potential irritants such as chlorobutanol and para-dichlorobenzene. Their use is contraindicated in the presence of otitis externa and patients should be warned to discontinue usage if any discomfort is felt.

It is difficult to assess the comparative efficacy of cerumenolytics from the literature, and many doctors hold the view that simple generic preparations, such as olive or almond oil, are satisfactory.

Removal of foreign bodies

Removal of foreign bodies from the ear (usually of a child) is best left to an expert unless the

CASE STUDIES

Case 1

A mother with her child of about 8 years asks the pharmacist for a bottle of paediatric paracetamol. She appears agitated and also enquires what the maximum dose is, and whether it could be exceeded.

How should the pharmacist respond?

Rather than a straightforward reply to her question, it will be important to determine the reason for her enquiry.

Obviously, before supplying the medication it is imperative that the patient understand the dosage, and the pharmacist must be confident she will respect it.

Commonly used medicines may carry the perception of being harmless.

This woman has just visited her GP, her child having had earache for 2 nights. She expected a prescription for antibiotics, but instead has been advised that there is 'no obvious infection'. The pain is less severe now, but she is concerned that it may worsen later.

A more detailed explanation may reinforce that of her doctor.

- There are several possible causes of earache. Pain which is worse at night on lying down may be due to catarrhal obstruction.
- Frequent repeated use of antibiotics has been implicated in the development of glue ear – chronic secretory otitis media, with associated hearing loss.
- Otitis media is often self-limiting, and some clinical trials have found little differences in outcome between groups treated with and without antibiotics.

This woman remained understandably anxious about the duration of the earache, and why she is given different treatments on different occasions.

Each episode must be judged separately, and in the context of a continuing problem.

Further symptomatic relief from eustachian tube dysfunction may be treated with decongestant nasal drops or inhalations.

Case 2

A young woman asks her pharmacist if she could obtain a small supply of antibiotics and cover this with a prescription from her doctor later. It is a Saturday morning. She works as airline cabin crew and is due to fly later that day. She has a cold and earache and needs to prevent any further damage or pain.

Is this reasonable?

Her GP may not be immediately available, and an unauthorised prescription is not permissible. She could be referred to a hospital emergency department, drop-in clinic or out-of-hours facility.

The young woman did not appear acutely ill, and wisely the pharmacist took a full history. She had suffered intermittent earache, with catarrh, over the last 2 days, and had experienced discomfort before when flying. She had taken time off work for this reason and was reluctant to do so again. While abroad she had obtained and taken antibiotics in the past; this had coincided with an improvement in her symptoms.

The pressurisation systems in modern aircraft are sufficient to make serious barotrauma unlikely, although a sudden descent in the presence of eustachian dysfunction may produce pain.

Antibiotics should not be used without a high suspicion of bacterial infection, and will not help here. Instead, treatment now with decongestants may relieve her discomfort and help protect her from barotrauma.

→

CASE STUDIES (continued)

This woman's condition may be affecting her career and her future health. She should be encouraged to consult her GP for an otoscopic examination as soon as possible, and possibly further investigation of her long-term management.

Case 3

A middle-aged man asks his pharmacist for some solvent to loosen ear wax.

What else needs to be known?

This man had several episodes of a build up of wax in the past, which had required syringing. He had no recent history of ear infection, but his hearing was diminishing in one ear more than the other, with a feeling that the canal was full up.

Accumulation of wax can be suspected from the recent and past history. Any suspicion of a perforated tympanic membrane needs to be explored.

He can safely be supplied with cerumenolytic ear drops, and as he has had ear syringing in the past he can make an appointment directly with his practice nurse. It would be wise for the pharmacist to ascertain which agent is used by his surgery to loosen wax, so that he can advise appropriately. It is unlikely his doctor will need to assess him.

There is a chance that the wax may be loosened and discharge itself in full, allowing the man to cancel the appointment.

11

Musculoskeletal disorders

The musculoskeletal system consists of the bony skeleton and associated soft tissues. The latter comprise ligaments, which are bands of tissue connecting bones, usually at a joint, imparting strength and stability to the latter and limiting abnormal movement; skeletal muscles, which shorten and lengthen to create movement; and tendons, which attach muscles to bone. Muscles and tendons function together as a unit. Small fluid-filled sacs called bursae reduce friction and serve a protective function between a bone and a tendon, between two tendons, or between a bone or tendon and the overlying skin.

Most musculoskeletal disorders are the result of wear, strain, overuse or trauma, resulting in inflammation or swelling and pain. The pharmacist may be presented with symptoms of chronic conditions such as rheumatoid arthritis and backache, or with acute injuries associated with falls or sporting activities.

Assessing symptoms

Neck

An ache in the neck can be caused by strain on the ligaments and muscles resulting from unaccustomed movements or positions, including lifting heavy weights or even sitting at a desk.

Pain in the neck may be felt in arthritis (usually in middle-aged to elderly patients) or when a disc prolapses (in both young and older age groups). Wry neck (acute torticollis) is a condition in which the neck is bent or twisted because of muscle spasm; it is often caused by unaccustomed or repeated movement, or after exposure to cold.

Onset, accompanying features and spread

A patient with wry neck will often complain of pain on one side of the neck and, if the powerful trapezius muscle is affected, down as far as the upper border of the scapula, close to the shoulder. (The trapezius is a triangular muscle with its base running along the spine between the occiput at the base of the skull and a point just below the scapula, converging to a point at the shoulder.) The condition often arises after sleeping in an awkward posture. It may also be traced to diving, heading a soccer ball or similar movements. There is usually no previous history of neck pain. Palpation of the tender area on the affected side results in spasm of the muscles.

In wry neck, the neck vertebrae are not tender. In contrast, in cervical spondylosis the vertebrae are often – but not always – tender to the touch. In wry neck the patient will be able to turn his or her head away from the affected side, but there will be difficulty and pain in turning towards the affected side. This is particularly the case if the sternomastoid muscles, which lie at the side and towards the front of the neck, are affected.

In arthritis or spondylosis movement is usually equally painful to both sides, but can be worse in one direction. If there is nerve root pain, movement brings a sharp pain down the shoulder and arm in the distribution of the affected nerve.

Viewed from the side, the normal cervical spine has a mild forward curve. In advanced degeneration or conditions of poor posture, this curve is exaggerated so that the head appears to have slipped forwards on the neck. This can be very painful.

Shoulder

The most common disorder affecting the shoulder joint, apart from trauma, is capsulitis (rotator cuff syndrome). This may be caused by overuse or unaccustomed movement resulting in inflammation in the ring of tendons attached to the shoulder muscles. Movement is restricted in one or all directions.

A common variant is the supraspinatus syndrome. The supraspinatus muscle, which lies on the upper border of the spine of the scapula, is responsible for abduction (raising) of the arm at the shoulder joint. In this syndrome the shoulder is particularly painful when the patient is asked to raise his arm laterally from the body. Palpation at the outermost point of the shoulder, just behind the lateral tip of the clavicle, will reveal an acutely tender supraspinatus tendon, confirming the diagnosis. In the more widespread rotator cuff syndrome the tenderness is slightly lower, around the neck of the humerus, and extends further.

After a painful disorder of the shoulder has apparently healed, it may become apparent some time afterwards that the arm cannot be raised above the head or behind the back. This is often due to scarring or fibrosis of the muscles, tendons and ligaments around the shoulder joint, which can occur to such an extent that the syndrome known as frozen shoulder develops, often with some degree of irreversibility.

Back

Thoracic spine and intercostal muscles

Thoracic spinal pain is uncommon and should be referred unless some obvious trivial cause can be found.

Pain arising in the intercostal muscles (between the ribs) may be due to a muscle strain, but must be distinguished from the pain of a myocardial infarction, pulmonary embolus or pleurisy.

Pain arising after straining, while lifting a heavy object or coughing, may be due to a muscle strain or tear, or to a prolapsed (slipped) disc, which will cause a ligament to be stretched and muscles to go into spasm. Such musculoskeletal damage must be differentiated from other serious causes of pain. Chest pain due to angina will usually disappear after resting or, if there is a history and the patient has medication, after glyceryl trinitrate. The pain of myocardial infarction lasts longer than 30 minutes and the patient will often be anxious, cyanosed and sweating, and in most cases will be obviously ill. A muscle strain or tear will cause a sharp pain in a small, defined area and will be exacerbated by coughing or deep inspiration. This is also the case with pleurisy or a pulmonary embolus, although in severe cases of these disorders the pain may be present continuously, with abnormal breathing.

If these latter diagnoses cannot be excluded, the patient should be referred.

Lumbar spine

Low back pain, often referred to as lumbago, may be mild or severe. In both types there will often be a strain of the spinal muscles and ligaments. In the more severe type the patient should be encouraged to rest to see whether the symptoms resolve. Sometimes the cause can be a prolapsed intervertebral disc, and in such cases harm can be done by the patient 'soldiering on'.

The pain of a prolapsed disc is constant but is exacerbated by movement. The patient will hold him- or herself rigid to avoid movement, and the gait will be stiff and awkward.

A prolapsed disc (Figure 11.1) will often impinge on the roots of nerves originating from the spinal cord, the most commonly affected being the sciatic nerve. In such cases the pressure on the nerve root will cause pain in the area supplied by the nerve. This is called sciatica. The pain may be intense and burning, radiating from the back to the buttock and the back of the leg, and sometimes to the front of the thigh. It may spread to below the knee. The patient with sciatica will limp and will be unable to flex the hip very far, making climbing stairs or sitting down uncomfortable. If a prolapsed disc is suspected, the patient should be referred.

Back pain which is worse after rest and improves with exercise may be due to ankylosing spondylitis, an inflammatory arthritis of the lumbar spine and sacroiliac joints. These joints

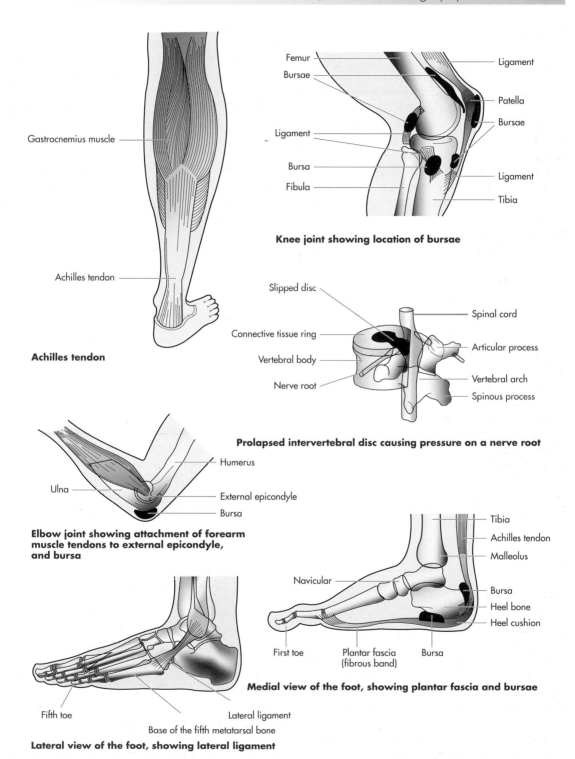

Gastrocnemius muscle

Achilles tendon

Achilles tendon

Femur
Bursae
Ligament
Bursa
Fibula

Ligament
Patella
Bursae
Ligament
Tibia

Knee joint showing location of bursae

Slipped disc
Connective tissue ring
Vertebral body
Nerve root

Spinal cord
Articular process
Vertebral arch
Spinous process

Prolapsed intervertebral disc causing pressure on a nerve root

Ulna

Humerus
External epicondyle
Bursa

Elbow joint showing attachment of forearm muscle tendons to external epicondyle, and bursa

Navicular

Tibia
Achilles tendon
Malleolus
Bursa
Heel bone
Heel cushion

First toe   Plantar fascia (fibrous band)   Bursa

Medial view of the foot, showing plantar fascia and bursae

Fifth toe   Lateral ligament
Base of the fifth metatarsal bone

Lateral view of the foot, showing lateral ligament

Figure 11.1   Diagrams showing parts of joints.

are often tender and there is notable restriction of flexion of the spine.

Acute soft tissue lumbago (strain of a ligament or muscle) can often be related to an event such as lifting or twisting. The pain may be experienced diffusely across both sides of the back at the level of the sacrum, or linearly and to one side in the vertically running spinal muscles. There is often no pain at rest or on slow movement. Chronic lumbago is common but very difficult to treat. Any history of a sporting, traffic or industrial injury, previous slipped disc or arthritis will require medical referral.

It should always be borne in mind that diseases of various organs can cause backache. Inquiry should be made to exclude discomfort on micturition or colicky abdominal pain, which may indicate a urinary tract infection or renal colic. In women, any cyclical low back pain should be viewed with caution, particularly if it occurs in the middle or second half of the menstrual cycle, as this warrants consideration of a non-musculoskeletal cause. Inquiry about any menstrual irregularity or abdominal pain should be made, but even in the absence of these symptoms recurrent cyclical pain requires referral.

Any change in bowel habit or any weight loss should be viewed with suspicion as it may reflect a disorder in the large bowel, which lies close to the sacral area of the lower back.

Persistent unexplained lumbar pain in middle age and beyond could indicate a malignant secondary tumour and must be investigated.

Coccygitis

Coccygitis produces a pain in the coccyx (tailbone) and is often caused by a fall on to a hard surface. The coccyx will be tender to the touch and painful, especially when sitting down. It takes a few weeks to heal.

Elbow

Various types of injury to the elbow or overuse of the associated muscles, which control wrist and finger movements, may be seen.

Location

Pain and tenderness to the touch around the small bony protuberance on the outer side of the elbow is characteristic of tennis elbow (see Figure 11.1). Similarly, pain and tenderness around the bony protuberance on the inner side of the elbow is known as golfer's elbow. These protuberances are the epicondyles, and the bony pains of tennis and golfer's elbow are known respectively as lateral and medial epicondylitis.

Pain and tenderness over the tip of the elbow (the olecranon) is popularly known as student's elbow.

Duration

The symptoms of any of these syndromes will last a varying amount of time, depending on the severity of the problem. Symptoms that persist for more than 1 or 2 weeks should be referred if they are particularly troublesome.

Onset, spread of symptoms and aggravating factors

Despite their popular names, it is not only golfers, tennis players and students who suffer these symptoms.

Student's elbow can be caused either by inflammation of, or bleeding into, a bursa at the tip of the elbow. It is fairly easy to diagnose without inquiry about its onset, although there may be a classic history of a blow to, or fall on to, the elbow, repeated flexing of the elbow, or persistent leaning on the elbow in such recreational pursuits as drinking or rifle shooting. Pain will be felt at rest and on movement of the elbow, and there may be swelling and redness. The swelling can extend to the forearm.

Tennis and golfer's elbow can be traced to overuse or unaccustomed movement, such as curling of the wrist as in powerful gripping and pulling actions, which strains the tendons of the forearm muscles attached to the outer (tennis) or the inner (golfer's) epicondyles at the elbow. The resulting stress on the elbow produces pain in both the elbow and the forearm muscles and a weakness of the wrist. Flexing the hand downwards at the wrist joint will cause pain in golfer's elbow, and bending the hand back at the wrist will cause pain in tennis elbow.

Pain may spread to the inner aspects of the forearm in golfer's elbow and to the outer forearm in tennis elbow.

Forearm, wrist and hand

Pain in the forearm, wrist and hand can be caused by entrapment of nerves. The most common presentations of this type of disorder are tenosynovitis and carpal tunnel syndrome. Both can produce pain and tenderness over the flexor surface of the forearm. If the pain is also felt in the palm of the hand, fingers and wrist, it suggests carpal tunnel involvement.

Treatment of mild cases of both conditions is similar, so that a definitive diagnosis is not important, but if suspected the patient should be referred.

Upper leg

Pain in the upper leg, apart from sciatica (see above), will probably be caused either by a strain or rupture of the thigh muscles or by cramp-like stiffness after unaccustomed exercise.

Onset and accompanying symptoms

A sudden stabbing pain in the anterior thigh after a rapid contraction of the muscles, e.g. when an athlete or sports player makes a forceful sudden movement, will most likely be due to a rupture of the quadriceps muscle. Pain at the back of the thigh will be caused by similar damage to the hamstring muscle. There will be tenderness, and often bruising and swelling.

Knee

In young people traumatic injuries to the knee are relatively common, whereas in older people a painful knee is often caused by osteoarthritis.

A swelling or lump on the back of the knee is likely to be due to a distended bursa, a condition known as Baker's cyst. The swelling is usually at least the size of a golf ball and is caused by leakage from an inflamed knee joint into the bursa at the back of the knee (see Figure 11.1).

Pain over the knee with swelling of the joint may be caused by prepatellar bursitis, popularly known as housemaid's knee.

Onset

Certain events, usually in sport, such as twisting, turning, or a lateral impact as in soccer, when two players kick the ball at the same time with the inside of their feet, may precipitate injuries to the joint capsule or its associated ligaments and the cartilages inside the joint itself.

Pain in the knee joint that is noticed for the first time when walking up and down hills or stairs (and is worse walking down) may be due to chondromalacia patellae. This condition involves thickening of the cartilage lining the kneecap, and is caused by overuse. A similar condition in young people causing pain and inflammation just below the kneecap, particularly on exercise, is called Osgood–Schlatter's disease.

Ankle

An ankle sprain is the most common soft tissue limb injury and commonly presents with a history of excessive movement on the joint.

The lateral ligament attaches the fibula (the thinner, outer bone in the lower leg) to the heel and foot bones on the outer side of the ankle joint (see Figure 11.1). The lateral ligament is weaker than the broader medial ligament, which attaches the tibia to the heel bone on the inner aspect of the ankle. Sprains are caused by an inversion injury to the lateral ligament. Swelling over the lateral ligament below the ankle is less significant than swelling over the lateral ankle joint.

There is usually swelling and tenderness around the front and side of the ankle. It is sometimes difficult to distinguish between a fracture and a ligament injury (sprain), and if there is any doubt the patient should be persuaded to have an X-ray. However, the following guidelines will be helpful:

- Refer if there is tenderness of either the bony protuberance of the ankle (malleolus), the navicular bone in the foot just below the ankle joint on the instep, or the base of the fifth metatarsal bone on the outer edge of the foot (see Figure 11.1 on p 143).
- Refer if the patient cannot weight bear for at least four steps.
- Refer if there is pain at rest.

Lower leg

Pain in the front middle part of the shin bone can be caused by an overuse injury. Other problems in the lower leg include sprained ankle, ruptured Achilles tendon (see Figure 11.1) and cramp in the calf.

Ruptures of muscles in the calf and of the Achilles tendon are common in sporting injuries, but can also occur in non-sporting day-to-day situations.

A sudden pain in the calf, as though hit on the back of the leg, with tenderness and difficulty in contracting the muscles, may be due to rupture of the calf muscles (the gastrocnemius and soleus).

A ruptured Achilles tendon is intensely painful over the Achilles area, which lies above the heel and below the calf muscles. There is often a classic history of a blow or a kick on the back of the leg, and the tendon can sometimes be heard to snap. Medical referral is necessary.

Where the tendon is totally ruptured, the patient will not be able to walk on the affected foot. Indentation may be noted in the tendon at the site of injury. In milder cases, such as partial rupture or tendinitis (inflammation of the tendon), there will be difficulty in standing on tiptoe. Even mild cases, where the injury to the tendon is slight, must be referred for proper examination and advice. The condition could otherwise result in scarring of the tendon, which is liable to become chronically inflamed.

Cramps are common in the calf muscles, not only during strenuous exercise but also at rest. They are experienced particularly by the elderly.

Foot

A painful heel may be the result of bursitis. Pain at the back of the heel may be due to inflammation of a deep bursa lying between the heel bone and the attachment of the Achilles tendon or a superficial tendon located under the skin (see Figure 11.1). There may be redness and swelling and it may become difficult to wear normal shoes.

In children up to the age of 18 fragmentation of the Achilles tendon attachment to the heel bone can occur, causing pain at the back of the heel during and for some time after walking or running.

Pain under the heel may be due to rupture of connective tissue below the heel. In such cases the heel bone becomes less firmly held and squeezes the cushion of fat normally beneath it to the side. This causes pressure on the skin, resulting in pain. There is also a bursa between the heel bone and the fat cushion, which may become inflamed.

Pain under the heel, often with pain in the sole, is commonly due to plantar fasciitis. This occurs where the arch ligaments (running under the foot from the toes to the heel) are stretched or damaged. The pain is relieved on rest, and is worse when on tiptoe or walking on the heels. There may be stiffness, particularly in the mornings.

Special considerations

Pregnancy

Because of the extra load placed on the skeleton by the growing fetus, lumbago is a common problem in pregnancy. Patients should be reassured, but if the pain is unbearable they are best referred. Musculoskeletal problems in pregnancy are commonly mechanical, the growing load being asymmetrically distributed. They may also be metabolic or related to pressure effects on the pelvic floor, blood vessels or other organs. Exercising opposing muscle groups to stretch the affected part may relieve the pain and spasm. If the condition is persistently troublesome, referral can be made.

Management

Treatment of acute soft tissue injury where there may be bleeding, for example in sports injuries and acute bursitis, should be immediate. The aim is to stop the bleeding, swelling, pain and tenderness. Bleeding can also delay healing, make infection more likely and distort scar tissue formation, producing a cosmetically poor result and possibly interfering with function.

The well-known mnemonic RICE comes into play here. This represents **r**est, **i**ce, **c**ompression and **e**levation, and may be combined with the use of NSAIDs as NICER.

Rest and elevation

Rest allows immobilisation, which enhances healing and reduces blood flow to the affected tissue. Rest should ideally be for 24–48 hours, but this is often difficult to achieve. Elevation of the affected part also reduces blood flow and leakage of fluid into the extracellular spaces.

Cooling

Ice packs are used to reduce blood flow to injured tissue and thus reduce bleeding and swelling. Cooling also has an analgesic effect. Ice packs should be separated from the skin by a thin towel or a handkerchief to prevent skin damage. To be effective, cooling should be continued for at least 30 minutes in, for example, a knee or ankle injury, and longer if the injury is particularly severe or when deep large muscles are involved, as in the thigh. One disadvantage of cooling is that it may encourage someone to begin exercising the affected part of the body too soon after an injury, thus causing more bleeding and delaying healing.

Cooling aerosol sprays can exert an analgesic effect if a bone that lies close to the skin, such as the ankle or shin, has been knocked.

Sprays only penetrate into the skin layer. They can, however, cause injury to the skin if they are not used carefully, and should not be applied to broken skin. Their brief and superficial action means that when cooling has ceased, the blood flow increases and any beneficial effect may be lost.

Compression

Compression of an acute injury allows haemostasis to occur and thereby reduces swelling. A supportive bandage, such as a crepe bandage or an elastocrepe, can be applied. Elasticated sports supports designed for specific areas are available.

Heat

Heat or massage will have the opposite effect to that of cooling on blood flow. It should therefore not be used until about 48 hours after an acute injury, i.e. when the risk of bleeding has disappeared. Heat offers relief from pain arising from inflammation or overuse.

As well as being of value in trauma heat is also effective in chronic joint pain, such as rheumatoid arthritis and osteoarthritis, wry neck, backache and deep muscle pain. Heat reduces joint stiffness and relieves muscle spasm. It increases the elasticity and plasticity of collagen fibres in tissues such as tendons, preventing them from becoming stiff, and also aids gentle exercise in the rehabilitation phase.

Heat may be generated in the form of topical medication (see below), infrared lamps, heating pads, hot baths or by ultrasound treatment, which is used by physiotherapists. Heat retainers commonly worn by sportsmen are supports made of synthetic materials that generate and retain heat as well as giving useful support and improving the mobility of joints and limbs.

Heat is useful in preventing injury, which explains the importance of warm-up exercises, especially in cold weather.

Topical medication

Topical medication applied to aches and pains is a traditional remedy and is generally effective.

Rubefacients

Most preparations cause vasodilatation and produce a sensation of warmth. They encourage healing and also provide analgesia. They are useful as a preventative and rehabilitative measure, but should not be used in the acute stage of injury, when there is a risk of bleeding.

The traditional constituent of embrocations and liniments is methyl salicylate, present in many proprietary balms, liniments and balsams. The concentration varies between different products, and the pharmacist should be aware of a possible difference in potencies because of this. Branded products also often include turpentine oil and a variety of salicylates and nicotinates. The efficacy of most topical medications is enhanced by massage during application, which will itself induce vasodilatation.

Topical non-steroidal inflammatory drugs (NSAIDs)

Topical preparations of the NSAIDs include ibuprofen, diclofenac and piroxicam, which are useful analgesic and anti-inflammatory agents. There has been considerable controversy about the efficacy of topical NSAIDs, but there is anecdotal evidence that they do provide symptomatic relief in some patients and can be used for muscular aches, sprains and strains, and rheumatoid symptoms. The reader is referred to the bibliography for reviews of the evidence of their effects. They can be used immediately after acute injury.

Oral analgesics and anti-inflammatory drugs

Simple analgesics such as paracetamol and NSAIDs such as ibuprofen can give effective relief of musculoskeletal pain when used either alone or in conjunction with other treatments, and they should be recommended as first-line treatment. Ibuprofen is particularly effective for symptomatic relief in musculoskeletal conditions. These drugs may be helpful in acute injury as well as more chronic conditions such as torticollis, sternocostal joint strain, frozen shoulder, carpal tunnel syndrome, back pain and coccygi-

tis. Care should be taken to inquire about any relative contraindications to NSAIDs, such as a history of peptic ulcer or upper gastrointestinal disorders and asthma.

Patients with chronic pain or stiffness should be referred for assessment. In some cases local steroid injections may be required.

It is helpful to give the patient an idea of the likely duration of the impairment of function caused by a sprain. For example, the time taken to recover from a sprained ankle varies from person to person, but as a guide most are noticeably better after 5–7 days and fully healed at 4–6 weeks. Gentle walking can be resumed a few days after injury, and jogging begun at 2–4 weeks.

Glucosamine

Glucosamine is a popular OTC remedy for arthritis and is believed to be localised in cartilage after oral ingestion. There is some evidence of a modest symptomatic effect in osteoarthritis, and thus it is reasonable to recommend it for chronic joint conditions.

Cod liver oil

Fish oils, particularly cod liver oil, taken orally are perceived to be helpful in the symptomatic relief of chronic joint pain such as arthritis.

Arnica

Arnica is an old herbal remedy. Topical arnica preparations have a traditional use for sprains and bruises. Arnica contains some terpenoids, which have pharmacological activity in animal models, but there is a paucity of clinical evidence.

Second opinion

Musculoskeletal problems are common in primary care and frequently present to GPs. Many will be recent in origin and self-limiting, although chronic conditions are also common. The incidence of osteoarthritis increases with age, although the suspicion of other conditions as mentioned can never be far away. Studies have shown a poor correlation between pain felt and radiographic changes, and so although radiology is often used to confirm the diagnosis, monitor progress or exclude other diagnoses, minimal changes on X-ray do not exclude clinical severity.

Examination is essential to localise the problem, but a detailed history is the cornerstone of both diagnosis and a management plan. Analgesia and perhaps anti-inflammatory agents are used for symptom control, and referral to physiotherapy for rehabilitation and longer-term help. Many patients will try osteopathy or chiropractic, although these are not commonly available on the NHS.

Blood tests for rheumatoid arthritis, ankylosing spondylitis and other specific arthropathies are useful, and finally it may be necessary to refer to either a rheumatologist or an orthopaedic surgeon. Even so, chronic conditions are still difficult to treat. Once established, arthritis is permanent and potentially disabling.

Bibliography

Anon (2002). Is glucosamine worth taking for osteoarthritis? *Drug Ther Bull* 40: 81–82.

Ernst E (1998). Over-the-counter complementary remedies used for arthritis. *Pharm J* 260: 830.

Lin J, Zhang W, Jones A, Doherty M (2004). Efficacy of topical non-steroidal anti-inflammatory drugs in the treatment of osteoarthritis: meta-analysis of randomised controlled trials. *Br Med J* 329: 324–326.

Moore RA, Tramer MR, Carroll D *et al* (1998). Quantitative systematic review of topically applied non-steroidal anti-inflammatory drugs. *Br Med J* 316: 33–38.

POEM (Patient-Oriented Evidence that Matters) (2003). Glucosamine improves joint mobility for 1 in 5 patients with osteoarthritis. *Br Med J* 2003 (6 December) 327; doi: 10.1136/327.7427. O-i (accessed through www.bmj.com, 10 March 2006).

Topical NSAIDs (2003). *Bandolier* 10; 6 (available through www.ebandolier.com)

 SUMMARY OF MUSCULOSKELETAL CONDITIONS

Achilles tendon injury

Inflammation of the Achilles tendon (tendinitis) may be a result of prolonged repeated loading and is common in athletes. It is provoked by cold weather or a change in ground surface, shoes or technique. Pain and swelling over the tendon occurs. It is treated in the acute phase by rest and cooling, and later by heat. If it does not improve within a few days, **refer.**

A rupture of the Achilles tendon can be partial or complete and is relatively common in many sports. It often occurs in athletes who resume training after a period out of training. There is intense pain at the time of rupture. Walking, particularly on tiptoe, is impaired. There may be swelling or bruising over the lower leg and foot. A ruptured Achilles tendon requires medical attention – **refer.**

Ankle sprain

A sprained ankle is the most common soft tissue limb injury. It is an injury to a ligament, usually the outer lateral ligament, which attaches the fibula to the heel and foot bones on the outer side of the ankle joint. This lateral ligament is weaker than the inner (medial) ligament, which attaches the larger tibia to the heel bone on the inner side of the ankle.

(continued overleaf)

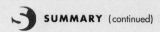

Ankylosing spondylitis

Ankylosing spondylitis is an inflammatory arthritis of the lower back and sacroiliac joints that has a genetic predisposition. It is more common in males, and starts in young adult life. The characteristic feature is of pain and stiffness, especially in the morning after rest. Specific exercises are important to prevent progression and deformity.

Bursitis

Bursae are small sacs of fluid. Their function is to reduce friction and protect adjacent structures from pressure. They are found between bones and tendons, between two tendons, and beneath the skin overlying a bone or tendon in particular parts of the body such as the hips, knees, feet, shoulders and elbows. Inflammation (bursitis) may be caused by friction (as in the Achilles tendon moving repetitively over a bursa), leading to inflammation and secretion of fluid into the bursa, resulting in swelling and tenderness, leakage of calcium deposits from inflamed or degenerating tendons into an adjacent bursa, and infection, especially of superficial bursae lying just beneath the skin in the elbows and knees. Bursitis is a painful condition and should be treated with rest and cooling, followed by heat after 48 hours. If pain or swelling is severe, **refer.**

Capsulitis

Capsulitis is inflammation of the fibrous supporting tissue surrounding the shoulder joint. If mobility is not restored with a programme of exercises (as soon as it is practical to do this), scarring and fibrosis of muscles, tendons and ligaments around the shoulder joint may occur, resulting in an inability (sometimes irreversible) to raise the arm above the head or behind the back (frozen shoulder) – **refer.**

Carpal tunnel syndrome

Where the tendons that control the movements of the hands and fingers cross the wrist, they are channelled through lubricating sheaths that cross the wrist in a narrow tunnel known as the carpal tunnel. Inflammation of the tendon sheaths at that point will reduce the space in the tunnel and compress the median nerve, which passes through it. Pain, and sometimes numbness, is felt in the forearm. The symptoms are often worse at night. The syndrome requires rest, NSAIDs, splinting, and occasionally either steroids (by local or systemic injection) or surgery to release the tendon sheaths – **refer.**

Cervical spondylosis

Cervical spondylosis is degeneration of the cervical spine, similar to osteoarthritis. In the early stages, X-rays can be normal. Nerve entrapment can occur.

Coccygitis

Injury to the small spur of the vertebrae at the tip of the spine (coccyx), as in a fall, causes a painful coccydynia and inflammation of the ligaments attached to the coccyx. The pain may last for several months. The best treatment is with analgesics, but the long duration of the symptoms should be borne in mind. It does not normally require referral, but if there is any doubt about the diagnosis in severe cases, **refer.**

Cramp

Muscle cramp is a common condition affecting active people during strenuous exercise as well as the inactive, usually at rest, and those with impaired peripheral circulation (claudication). The cause is unknown, although it is thought to be due to an accumulation of lactic acid. Immediate treatment is to rest the limb, although the spasm of nocturnal cramp may be helped by weightbearing and by massage to stimulate the circulation. If persistent or recurrent, **refer.**

→

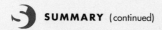 **SUMMARY** (continued)

Golfer's elbow

The lower end of the humerus broadens into two bony protrusions (epicondyles). One is located on the inner (medial) side of the elbow and one on the outer (lateral) side. The epicondyles are the points of insertion of the forearm muscles that move the fingers and wrist. The muscles are joined to the epicondyles by narrow tendons. Considerable force to, and vibration in, the muscles, as in some sports or some occupations, can cause disruption of the tendons from the epicondyles. Symptoms are pain and tenderness in the inner aspect of the elbow, which may radiate along the forearm. The wrist is weak and simple clenching movements of the hand are painful. If mild, the condition responds to rest and analgesics or NSAIDs, but symptoms can take weeks or months to resolve. In more painful presentations local steroid injections may be required. If severe, **refer.**

Lumbago

Lumbago is low back pain, most common in the third and fourth decades. It can be caused by strains of the spinal muscles and ligaments (soft tissue lumbago), or more seriously by disorders of the vertebrae, intervertebral discs and their associated joints. If the intervertebral discs are squeezed outwards and prolapse (slipped disc), there will be sudden severe backache. The patient will hold him- or herself rigid to avoid movement and will find sitting down painful and difficult. Such cases require rest.

The decision to refer depends on the course of previous episodes, but in cases where prolapse is suspected, **refer.**

Osteoarthritis

Osteoarthritis is degeneration and excessive wear of the cartilage covering the surface of bones in a joint. Its incidence is greater in the elderly. Osteoarthritis may be primary (cause unknown) or secondary (due to injury or an inappropriate load on a joint). There is joint pain, tenderness, swelling, reduced mobility and stiffness – **refer.**

Plantar fasciitis

The plantar fascia comprises two arch ligaments and a band of fibrous tissue overlying them, and runs over the heel bone (where it forms the heel cushion) to the toes. Stretching of the fascia can cause inflammation, resulting in pain and stiffness in the sole and heel. It can be treated with rest, anti-inflammatory measures and, if necessary, arch supports. If treatment fails, **refer.**

Rheumatoid arthritis

Rheumatoid arthritis is a chronic inflammatory condition of the synovial membrane in joints, causing inflammation, pain, swelling and reduced mobility. It may also affect soft tissues such as tendons, tendon sheaths, muscles and bursae. If suspected, **refer.**

Sciatica

Sciatica is often caused by a prolapsed disc that compresses the roots of the sciatic nerve. It may be preceded by lumbago in some cases. Pain radiates from the back down one leg and there may be numbness and weakness of that leg. The back of the leg, from the buttock down the thigh as far as the calf, is the most commonly affected area, but the front of the leg can also be involved. The best treatment is rest, analgesics or NSAIDs, and heat. If the pain is severe and persists for more than a few days, **refer.**

Sprain

A sprain is an injury to a ligament or joint capsule usually caused by a forceful movement. It is characterised by pain, swelling, and some loss of function.

(continued overleaf)

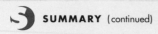

SUMMARY (continued)

Strain

A strain is an injury to a muscle usually caused by excessive stretching or overuse.

Tennis elbow

Tennis elbow is caused by excessive force acting on the insertion of the tendons of the forearm muscles at the outer (lateral) epicondyle (see Golfer's elbow). This is common in racquet sports and also in activities involving repetitive twisting movements, such as turning a screwdriver. Symptoms are similar to those of golfer's elbow, but pain is felt in the outer part of the forearm and may spread to the upper arm. The pain is worse when the hand is clenched or is bent backwards at the wrist.

   The course of the condition is similar to that of golfer's elbow, and the indications for referral are the same.

Tenosynovitis

Tenosynovitis is a painful inflammation of the muscles, tendons and tendon sheaths that commonly occurs in the forearm. It often results from overuse (as in the popularly named 'pudding stirrer's thumb') and produces pain and tenderness in the flexor muscles of the forearm. It is easily confused with carpal tunnel syndrome (see above), but the latter is usually more recurrent and chronic. Treatment involves a sling to rest the arm or wrist. If this is ineffective, a splint or even a plaster cast can be used – **refer.**

Wry neck

Wry neck (torticollis) is a painful condition in which there is spasm of one or more muscles in the neck. It occurs after straining muscles with repeated or unaccustomed movement, or on exposure to cold.

   There will be pain in the neck, sometimes extending to the top inner edge of the scapula, triggered by neck movement. The neck is tender and tense. Treatment should involve immobilisation of the neck, as far as is convenient, and analgesia. If there is no improvement in 1 week or if the pain is severe, **refer.**

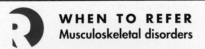

WHEN TO REFER
Musculoskeletal disorders

- There have been substantial impact forces and a fracture cannot be ruled out
- There is pain at rest
- Pain is not being relieved by OTC medicines
- Improvement in function of the affected limb is not obvious in 5–7 days
- Patient is elderly or a child
- There is a bony abnormality or tenderness (by observation or touch)
- The patient cannot weight bear for four steps
- There is obvious deformity

CASE STUDIES

Case 1

A woman asks the pharmacy assistant for two crepe bandages, of a size suitable for a child of 8. Should the pharmacist intervene?

There are many requests that could benefit from professional advice, but if, as here, there is no obvious reason apparent, it is wise to enquire.

There is always difficulty in assessing people who are not present in the pharmacy, and staff need to be aware of this.

In this instance the child had just tripped on a paving stone and twisted her ankle. She remained resting at home, and although she could weight-bear it was painful, resulting in a limp.

The chances of a fracture are small and the nature of the incident common. Even so, only an X-ray will provide a definite diagnosis; this requires a visit to the Accident and Emergency department.

In minor injuries, the clinical condition and mobility may improve within a few hours. A medical examination that does not elicit tenderness over the lateral malleolus and with no excessive swelling or bruising at the site may be treated conservatively with rest, elevation and a cold compress, although failure to improve will require an X-ray.

Injuries to the medial side of the ankle should always be referred, being considerably less common, and with simple sprains consequently less likely.

Many people may be reluctant to take frequent or minor conditions to an already overburdened hospital department, with the prospect of a substantial waiting time. The decision is difficult, and many X-rays of normal ankles are taken every day, but it remains the only way to be completely confident. To risk a late diagnosis, with a poor fusion of the fracture in a young person, is unwise. Even if the injury is to the ligaments alone, immobilising the joint for several weeks followed by remobilisation through physiotherapy may still be needed for a complete recovery.

Case 2

A man in his 40s was a semi-regular visitor to the pharmacy, usually to request a small supply of an analgesic or a topical anti-inflammatory preparation. He had purchased this two or three times in the last 6 months, and is now asking again.

Is it appropriate to enquire further?

The supply of these medicines requires some routine questioning about their use, but the frequency of these requests should invite a fuller history.

It is important to offer advice, making it apparent that help rather than some sort of control is motivating it.

This man was employed in a strenuous manual job, and regarded his frequent episodes of back pain as nothing more than an occupational hazard. He may even initially resent deeper enquiries, choosing to use the pharmacy for his medication as he sees no reason to consult his GP.

A fuller history reveals episodes of back pain often associated with or aggravated by lifting or straining. He also suffers pain down the left leg, which can be incapacitating and is not always effort related. He had had these pains ever since a motorcycle accident some 20 years ago.

There is a possibility of degenerative arthritis, perhaps consequent on previous injury.

The leg pain suggests sciatic pain.

The reason why this man chooses to manage his problems in this way needs to be sensitively explored. He may simply be denying the severity of his condition, or be ignorant of the treatment options available.

(continued overleaf)

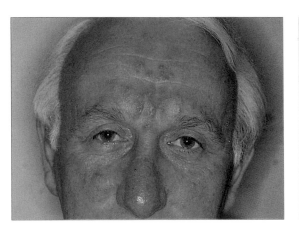

Figure 12.1   Rosacea. (Reproduced by permission from the Science Photo Library.)

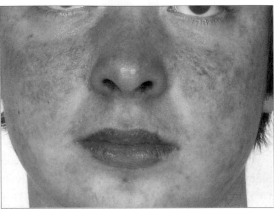

Figure 12.2   Systemic lupus erythematosus. (Reproduced with permission from the Wellcome Trust Medical Photographic Library.)

This starts as a red rash or flushing, particularly over the cheeks and bridge of the nose. It often progresses to a papular acne-like rash. The rash may appear symmetrically and is often described as a butterfly rash because of its shape and distribution. If this condition is suspected, the patient should be referred for appropriate antibiotic treatment.

Another rash that causes a butterfly appearance over the nose and cheeks is that of systemic lupus erythematosus (Figure 12.2). This is a relatively rare condition, sometimes precipitated by drugs, in which the lesions are more scaly than in rosacea. Drugs associated with this disorder include beta-blockers, chlorpromazine, hydralazine, isoniazid, lithium, methyldopa, penicillamine, phenytoin, procainamide, sulfasalazine and thiouracils.

Mitral valve disease, another relatively rare condition, may also be associated with a butterfly rash. In summary, any rash with a butterfly distribution over the face should be referred for a medical opinion.

The presence of red papules or pustules in the beard area is characteristic of a staphylococcal infection of the hair follicles called sycosis barbae (Figure 12.3). It may sometimes be caused by a tinea (ringworm) infection. It is most commonly seen in middle-aged men. Mild cases may resolve if shaving is stopped for a few days, but failure to resolve requires referral.

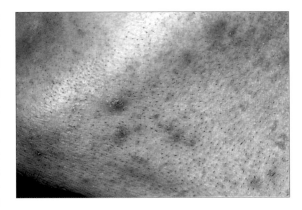

Figure 12.3   Sycosis barbae. (Reproduced with permission from the Science Photo Library.)

A scaly rash with mild erythema affecting the scalp and forehead, eyebrows, nose and pinna of the ear will probably be seborrhoeic eczema (Figure 12.4). It may also be associated with scaling on the edge of the eyelids (blepharitis), sometimes with loss of eyelashes. In babies during the first few months of life it may present as cradle cap, producing yellowish crusts, chiefly on the scalp but sometimes also on the ears and eyebrows (see Figure 12.13).

A red, dry scaly rash appearing on the cheeks of babies will probably be atopic eczema (Figure 12.5). It often spreads to flexures in the neck, wrists, elbows, and behind the knees. It is very

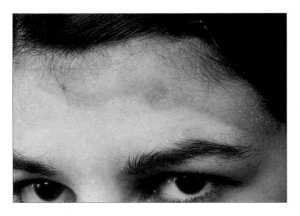

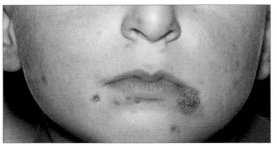

Figure 12.6   Impetigo. (Reproduced with permission from the Wellcome Trust Medical Photographic Library.)

Figure 12.4   Seborrhoeic eczema. (Reproduced with permission from the Wellcome Trust Medical Photographic Library.)

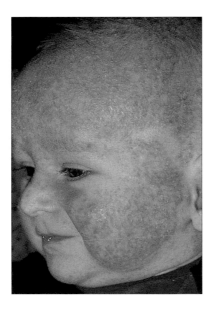

Figure 12.5   Atopic eczema. (Reproduced with permission from the Science Photo Library/Dr P. Marazzi.)

irritant and the scratching that ensues can cause marked excoriation of the skin and increases the risk of infection. In older children and adults atopic eczema appears as lichenification, which is a dry, crusty thickening of the skin that often becomes cracked.

Erythema around the nose and mouth with vesicles that weep and then produce yellow or brown crusty scabs suggests impetigo (Figure 12.6). This occurs most commonly in children during the early school years. It may be difficult to differentiate from infective eczema in some cases, although the crusts of impetigo are very characteristic. In either case, a referral is necessary.

Lesions on the lips may be caused by infection with the herpes simplex virus, which causes cold sores. These are often self-diagnosed by the patient. There is usually a tingling or pricking sensation in the early stages, and it is at this time that treatment with over-the-counter (OTC) medication should be started for best effect.

A tender, red swollen area of skin may herald a furuncle (boil), which is an abscess with a single pus-filled or discharging centre. Boils are commonly seen on the nose or chin, but can also occur on the nape of the neck, particularly in adolescent males. Sometimes such a red area may be the result of an insect bite and, rarely, it will be a streptococcal or staphylococcal skin infection called cellulitis (Figure 12.7).

Large urticarial weals should be observed with caution. If there is any suggestion that they are spreading quickly and becoming confluent, or if they are accompanied by swelling of the eyelids or lips (angio-oedema), the patient should be referred swiftly to an Accident and Emergency department.

A small, discrete, raised nodular lesion that eventually ruptures to form a small, red or purple wart-like ulcer should be viewed with suspicion, as this is how rodent ulcers (basal cell carcinoma) present (Figure 12.8). They can occur anywhere on the face, but are most common on the nose, cheeks and pinna of the ear. Any suspicion requires a referral.

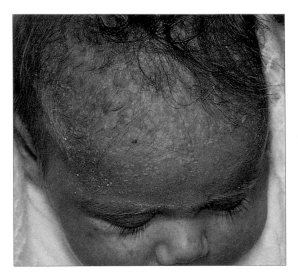

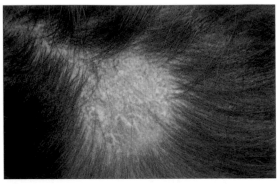

Figure 12.14   Tinea capitis. (Reproduced with permission from the Science Photo Library.)

Figure 12.13   Cradle cap. (Reproduced with permission from the Wellcome Trust Medical Photographic Library.)

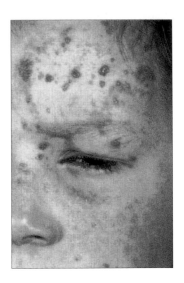

lice infection can, however, only be made when lice are detected by combing dampened hair with a fine-toothed comb over a sheet of white paper. Outbreaks of head lice often occur in schools, nurseries etc., and parents will often diagnose the condition themselves. Treatment and prophylaxis can be undertaken with appropriate OTC medication. More details of head lice infection appear in Chapter 14.

A bald patch on the scalp may be caused either by alopecia areata or by scalp ringworm (tinea capitis; Figure 12.14). The latter tends to present as scaly itching lesions, the former without scales and with no irritation. Both should be referred, if suspected.

Severe scaling of the scalp may be due to psoriasis. Psoriasis rarely affects the face, but it may be found elsewhere on the body, giving a clue to the diagnosis of any scalp lesions. On the scalp it usually appears as a scaly or red rash and there may be some loss of hair.

A rash occurring unilaterally over the scalp and forehead, extending to the eye, should be suspected as shingles (Figure 12.15). The rash may be macular at first, changing to vesicles and it can be very painful. The patient should be referred immediately.

Figure 12.15   Shingles: ophthalmic. (Reproduced with permission from the Wellcome Trust Medical Photographic Library.)

Duration and onset

Many skin conditions are chronic, and the patient will report a long-standing lesion or rash. In such cases time is not of the essence, and even if referral is thought to be appropriate it can in most cases be arranged at the patient's convenience. Examples of such conditions are acne vulgaris and rosacea, seborrhoea, most cases of eczema, vitiligo, telangiectasia, psoriasis, and even a suspected rodent ulcer, although in the last case the importance of seeing a doctor should be emphasised to the patient. More acute situations will require more urgent referral, the timescale depending on the severity of the signs and symptoms. Thus, infections such as cellulitis and drug-related photosensitivity may need an opinion within a day or two, whereas angio-oedema or jaundice, particularly where the patient has other significant symptoms or is feeling unwell, require more urgent attention. Angio-oedema should be regarded as a medical emergency.

The onset of a skin rash can often be related in time to likely causative factors, such as the use of a hair colorant or cosmetics, or concomitant drug therapy.

Reference has already been made to the age of the patient, which may give some clue as to the likelihood of particular diagnoses. Thus, acne vulgaris usually starts in adolescence and has generally disappeared by young adulthood. Impetigo and head lice are less likely to be seen in adults than in young children.

Accompanying symptoms

Swelling of the lips or tongue, especially in the case of an urticarial rash, requires immediate medical attention.

Itching (pruritus) is a common accompaniment to eczema, and also to scalp infections and infestations. Generalised itching over most of the body without the appearance of a rash may be a sign of systemic disease, such as liver or kidney disease, and the patient should be referred. Headache, fever, malaise and lymphadenopathy (swollen glands, seen or easily felt in the neck) suggest systemic disease or infection and require referral.

Spread

Acne vulgaris, although occurring most noticeably on the face, is often found also on the neck, upper chest and back. In acne rosacea there may eventually be involvement of the nose, resulting in rhinophyma, in which the nose becomes enlarged, rounded and red.

Photosensitivity rashes will be seen on other sites exposed to light, besides the face, such as the backs of the hands, neck and upper chest. Non-photosensitive drug rashes will often appear as a morbilliform rash, usually involving the trunk and sometimes the limbs, as well as the face.

The rashes of measles and German measles (rubella) characteristically begin on the face or the back of the neck and spread down the trunk.

Psoriasis and eczema both appear on other parts of the body. Psoriasis occurs usually as individual plaques of scaly, silvery lesions, particularly on the knees, elbows and forearms. Eczema may be localised to sites where there is contact with irritants or sensitising agents, and atopic eczema to sites where there are flexures in the skin, such as the wrists, and behind the knees and elbows.

Recurrence

Some skin lesions will recur after a relatively symptom-free interval. This may represent a chronic condition that spontaneously resolves and relapses (e.g. seborrhoeic eczema or atopic eczema), repeated exposure to the chemical irritant or allergen (as may occur in contact irritant or allergic eczema), or reinfection and reinfestation from close human contact (e.g. impetigo or head lice).

Repeated bacterial infections, such as boils or cellulitis, can occur in patients with diabetes. Patients with this condition should be questioned about their blood glucose control, whereas those who have never been diagnosed as having diabetes should be asked about the presence of nocturia, thirst and weight loss.

Management

Eczema

Emollient creams and ointments are useful to hydrate the skin and form an occlusive barrier that prevents further evaporation of moisture. This action is particularly appropriate in dry lesions, such as atopic eczema on the face. Non-proprietary preparations such as oily creams are suitable, and there is also an array of proprietary emollient products. The use of emollients is discussed in more detail in Chapter 13.

If irritants or sensitising agents are thought to be the cause of an eczematous reaction, it is obvious that these should be removed or the skin protected from them before any treatment can be successful. In the case of sensitivity to nickel earrings, proprietary lacquers are available to coat the earrings and prevent contact with the skin. Topical hydrocortisone may be applied to the ears and neck, but is not licensed for OTC use on the face.

Wet eczematous lesions can be treated with potassium permanganate soaks or compresses. These may be particularly useful when lesions are crusting and weeping. A few crystals of potassium permanganate should be dissolved in a cupful of water and the solution applied for about 15 minutes two or three times daily. The mechanism of action is not clear, but this is a method traditionally used by dermatologists to treat weeping eczema.

Acne

The most common constituent of proprietary creams and gels for acne treatment is benzoyl peroxide. It has been shown to be effective in clinical trials for the treatment of mild to moderate facial acne. It is bactericidal to *Propionibacterium acnes* and is also thought to act partly by reducing the breakdown of sebum into irritant fatty acids, which cause inflammation in the sebaceous ducts. Benzoyl peroxide is also keratolytic, and is thereby thought to unplug the ducts and drain the sebum from the sebaceous glands. It thus has an action on the pre-inflammatory stage of acne (comedones) as well as the inflammatory stage (papules and pustules). It often causes an irritant dermatitis characterised by dryness, erythema, peeling and stinging after the first few applications. Patients should be warned of this and advised to use products cautiously at first, perhaps just once a day. If usage proves to be too unpleasant, the patient should be told to stop application for a few days and then start again, perhaps on alternate days at first. Application should be to all the affected area and not just to the comedones. Benzoyl peroxide is also well known for its bleaching action on clothes and hair, and this should be pointed out to patients before use. In common with most acne remedies, there may be no apparent benefit for several weeks or months after starting treatment and it is wise to ensure that patients are aware of this. Products containing a low concentration (5 per cent) should be used at first, and if no improvement is seen after 4 weeks a higher concentration can be substituted.

Salicylic acid is an old-established keratolytic agent which is present in various proprietary products as well as in official preparations such as salicylic acid ointment. It is thought by some to have dubious efficacy in acne, and its use is falling out of favour.

Other traditional keratolytics include sulphur and potassium hydroxyquinoline, and these are found in combination with benzoyl peroxide in some products.

Frequent washing and degreasing improves acne, and various cleansing lotions and skin washes are marketed for this purpose. Patients should be advised to take advantage of sunlight, as this removes excess oil from the skin and appears to be beneficial.

Cold sores

Cold sores can be treated with an antiviral cream containing 5 per cent aciclovir. It should be applied to the lesion as early as possible, at the time when a tingling sensation is felt. Patients should be warned that it may cause initial stinging when applied.

Scalp treatments

Seborrhoea capitis may be treated with an anti-dandruff shampoo, such as a product containing selenium or zinc pyrithione. Ketoconazole shampoo, which attacks the yeast *Pityrosporum ovale*, a causative factor in seborrhoea, is effective, especially in difficult cases. Tar-based shampoos may also be useful. Severe or chronic cases may need to be referred.

In babies, cradle cap can be managed by rubbing in olive oil or emulsifying ointment to loosen the scales and then shampooing with a standard baby shampoo.

Mild cases of psoriasis on the scalp can be treated with shampoos containing coal tar, but more severe cases are best referred.

The prevention and treatment of head lice is a common problem that pharmacists are asked to deal with. First, there are various important health education messages to convey, such as eliminating the view that head lice are associated with a lack of hygiene or care, and that short hair is less likely to be infested than long hair. Indeed, the term 'infestation' should be replaced with 'infection' when referring to head lice, to remove the pejorative overtones that exist among the public. The prophylactic use of a pesticide shampoo or lotion should be discouraged, as it will be largely ineffective and may give rise to resistance. Treatment of head lice can be with an anticholinesterase such as malathion or a pyrethroid such as phenothrin or permethrin. Treatment should be with a lotion rather than a shampoo.

Resistance to insecticidal preparations has developed, and the former practice of rotating the use of insecticides across a district has now lost favour. The current maxim 'no louse, no treatment' may help to reduce the indiscriminate use of insecticides and thereby lessen the prevalence of apparent resistance. Criteria for diagnosis of infection are described in detail in Chapter 14, and pharmacists should become more confident in confirming cases and starting treatment.

It is also important for pharmacists to educate parents about the pathogenesis of the condition, pointing out particularly that the symptom of an itchy scalp is an allergic reaction to lice. The itchiness usually manifests itself several weeks after the scalp has become infected and, in similar fashion, may not disappear until several days or weeks after all lice have been removed. Before a course of treatment with two applications of insecticide is deemed to have failed, on the whim of an anxious parent who believes that a child who persists in scratching its scalp must still be infected, evidence for the continued presence of lice must be produced. Until detection combing produces such evidence, consideration cannot be given to further chemical treatment using other insecticides.

Full details of techniques for detection and treatment are given in Chapter 14.

Second opinion

In most patients presenting to GPs with problems of the skin on the face and head, the condition is easily examined and the treatment straightforward. A small proportion may be puzzling, particularly eruptions that may be irritant or allergic in origin. The face is exposed to many chemicals, some of them self-applied, and the delay between exposure and reaction can make identification difficult. Persistent cases may need referral for a dermatological opinion and perhaps skin testing.

Conditions on the scalp and in the hair may be less easy to visualise. Head lice are common but may still be overestimated, and good practice suggests treatment only when living lice have been seen.

There are occasional conditions that demand a swift intervention and thus a high level of awareness, such as angio-oedema, herpes zoster and cellulitis. Patients will need close and frequent monitoring, and possibly hospital admission if they do not respond. In addition, any significant condition that threatens to involve the eye will raise anxieties in both doctor and patient.

With allergic and irritant reactions common, topical steroids are often prescribed for conditions on the face. The dangers of prolonged or potent exposure are well recognised, and fluorinated preparations will be avoided except in exceptional circumstances and for short-term use only.

Bibliography

Barnetson R St C, Rogers M (2002). Childhood atopic eczema. *Br Med J* 324: 1376–1379.

Ozolins M, Eady EA, Avery AJ *et al* (2004). Comparison of five antimicrobial regimens for treatment of mild to moderate inflammatory facial acne vulgaris in the community: randomised clinical trial. *Lancet* 364: 2188–2195.

Webster GF (2002). Acne vulgaris. *Br Med J* 325: 475–479.

 SUMMARY OF CONDITIONS PRODUCING FACE AND SCALP LESIONS

Acne vulgaris

Acne is caused by inflammation and blockage of the sebaceous glands and hair follicles. It is associated with the bacterium *Propionibacterium acnes*, which is thought to split the triglycerides in sebum into fatty acids, which are irritant to the pilosebaceous unit. The condition is recognised by the familiar comedones (whiteheads and blackheads), which often become pustular. There is no pruritus, but the rash causes embarrassment and self-consciousness in young people. It occurs predominantly on the face, but also appears on the nape of the neck, shoulders and the upper trunk. In severe cases scarring may result. Acne is most common in adolescents (Figure 12.16), classically appearing around the time of puberty, although it can persist into adulthood.

Acne rosacea

Acne rosacea is a skin condition of uncertain origin. It appears with a characteristic pattern of flushing over the bridge of the nose and the cheeks (see Figure 12.1), often referred to as a butterfly rash, and may progress to acne-like papules – **refer.**

Allergic eczema

Contact between an allergen and the skin may produce an eczematous reaction at the site of contact, and sometimes at a site distant from it. The most common examples on the head are nickel allergy (from earrings) and sensitisation to perfumes and cosmetics.

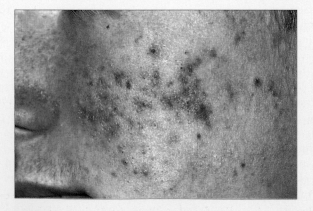

Figure 12.16 Adolescent acne vulgaris. (Reproduced with permission from Dr P. Marazzi/Science Photo Library.)

→

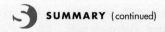 **SUMMARY** (continued)

Atopic eczema
Atopy is an inherited predisposition to develop asthma, hay fever and eczema. Atopic eczema is a constitutional eczema that usually occurs in patients with a family history of atopy. It commonly begins after the first few months of life, and although it often resolves spontaneously it can persist into adulthood. The lesions are erythematous, papular, and either dry or weeping. They are commonly seen on the face, for example on the cheeks (see Figure 12.5), and also on the wrists, arms and knee flexures. They are accompanied by intense pruritus, leading to frenzied scratching in some children.

Cellulitis
Cellulitis is a bacterial infection of the skin caused by either Streptococci or Staphylococci, and sometimes both together. The infection may arise at the site of trauma, but it can also affect previously healthy skin. A similar condition caused by Streptococci is called erysipelas. The rash is red, and often hot and oedematous (see Figure 12.7). It is seen commonly on the face, arms or legs. There is often headache, fever and malaise – **refer.**

Furuncles
A furuncle (boil) is a superficial abscess, usually caused by *Staphylococcus aureus*, which has a single discharging centre. Males and adolescents are most commonly affected. Furuncles are mostly sited on the face, nape of the neck, ears and nose. Patients with recurrent boils should be checked for diabetes.

Impetigo
Impetigo is a contagious bacterial infection of the epidermis caused by either Staphylococci or Streptococci. It mostly affects the face of children of school age and causes a weeping, vesicular rash which eventually dries to form yellowish-brown crusted lesions (see Figure 12.6). Itching results in scratching, which spreads the infection on the skin – **refer.**

Irritant contact eczema
Irritant chemicals can cause trauma to the skin, resulting in an inflamed area at the point of contact. The most common irritants are soaps, detergents, shampoos, bleaches, and various substances used in the workplace. The rash usually resolves when the irritant is removed.

Photosensitive dermatitis
Photosensitivity causes a rash with a characteristic appearance on the face, neck, back of the hands and upper chest. It may be aggravated by various drugs (see Table 12.3).

Psoriasis
Psoriatic lesions rarely occur on the face, but may be seen on the scalp and at other sites. Psoriatic plaques, recognised as red lesions covered with silvery scales, may be found on the elbows, knees and the lower back. On the scalp the lesions appear as a thick mat of dandruff, with loss of hair. It is a chronic recurrent disorder – **refer.**

Scalp ringworm
Scalp ringworm (tinea capitis) appears as a round, scaly, bald patch in and around which may be seen the broken stumps of hair follicles (see Figure 12.14). Treatment is often systemic – **refer.**

(continued overleaf)

CASE STUDIES

Case 1

The man in his early 60s in the pharmacy is well known and has worked as a builder all his life. A rugged, outdoor man, he wears his hair long, often with a cap on top, but sometimes revealing a nodular lesion on the pinna of his right ear which is sometimes covered with a plaster.

Should the pharmacist draw attention to this lesion?

Medicine remains for the most part a responsive profession, although in recent years the trend has been to encourage early screening procedures. The patient of course retains the right to refuse absolutely.

A casual reference and offer to examine the lesion may be appropriate.

On close inspection this lesion was a rounded, pearly, and dimpled in its centre. The patient referred to it as a wart that had been present for years and was of no consequence.

The clinical appearance suggests a basal cell carcinoma (BCC). This man's outdoor life and probable sunlight exposure make the diagnosis more likely.

This can be an awkward diagnosis to communicate to the patient. Having discovered a progressive and thus potentially serious condition the onus on the pharmacist now is to encourage a medical opinion and appropriate treatment.

Although technically this is a 'cancer', to talk in these terms may produce unnecessary anxiety for a condition that never metastasises and which can be completely treated. Even so, advanced lesions may require radiotherapy and even skin grafting. Untreated BCCs will progress at a variable speed and cause tissue damage and erosion, making the condition harder to treat.

Case 2

A woman in her mid-50s presented the pharmacist with a repeat prescription. He asked if all was well – his usual courtesy – and she replied that on her last blood pressure check with the practice nurse she mentioned a rash over her nose and cheeks, which although disguised with make-up was bothering her somewhat. She was fairly abruptly told it was most likely due to excessive alcohol intake. She embarked on a detailed description of her drinking habits, which seemed very moderate and designed to convince the pharmacist of the injustice she has suffered.

How should the pharmacist handle this situation?

It seems unlikely that the explanation offered by the nurse is correct, although there is no practical way of checking her story.

Respecting this woman's confidence while supporting a colleague, when there has clearly been a conflict of opinion, is difficult. One strategy is to make little comment on what has happened, and to start again.

The pharmacist reviewed the calendar of alcohol use and compared it with the recommended maximum, which it was considerably below. He then offered his opinion on the rash. Using a tissue to remove the camouflage, a red, thickened area of skin was revealed in a symmetrical pattern over the bridge of her nose.

This woman may have been keen to accept an alternative explanation for her rash, and it is important not to make a diagnosis unless it can be substantiated. She was advised that alcohol was unlikely to be the cause, and to see her GP.

The doctor agreed with the likely diagnosis of acne rosacea and to a trial of low-dose antibiotics. She responded very well.

→

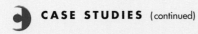 **CASE STUDIES** (continued)

Case 3

A man in his early 60s comes into the pharmacy requesting something for migraine.

How should the pharmacist respond?

A standard history was taken. This was the first occasion, and for 2 days he had had a constant but increasing pain over the left temple and side of his face, with odd sensations of tingling and hot and cold. Examination showed nothing obvious on the skin, although it was tender to touch.

With no nausea, visual disturbance or previous history, the diagnosis of migraine must be questioned. Sinus problems, temporal arteritis and other possibilities were explored, but again there was no objective evidence.

Should the patient be referred at this stage?

Without a definitive diagnosis, referral should be recommended.

A small quantity of analgesics may be supplied if there is a likely delay before he can be seen by the doctor.

The man was seen by his GP the same day, although with no further evidence to draw upon he was advised to monitor the condition closely. The following day he returned to his doctor with the appearance of an erythematous rash over the affected area. An early herpes zoster eruption was confirmed, and he returned to the pharmacy with a prescription for antiviral medication. The attention of two professionals who could not make a diagnosis, but who were prepared to watch closely, enabled its detection in time for treatment.

On the face, ophthalmic involvement is a possibility and he had an urgent referral to an ophthalmologist. The rash developed and could have threatened to involve the left eye, with the prospect of many months of pain and possible blindness with it. However, after the first 2 days of treatment the spread was contained and resolution occurred over the following 3 weeks.

13

Skin disorders: trunk and limbs

Assessing symptoms

Location and spread

Hands and arms

The hands are particularly susceptible to traumatic or contact irritant eczema. Common irritants include detergents, mineral oils and various degreasing agents. The backs of the hands and fingers are often affected first, as the skin here is less protected than on the palms, but if the irritant is being gripped or held (e.g. tools) the eczema appears on the palm. In cases of contact eczema caused by immersion of the hands in an irritant, such as washing-up liquid, both hands will be affected. The skin will usually appear red and will be sore.

An eczematous reaction caused by contact with sensitising agents such as dyes, cement or rubber gloves may involve the palms, depending on the specific site of contact with the skin. Psoriasis may occur as red lesions on the palms and is difficult to distinguish from chronic eczema at this site.

Lesions on the palms of the hands appearing as vesicles (small blisters) are characteristic of pompholyx (Figure 13.1), an endogenous condition (i.e. not caused by specific irritant agents or chemicals). Pompholyx often affects the feet as well. The condition is very itchy, and can be chronic or recurrent. If the pruritus is severe, referral is advisable for topical steroids to be considered.

Itching in the finger webs with discrete small red lesions is a classic symptom of scabies (Figure 13.2). The lesions may spread to the palms, wrists, armpits, genitalia, buttocks and abdomen. The itching is worse at night. Burrows (tracks made by the mite burrowing through the skin) may be identified as small (up to 1 cm) grey curved lines in the skin, but it is not always possible to see them. Family members and any sexual contacts will sometimes also be affected.

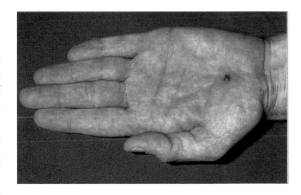

Figure 13.1 Pompholyx. (Reproduced with permission from Dr P. Marazzi/Science Photo Library.)

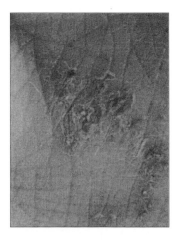

Figure 13.2 Scabies skin infection. (Reproduced with permission from the Wellcome Trust Medical Photographic Library.)

Wrists and elbows

Besides being a site for scabies, the wrists are also a common site for allergies to watch straps or nickel in jewellery.

The outside of the elbows is a common site for the characteristic appearance of psoriasis as red plaques with silvery scales (Figure 13.3).

Fingernails

Psoriasis can affect the fingernails, producing characteristic pitting or denting on the surface of the nail (Figure 13.4). This may be ignored for some time by the sufferer, who often does not associate the nail lesion with the psoriasis that is affecting the skin elsewhere. It is relatively difficult to treat and requires referral.

Fungal nail infection (onychomycosis) may present as painful inflammation in the skin around the base of the nails as well as involvement of the nail itself. It affects one or two nails initially, but can spread to involve others. It may progress so that the nail appears thickened or yellow, although this is more common in toenails. Topical antifungal agents may be effective and should be tried as a first-line treatment in mild cases in normally immunocompetent patients. However, in susceptible groups, such as diabetic and immunocompromised patients, and in more severe cases, early referral is recommended to avoid complications so that oral antifungal agents can be prescribed if appropriate.

A paronychia (whitlow) is similar to onychomycosis, but is usually caused by candidal infection and affects chiefly the skin around the base of the nail. Paronychias tend to be more acute and have pus in them, which may require draining.

The appearance of the fingernail may be changed with no known – or at least no significant – cause. For example, white spots on fingernails are traditionally associated by the layperson with dietary deficiencies such as calcium, etc. This is not the case, and the cause is more likely to be normal wear and tear. Patients should be assured that they will grow out or lessen in time. Similarly, vertical or horizontal ridging of the nails is of little consequence, particularly in older patients, and will often disappear over several months, provided the nail is not thickened and horny (onychogryposis).

Trauma to the nail bed can produce a black nail, which is a haematoma or bruise under the nail. It will clear in time, although the damaged nail may eventually separate as the new one grows. Occasionally it may be necessary for the doctor to bore a hole in the nail to drain the blood and fluid beneath if the pressure caused by the inflammatory process is causing pain that does not disappear over a few days.

Splitting along the vertical axis of the nails may be caused by exposure to excess water or

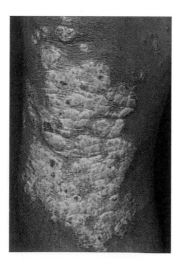

Figure 13.3 Psoriasis. (Reproduced with permission from Glaxo Wellcome.)

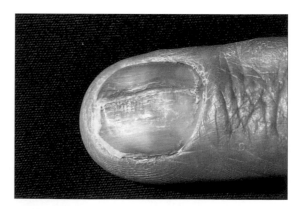

Figure 13.4 Psoriasis of the nail. (Reproduced with permission from Dr P. Marazzi/Science Photo Library.)

detergents, as may the condition known as 'hangnail' or ragged cuticles.

Splinter haemorrhages are rare and appear as tiny vertical dark lines in the nail. If there has been no trauma to the nail referral is necessary, as they can sometimes be a sign of systemic disease.

Feet

The foot is a site for allergic contact eczema caused by leather shoes or the dye in stockings and socks. The soles may be affected by psoriasis, which can also affect the nails. Psoriasis may be recognised by the concurrent appearance of lesions elsewhere.

Perhaps the most common skin condition affecting the feet that will present to the pharmacist is tinea pedis (athlete's foot; Figure 13.5). This usually starts between the toes (classically between the fourth and fifth digit) and can spread to the sole and upper part of the foot. It often appears red and itchy at first, and later turns white with maceration and soreness between the toes. Involvement of the interdigital space helps to distinguish athlete's foot from eczematous or psoriatic conditions.

Fungal infections of the toenail may be a consequence of the spread of infection from the surrounding skin or may represent isolated lesions, as can occur in the fingernail (see above).

Other conditions affecting the feet are described in Chapter 15.

Legs

Itchy papules or larger lumps on the lower leg are often the result of insect bites, including from pet fleas. Fleas may also attack the trunk and neck. The diagnosis can generally be confirmed by an appropriate history. If scabies can be identified elsewhere on the skin, it may manifest itself here too. Inquiry as to whether other family members are similarly affected may provide a helpful clue, although individuals react differently to insect bites.

The plaques of psoriasis (red with silvery scales) are classically seen on the knee and are quite distinctive and relatively easy to recognise. An itching rash behind the knee is likely to be atopic eczema (Figure 13.6), particularly in children.

A rash around the ankles, particularly in elderly patients, may be varicose or stasis eczema, caused by poor circulation in the lower limbs. It is often sore, dry and lichenified, and may lead to oedema and eventually to leg ulcers.

Lichen planus is an eruption of small, itchy, papules which are often a purplish colour initially, later turning brown (Figure 13.7). Sometimes a white lace-like pattern may be seen on the papules. The condition often affects the mouth at the same time, producing characteristic white lacy streaks on the buccal mucosa. As well as the legs, this condition can also occur on the wrists, back and abdomen. It is usually symmetrical, occurring at similar sites on both legs.

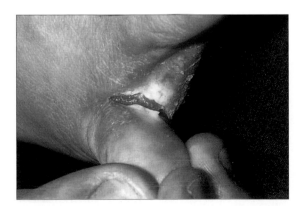

Figure 13.5 Tinea pedis (athlete's foot). (Reproduced with permission from Dr P. Marazzi/Science Photo Library.)

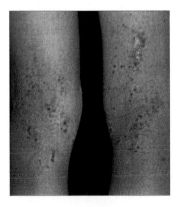

Figure 13.6 Atopic eczema. (Reproduced with permission from Glaxo Wellcome.)

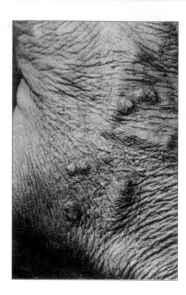

Figure 13.7 Lichen planus. (Reproduced with permission from Glaxo Wellcome.)

It is seen in young and middle-aged adults, but is rarer in the elderly and in children.

Skin conditions affecting the groin and genital area are generally very irritating. Scabies may appear as red papules. Pubic lice have a characteristic appearance, which leads to them being referred to by the layperson as 'crabs'. They lay eggs, in a similar way to head lice, which may be detected on pubic hair. Both scabies and pubic lice may be spread to others by close physical and sexual contact. Scabies is commonly transferred by holding hands, and lice can be transferred from unwashed clothing, towels and bedlinen.

The groin is a site where intertrigo may occur. This is an eruption caused by friction between opposing folds of skin. The moist warm conditions at such sites are conducive to infection by *Tinea* and *Candida*. Tinea infection of the groin (tinea cruris) is relatively common, especially in men. It appears as a red, itchy rash on the inner thighs, adjacent to but rarely involving the scrotum. The rash is typical of tinea infections, with a well-defined edge that is generally redder than the centre of the lesion and spreading outwards.

The rash of candidiasis in the groin can be differentiated from tinea by its less well-defined edges; also, there are often satellite lesions (sometimes vesicular) beyond the rim of the rash.

The groin is also the site for pubic lice infection. This will usually be self-diagnosed by the patient but may be described as intense, continuous itching. In hairy males pubic lice may spread and may even affect the eyelashes. In children without body hair, it is the scalp margins and eyelashes that are principally affected.

Trunk

Rashes that cover large areas of the body are probably best referred for a medical opinion. Sometimes the cause may be obvious, as when associated with drug treatment or when the patient is sensitive to certain foodstuffs. If urticaria appears shortly after exposure to drug or food allergens, care should be taken that swelling of the eyelids or of the tongue or airways (angio-oedema) does not occur. If there is any suspicion of this, the patient should be directed to a hospital Accident and Emergency department as a matter of urgency. Other reactions generally require less urgent referral, but a medical opinion is desirable, if only to make the GP aware of a possible adverse drug reaction so that treatment can be reviewed.

Herpes zoster infection (shingles) manifests itself as a unilateral rash following the course of a nerve tract, which is commonly described as a belt of erythema followed by small blisters (Figure 13.8). The rash may run from the back across the chest, along the course of an intercostal nerve (between two ribs) or around the abdomen, always stopping at the midline. The condition can be very painful, both before the rash appears and after it has gone.

The plaques of psoriasis can be found in the sacral area of the back.

Tinea corporis occurs as isolated lesions or clusters of round or oval red patches on the trunk or limbs (Figure 13.9). The well-defined edges are helpful if the diagnosis is in doubt.

Vagrants and people with low standards of personal and domestic hygiene who present with severe itching may have body lice. These mites live in clothes and bedding, and bite the trunk, buttocks and shoulders. Questioning about the site of the initial skin irritation can sometimes help to distinguish this condition from scabies. However, the precise diagnosis is of little con-

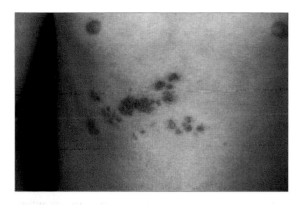

Figure 13.8 Shingles. (Reproduced with permission of Dr P. Marazzi/Science Photo Library.)

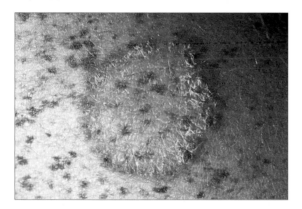

Figure 13.9 Tinea corporis (ringworm rash) on an arm. (Reproduced with permission from Dr P. Marazzi/Science Photo Library.)

with tiny discrete nodules under each sweat gland.

Another type of sweat rash may be caused by candidal infection, especially in intertriginous areas where folds of skin overlap to produce a moist, warm environment. Usual sites are under the breasts, the axillae and the back. The groin has already been mentioned as another area that may be infected.

Although classically affecting the face, seborrhoeic eczema and acne can also affect the chest. The diagnosis can be confirmed by the presence of lesions on the face.

Duration

Skin conditions vary in timescale from a few hours to chronic disease lasting a lifetime. If a new skin condition does not show improvement within 1 or 2 weeks, then as a general rule it is wise to refer the patient. Sometimes a topical steroid will clear a mild eczema, which if otherwise left might progress to a more severe or chronic condition.

The early recognition and referral of patients with shingles will optimise the effects of therapy, which should be instigated early to reduce the unpleasant sequelae that can occur.

Accompanying symptoms

The location and appearance of a rash are the principal pointers to diagnosis. Some other factors can, however, be helpful, although their presence or absence should not be used as absolute criteria to exclude any conditions. Most rashes are accompanied by pruritus, and this is particularly true for most types of eczema. Sometimes psoriasis does not itch. This may be useful when differentiating between a chronic eczema and psoriasis of the palms, or between an intertriginous psoriasis (such as in the groin) and a tinea or candidal infection at the same site.

It should be remembered that pruritus may, rarely, be a sign of systemic disease, often in the absence of a rash. Patients complaining of pruritus without an obvious skin lesion should therefore be referred. In many cases, scratching and

sequence as the treatment is similar for both conditions.

Rashes on sun- or light-exposed areas of the limbs and trunk (e.g. upper chest and neck), in conjunction with a similar problem on the face, will suggest a possible light sensitivity reaction. This may be precipitated by drugs (see Chapter 12), or may be due to polymorphic light eruption. The latter appears as erythema, with small macules, papules or vesicles, is very itchy, and often appears during sudden exposure to hot climates, e.g. on foreign holidays.

Prickly heat or sweat rash occurs at sites where sweat ducts are occluded, particularly under clothing. The blocked follicles produce a reddened and often highly irritant skin surface, excoriation in response to pruritus may cause marks on the skin that can be mistaken for genuine lesions.

Malaise, fever or other systemic symptoms may accompany infections such as shingles and some other serious skin disorders, and such cases should be referred.

Any peeling of the skin, apart from that commonly associated with sunburn, requires referral, as this may indicate an unusual or serious disorder. This should not be confused with the shedding of scales that may occur in some eczemas and psoriasis.

It should be remembered that psoriasis can involve the scalp and nails, and enquiry should be made in someone who has a rash on the body, particularly about pitting of the nails, which the patient may not appreciate is due to the same condition as the psoriatic rash.

Onset and aggravating factors

A pertinent history can often unravel a potential causative agent for skin conditions. Examples include a patient lying on a sunbed after being prescribed a photosensitising drug, ingestion of seafood prior to the appearance of an urticarial rash, a picnic in a meadow followed by itchy red lumps on the lower legs (insect bites), or a comment that other family members have similar papular lesions and itching is worse at night (scabies).

Exposure to chemical irritants in the workplace or to contact allergens will often give a valuable clue in the diagnosis of contact eczemas. Constant wetting of the hands, as occurs in housewives, hairdressers etc., increases susceptibility to contact eczema as well as to candidal infection and paronychia. As an adjunct to any treatment that may be given, patients should be advised to keep their hands dry by wearing rubber gloves.

Some conditions are thought to have a genetic association. Atopic eczema is a classic example of this, and there may be a family history of eczema, hay fever or asthma. In patients with psoriasis, a history of the disease in another close family member is not unusual.

The onset of guttate psoriasis often follows a streptococcal infection such as a sore throat.

Cold weather, stress and drugs such as lithium, beta-blockers and non-steroidal anti-inflammatory drugs can provoke an attack of psoriasis.

Recurrence

Many common skin conditions are chronic, for example eczema and psoriasis, and will resolve and reappear at intervals. Patients should be warned of this.

It is important that the skin be treated with emollients in conditions where drying and fissuring may occur between the acute exacerbations. Most emollients are underused, and the frequent correct application may often reduce exacerbations and the need for other therapy.

Management

Antipruritics

Itching is a symptom that will be reduced as the skin lesion causing it is resolved. In this respect, topical steroids are powerful agents. Hydrocortisone 1 per cent will effectively reduce the inflammation and associated itching of mild eczemas and insect bites. Flea bites may be treated with topical hydrocortisone, but attention should also be drawn to the treatment of household furnishings (see Parasiticidal agents).

Topical antihistamines have fallen out of favour with dermatologists because of their tendency to cause sensitisation. However, although they should not be used in eczemas and psoriasis, they can be recommended for short-term treatment for insect bites, sunburn and urticarial eruptions, and cause problems in only a very small number of patients. Calamine lotion is a cheap, traditional antipruritic preparation and has long been used, especially for the relief of sunburn.

Sedating oral antihistamines are also useful for pruritus. They can be taken at night to relieve night-time pruritus, as well as having a carry-over effect into the next day.

Emollients

Emollients, such as emulsifying ointment and a large number of proprietary products, are extremely important in the treatment of chronic eczema and psoriasis. They maintain hydration of the stratum corneum and are effective in preventing drying and cracking of the skin, which can be very painful. They should be applied after washing or bathing, when the skin is still moist.

The choice between the different products available is largely one of cosmetic acceptability. Ointments such as emulsifying ointment tend to be most effective, but creams are less greasy and more acceptable to patients. However, where dry skin is a particular problem in a non-visible part of the body, such as the feet, priority should be given to efficacy rather than cosmetic tolerance.

The epidermis of healthy skin is covered with a hydrolipid layer, which acts to control water loss from the skin. Greasy ointments such as emulsifying ointment form a protective layer that prevents evaporation of moisture from dry skin, as occurs in eczema when the hydrolipid layer is not functioning properly and abnormal water loss from the epidermis occurs. Emollients should be applied liberally and frequently. An appropriate treatment regimen would be to use a greasy ointment at night and a more cosmetically acceptable cream by day.

For an enhanced effect, the use of preparations containing a humectant may be appropriate. Urea, glycerine and polyethylene glycol are humectants and absorb water from the dermis into the epidermis, thereby helping to maximise the water-retaining properties of occlusive ingredients such as soft paraffin. Ingredients such as wool fat (lanolin) and wool alcohols also act as moisture absorbents. Pharmacists can select a suitable emollient according to the severity of the problem and the convenience of the patient.

Aqueous cream has fallen from favour because of its irritant properties and should only be used for short periods on the skin, or preferably as a wash-off soap substitute.

Eczematous patients should be discouraged from using perfumed soap and bath additives, as these may cause sensitisation as well as having a degreasing effect on the skin, causing it to dry out after bathing. Instead, a proprietary bath emollient or emulsifying ointment can be used. The latter can be used in the bath by mixing about 100 g in a bowl of hot water before adding to the bath water, or alternatively mixing this amount thoroughly, a little at a time, in the water under the tap. Most bath emollients contain light liquid paraffin as the active constituent, and although their effectiveness is matched by emulsifying ointment they tend to be more cosmetically acceptable, despite their higher cost.

Topical steroids

OTC topical hydrocortisone 1 per cent is licensed for short-term use in the treatment of mild to moderate eczema flare-ups in known sufferers, as well as for contact eczema and insect bites. It is effective for mild, uncomplicated contact eczemas.

Clobetasone 0.05 per cent is a more potent steroid than 1 per cent hydrocortisone and is more suitable for the short-term treatment of flare-ups of eczema of a more severe nature in adults.

Where the skin is thickened and lichenified, referral is probably best so that consideration can be given to the prescription of more potent topical steroids.

The fingertip unit

In contrast to the liberal use of emollients, users of topical steroids should be instructed to apply these preparations more carefully and economically. The fingertip unit is an arbitrary but convenient measurement for instructing patients as to how much to apply. The unit is the amount of product that can be squeezed out from the tip of the finger to the first crease (Figure 13.10). For example, half a unit will be sufficient to apply to an area the same size as the palm of one hand.

Weeping lesions

Wet lesions may or may not be infected. Provided the exudate is clear and watery, as

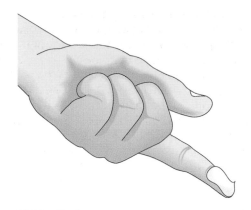

Figure 13.10 The finger tip unit.

occurs in some cases of eczema, the application of potassium permanganate soaks (see p 162) for about 15 minutes three times a day can sometimes produce good results. Patients with any purulent or unusual discharge should be referred.

Antifungal agents

The imidazoles, e.g. clotrimazole, miconazole and ketoconazole, are effective topical antifungal agents and have largely superseded more traditional preparations such as Whitfield's ointment (benzoic acid and salicylic acid). They are effective against tinea cruris, tinea corporis and tinea pedis, as well as candidiasis. This broad spectrum of activity makes them particularly suitable for the treatment of intertriginous rashes, where the exact causative infective agent may not be clear. Where the rash is particularly irritant they may be used in a combination product with hydrocortisone.

Terbinafine cream is an effective treatment for tinea pedis and tinea cruris.

Tolnaftate is effective against tinea but has little activity against *Candida*.

Treatment for tinea and *Candida* infections must be continued for at least 1 week (and preferably longer) after symptoms have subsided to ensure complete eradication of the infection.

Potassium permanganate soaks are also a useful supplement in moist areas and where the skin is macerated, as in the toe webs in tinea pedis (see Figure 13.5).

Parasiticidal agents

Treatment of scabies

The scabies mite, *Sarcoptes scabiei*, burrows into the epidermis and leaves eggs and faeces behind it. Protein in the faeces causes an allergic reaction in the skin. Patients should be advised that itching occurs several weeks after infection has occurred and may not disappear until a similar period after successful eradication of the mite. This is important to convey, first because symptomatic treatment with topical hydrocortisone or an oral antihistamine after using a scabicide may be appropriate, and second because other individuals in close contact with the patient will also probably be already infected by the time the patient has symptoms. Infection is spread by close physical contact, and hence it is necessary to treat all family members and sexual contacts at the same time.

As with head lice, it is both diplomatic and less stigmatising for pharmacists to use the word 'infection' rather than 'infestation' when discussing scabies with patients.

There is now a wide range of proprietary products for the treatment of scabies that has largely supplanted the traditional application of benzyl benzoate. The latter is irritant, and this might also be a potential problem with alcoholic formulations. Thus, a non-alcoholic lotion of malathion (0.5 per cent) or a cream containing permethrin (5 per cent) are the best recommendations.

Traditionally, patients were told to take a hot bath before applying a scabicide. This is no longer deemed necessary, but the skin should be clean, cool and dry before application. The scabicide should be applied with cotton wool or a piece of sponge to the whole body, from the soles of the feet upwards, but excluding the head and neck. Children under 2 years of age should not be treated without a referral first.

The scabicide penetrates the skin to kill the mite and eggs in the basal layer of the epidermis. Care should be taken to apply it between the fingers and toes and under the nails. Aqueous applications should be left on for 24 hours and creams for about 12 hours. It is important to tell the patient that if the hands are inadvertently washed or immersed in water during this period, the scabicide should be reapplied.

It is not necessary to repeat the application. Because of residual itching, it may take up to 3 weeks before treatment can be deemed successful. During this period when the skin is still irritated, treatment with 1 per cent topical hydrocortisone or crotamiton may give symptomatic relief.

If the patient is still symptomatic after this time, a referral to confirm the diagnosis is advisable.

Because the scabies mite cannot survive outside the human body, it is not necessary to make special arrangements for laundering or washing clothes and bed linen.

Treatment of body lice

Pubic lice are treated in a similar way to head lice with a lotion containing malathion or phenothrin (see Chapter 12). Where the eyelashes are affected, white soft paraffin can be smeared lightly over the lids and lashes twice daily for 2 or 3 weeks. This prevents the lice from respiring normally.

Body lice are treated in the same way as scabies (see above). The clothes and bedding should be washed.

Treatment of fleas

As already mentioned, the itchy skin lesions caused by flea bites can be treated with topical hydrocortisone or antihistamines, or oral antihistamines. However, attention to household furnishings is also necessary, and it is useful to explain the lifecycle of the flea to patients to gain their cooperation and compliance in eradicating the problem. Cats and dogs harbour adult fleas in their coats. The fleas feed by sucking blood from the skin of their host and lay their eggs in the animal's fur. The eggs drop from the animal on to carpets, pet bedding, soft furnishings etc. and hatch into larvae, which then migrate away from light under carpets, rugs and furniture. The larvae pupate before eventually hatching into the next generation of fleas, which search for a host (animal or human) to start the cycle again. Humans are usually bitten when fleas jump from their pets.

One of the available proprietary insecticidal products should be applied about the home to kill the adult fleas and prevent metamorphosis, with special attention to soft furnishings and areas under carpets and furniture. This should be accompanied by regular vacuuming, including under rugs and furniture, and cleaning of pet bedding. Finally, the pet itself should be treated by applying one of the proprietary topical insecticides available from pet supply shops, on a regular basis to prevent reinfestation.

Sunscreens

Although at one time the efficacy of sunscreens was judged by their ability to protect against UVB light, which is the part of the ultraviolet spectrum mainly responsible for sunburn, the importance of UVA in the pathogenesis of skin ageing and skin cancer has resulted in a requirement to protect the skin from both UVA and UVB. Products should be chosen that have a high sun protection factor (SPF) for UVB and a high star rating for UVA. This is also important with respect to drug-induced photosensitivity (largely mediated through UVA) and polymorphic light eruption (mediated through UVA and UVB).

Self-tanning agents

Most self-tanning products contain dihydroxyacetone, which acts on acids in the skin to form a brown colour. However, this agent alone offers no protection from UV light and users still need to use a sunscreen.

These agents may be used by patients with vitiligo, which is characterised by patches of skin contaning no melanin pigment, but the warning about the use of a concomitant sunscreen should not be forgotten.

Evening primrose oil

Many clinical trials have been carried out on the effect of evening primrose oil capsules (containing gamma-linolenic acid) on eczema. The results are conflicting and the overall evidence is not convincing.

Wart solvents

So-called wart solvents generally contain high concentrations of salicylic acid, a keratolytic agent, which will reduce the size of the wart. Clinical trials have shown that topical salicylic acid has a significant cure rate for warts and compares favourably with cryotherapy. Although warts will usually resolve spontaneously within 2 years or so, they are cosmetically unacceptable to many patients. If a proprietary solvent does not achieve the desired effect, a referral should be made so that cryotherapy can be considered.

Second opinion

Rashes often appear far less well presented 'in the flesh' than in textbooks, and are the cause of as much confusion to doctors as to everyone else. With experience they may rely upon experience and pattern recognition to diagnose common rashes, but to start with doctors are taught the value of noting features carefully and comparing them to standard descriptions.

Most dermatological conditions can be treated without specialist investigations or opinion. Topical steroids are used sparingly and often in combination with other, more bland, agents such as emollients. Some GPs are happy to include punch biopsies in their range of minor surgical procedures, sampling for histology in chronic eruptions where the diagnosis is in doubt.

Urgent referral is necessary when malignancy is suspected and routine referral when the diagnosis evades the clinician, the response to treatment is unsatisfactory, or the patient requires specialist therapy.

Occasionally, when the diagnosis is in doubt but there is no suspicion of a serious problem, a short trial of treatment may be valuable in moving a hypothesis towards a conclusion.

Bibliography

British Association for Sexual Health and HIV (2001). *National Guideline on the Management of Scabies.* www.bashh.org/guidelines/2002/scabies_0901b.pdf (accessed 9 March 2006).

Clark C (2004). How to choose a suitable emollient. *Pharm J* 273: 351–354.

Cox NH (2000). Permethrin treatment in scabies infestation: importance of the correct formulation. *Br Med J* 320: 37–38.

Gibbs S, Harvey I, Sterling J, Stark R (2002). Local treatments for cutaneous warts: systematic review. *Br Med J* 325: 461–463.

Williams HC (2003). Evening primrose oil for atopic dermatitis. *Br Med J* 327: 1358–1359.

SUMMARY OF CONDITIONS PRODUCING TRUNK AND LIMB LESIONS

Allergic contact eczema

Allergic contact eczema produces an erythematous rash, often localised to the contact point with the causative agent. Common causes are nickel (metal jewellery, buckles and jeans studs), leather (shoes and watchstraps) and dyes (clothing).

Atopic eczema

Atopic eczema is often associated with a personal or family history of atopy (eczema, asthma, hay fever or urticaria). It appears as a dry, often scaly, erythematous rash (see Figure 13.6). It is very itchy, and evidence of this is apparent in the form of visible scratch marks (excoriations) in some patients. It is the commonest form of eczema in babies from 3 months of age. Although atopic eczema often resolves in childhood, it can continue into adulthood. It is common on the face and in skin flexures, as in the wrists, the crease of the elbows and behind the knees. In some instances it may be vesicular. If eczema becomes a chronic condition, it runs a fluctuating course. Between acute exacerbations the skin will become dry, leading to cracking, which can be painful.

Cancer

There are three main types of skin cancer. The most common, basal cell carcinomas, are usually ulcerating (rodent ulcers), relatively slow growing and never metastasise. They are commonly seen on exposed skin. They arise from the basal cell layer of the skin or in hair follicles. Initially they may appear as a small, innocent-looking, isolated red papule, but eventually they develop raised or rolled edges, giving the typical appearance of an ulcer – **refer.**

Squamous cell carcinoma is common on exposed sites such as the face and arms. It may present as a rapidly growing or a slowly growing nodule that does not resolve – **refer.**

A melanoma can be malignant if not checked early. It is derived from collections of pigment cells in the skin (moles). Moles are common on healthy skin and are normally harmless. However, damage, such as from excessive sunlight, can trigger a change in both nature and appearance. At this stage a medical opinion should be sought. Any sudden increase in size or colour change, bleeding, ulceration, pain or irritation indicates the need to **refer.**

Cellulitis

Cellulitis is a bacterial infection of the skin caused by either Streptococci or Staphylococci, and sometimes both together. The infection may arise at the site of trauma, but it can also affect previously healthy skin. A similar condition caused by Streptococci is called erysipelas. The rash is red and often hot and oedematous (see Figure 12.7). It is seen commonly on the face, arms or legs. There is often headache, fever and malaise – **refer.**

Drug eruptions

Drug rashes can take many different forms but the most common types are macular and maculopapular rashes, urticaria and photosensitivity (Figure 13.11). The first two types may be widespread in their distribution or confined to small areas on the limbs. They typically appear about 3–7 days after starting the drug, but can occur much earlier (on the same day) if the patient has been exposed to the drug on a previous occasion. Drug-induced urticaria occurs relatively rapidly, within hours of administration. Photosensitive rashes induced by drugs resemble sunburn on light-exposed areas of the skin. They can be either rapid or slow in onset. As the patient's GP should be aware of such reactions to drugs, **refer.**

(continued overleaf)

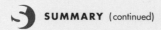

SUMMARY (continued)

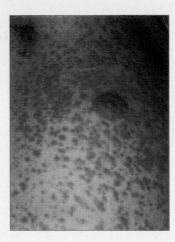

Figure 13.11 Antibiotic-induced rash. (Reproduced with permission from the Wellcome Trust Medical Photographic Library.)

Irritant contact eczema

Irritant chemicals can cause trauma to the skin, resulting in an inflamed area at the point of contact. The condition is particularly common on the hands. Causes include oils, lubricants, inks etc. at work, and detergents and washing-up liquids at home.

Intertrigo

Intertrigo is a rash between occlusive or opposing folds of skin in which a moist warm environment favours the growth of *Candida* and *Tinea*. It is more likely to occur in obese people, under the breasts in women, in the axilla and in the groin. The rash is often sore. It may respond to topical antifungal preparations, but severe cases may require referral.

Lichen planus

Lichen planus presents as small, flat-topped, pruritic shiny papules, often with a purple colour initially (see Figure 13.7). White streaks may be seen on the surface. Sometimes its appearance may be similar to that of eczema. It affects the flexor aspects of the wrists, limbs, and sometimes the trunk and genitalia. Lesions may sometimes be seen in the mouth, where a white lace-like or streaky pattern can be seen on the buccal mucosa. The condition, which is of unknown aetiology, is self-limiting over several months. As it subsides, post-inflammatory hyperpigmentation imparts a brown colour to the lesions, and in some cases this can appear without any obvious preceding inflammation. If the accompanying pruritus cannot be relieved with oral antihistamines, topical steroids may be required, in which case **refer.**

Lichen simplex

Lichen simplex can be regarded either as a form of atopic eczema or as a consequence of it. Intense itching causes skin thickening (lichenification; Figure 13.12). Scratching perpetuates the condition. If the pruritus is severe, **refer.**

→

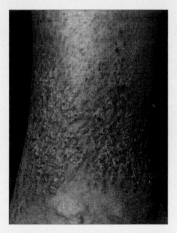

Figure 13.12   Lichen simplex. (Reproduced with permission from Glaxo Wellcome.)

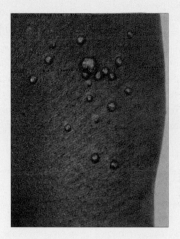

Figure 13.13   Molluscum contagiosum. (Reproduced with permission from the Wellcome Trust Medical Photographic Library.)

Molluscum contagiosum

This condition occurs predominantly in children and is caused by a pox virus. Small, smooth, shiny pearl- or flesh-coloured papules occur on the trunk, face or limbs (water warts; Figure 13.13). The lesions may be isolated or appear in groups, and there are no symptoms. The condition eventually resolves and there is no satisfactory medical treatment.

Polymorphic light eruption

Polymorphic light eruption is a reaction to sunlight and is often referred to as heat rash by the lay public. It appears on light-exposed areas as erythema, with small macules, papules or vesicles. It occurs in the spring and the summer. Sites frequently exposed to sunlight, such as the face and hands, are usually spared. The condition is most common in adolescents, particularly females, and appears within 24 hours of sun exposure. It is very itchy and is thought to be due to both UVA and UVB light. Sunscreens or a carefully developed suntan may help to protect the skin.

Pompholyx

Pompholyx is the name given to endogenous eczema (i.e. not contact eczema) of the hands (see Figure 13.1) or feet. Often the two sites are affected together. The condition starts as small vesicles (blisters), which may become bullae and burst. On the hands, the palms are usually affected. There is pruritus. Topical steroids are usually required – **refer.**

Prickly heat (miliaria)

Often referred to as sweat rash, prickly heat is an itchy rash occurring at sites of friction from clothing or following the application of topical preparations that occlude the sweat ducts. Treatment involves avoiding tight clothing or offending materials.

(continued overleaf)

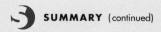

SUMMARY (continued)

Psoriasis
Psoriasis is a condition in which the rate of turnover of epidermal cells increases tenfold and the epidermis thickens. In its most common form, it presents as raised erythematous plaques covered with white or silvery scales (see Figure 13.3). The lesions vary in size and are often circular or oval. Common sites are the elbows, knees, scalp, sacrum, nails, intertriginous areas, and sometimes the hands and feet. Psoriasis occurs most frequently in young adults, and is usually a chronic condition that waxes and wanes in severity. The condition is often asymptomatic, but there may be pruritus. The appearance of the rash and the exfoliation is the cause of much distress – **refer.**

Scabies
The scabies mite burrows into the skin and causes pruritus, leading to excoriation and sometimes secondary infection. Sometimes thin greyish burrows, about 0.5 cm long, can be seen, although the mite itself is too small to see. The skin erupts in small red papules (see Figure 13.2). The finger webs are classically affected first, and then the wrists, axillae, genitalia, buttocks and abdomen. The chest and upper back are rarely affected. Although the mite is found on the face and head, in adults the rash and pruritus do not occur at these sites. In young children and the elderly, however, the rash can involve the face (this condition is called crusted scabies). The scabies mite is spread by skin contact and often occurs in epidemics, particularly in care homes for the elderly.

Shingles
Shingles is caused by reactivation of the herpes zoster (chickenpox) virus which has lain dormant in a sensory root ganglion. The virus travels along the course of a nerve, producing the characteristic eruption of the skin and acute pain (see Figure 13.8). The rash may run from the back across the chest or around the abdomen. It is classically unilateral and finishes at the midline – **refer.**

Sunburn
Sunburn is a well-recognised acute, erythematous, inflammatory eruption occurring a few hours after excessive exposure to ultraviolet light. It is chiefly due to UVB; in severe cases, burns and blistering can occur. Sunburn may be accompanied by shivering, fever and nausea. Chronic exposure to sunlight can cause premature ageing of the skin and predispose to cancer – this is largely due to UVA.

Tinea cruris
Tinea (ringworm) infection of the groin area (dhobi itch) is more common in men than women. It results in a circular, scaly, erythematous lesion characterised by well-defined edges. The rash, which is symmetrical, appears to clear from the centre, is redder at the edges and spreads outwards. Pruritus is often present. The patient often also has tinea pedis. The condition may be treated with topical antifungal agents.

Tinea corporis
Ringworm infection of the trunk or limbs may be contracted from animals or humans. Typically there are isolated erythematous and scaly lesions, often round or oval in shape (see Figure 13.9). As for tinea cruris, the lesions have characteristic defined edges and central healing, and these features are useful in distinguishing tinea from eczema. The distribution is not symmetrical.

→

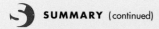 **SUMMARY** (continued)

Tinea pedis

Tinea infection of the foot (athlete's foot) appears in the toe clefts (classically between the fourth and fifth toes). It usually presents with itching, as a red, scaly eruption, and there may later be maceration and fissuring (see Figure 13.5). The condition can spread to other parts of the foot. Treatment is with topical antifungal agents.

Urticaria

An urticarial rash (Figure 13.14) has characteristic weals and erythema, and pruritus is usually present. It may occur on any part of the body. It is often part of an allergic reaction to drugs, foods, preservatives and colourants, although it is sometimes triggered by changes in temperature and fever. It generally only lasts about 24 hours, and if mild can be treated with oral antihistamines. If the patient has considerable oedema, and especially if the oedema spreads to the eyelids and lips and occludes the upper airway (angio-oedema), the condition should be treated as a medical emergency. A tracheostomy can be lifesaving in such circumstances.

Vitiligo

Vitiligo presents as patches of depigmented skin. There may be a hereditary link. The condition can affect the trunk and limbs as well as the face, and is often distributed symmetrically on both sides of the body. It is generally symptomless and of no consequence, but care should be taken to protect lesions from an increased susceptibility to sunburn.

Warts

Warts are well-defined, benign epithelial outgrowths associated with a virus. They are most common on the hands and fingers and the soles of the feet (verrucae). They may occur singly or in crops. Verrucae are painful when pressure is applied to them. Warts generally resolve spontaneously within 2 years. If they are particularly unsightly or unacceptable to the patient they can be removed by freezing with liquid nitrogen. In such cases, **refer.**

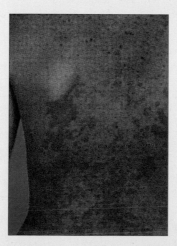

Figure 13.14   Urticaria. (Reproduced with permission from the Wellcome Trust Medical Photographic Library.)

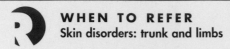

WHEN TO REFER
Skin disorders: trunk and limbs

- Any skin rash, lesion or pruritus that does not respond to OTC management

Hands
- Erythema or vesicles on palms
- Inflamed, painful skin surrounding the nail
- Pitting of fingernails

Legs
- Erythematous rash or ulceration on the lower leg or ankles in an elderly person

Trunk
- Unilateral rash on the chest or abdomen that stops at the midline
- Photosensitive rash or urticaria in a patient taking prescribed medication
- Chickenpox in special cases such as in pregnancy or in a mother less than 4 weeks after childbirth, or if the patient either is prescribed steroids, is immunocompromised or is unwell
- Moles with two of the following characteristics:
  - Increasing in size
  - Change in shape or outline from regular to irregular
  - Change in colour or mixed colour in the same mole
  - Itching
  - Bleeding
  - Crusting
  - Inflammation

Genitalia
- Sores or blisters

Accompanying symptoms
- Skin lesions accompanied by: malaise, fever or swollen lymph glands
- Urticaria accompanied by swelling of eyelids, lips or difficulty in breathing – emergency referral
- Urticaria or photosensitivity rash in a patient taking prescribed medication

CASE STUDIES

Case 1

A young man has presented a prescription for malathion lotion. He appears anxious and asks to speak to the pharmacist. He has come straight from his GP appointment but cannot agree with the diagnosis. He is a university student, home for the summer holiday, and the idea of scabies is completely alien to him.

How would the pharmacist respond?

There remains a widespread belief that scabies, lice and similar infections are the sole province of the dirty and unkempt. A detailed explanation of the epidemiology and infectivity, with suitable reassurance, may be necessary, and will increase the compliance needed for successful use of the medication.

It may be worth exploring his understanding of his parents' attitudes. If they share his prejudices, and find their son returning from his university accommodation with this infection, their fears may be heightened.

The young man was scratching even in the pharmacy, and in considerable discomfort. A second opinion may help his acceptance of the diagnosis.

The diagnosis of scabies can be difficult to make, the characteristic appearances often difficult to find. Examination of the webs between the fingers may reveal fine red lines.

On dark skins the diagnosis is even more difficult.

The history is often the most helpful diagnostic aid, and a trial of treatment may be the final arbitrator.

He returned to the pharmacy about 10 days later to report that the treatment had failed.

The intense irritation associated with scabies is due in part to the excrement of the mite, which is deposited in the subcutaneous burrows. This persists after the infection has been eradicated, and will not cease until the epidermis has been replaced, a process that takes several weeks.

It is important to make sufferers aware of the timescale of resolution, the other uncertainties around diagnosis and treatment being compounded by a perceived failure of treatment.

Case 2

A woman in her early 30s requests a recommendation for head lice.

What else does the pharmacist need to know?

Ideally, and to reduce resistance to insecticides, medication should only be provided for those in whom live lice have been found. This may be difficult, many children having symptoms with relatively few lice in their hair.

Nits, the egg cases of hatched lice, are evidence of past but not current infection.

Enquiry is needed as to the likely source of the infection, to minimise the chance of recurrence. This may be children at school, but is often asymptomatic in adult carriers.

In this case the 'patient' is this woman's partner, who has been abroad backpacking and returned with lice. This woman's request for treatment ostensibly for head lice could have caused confusion, and a recommended course of treatment could have failed if the pharmacist had not asked for sight of a head louse. In fact, the question did cause the woman to confess – embarrassingly – that the lice had been found on her partner's body and not his head, and he had suffered from intense itching.

Body lice will be killed by suitable insecticides, although this may not eradicate the infection. They live in clothing, and the irritation is from biting their host in search of blood.

Treatment to the body, as for scabies, will remove any lice, but clothing and bedding where the eggs are laid must be treated too. Washing in hot water is usually effective, and, as the lice are heat sensitive, ironing afterwards is also useful. Particular attention should be paid to the seams of the material, where eggs are often found.

(continued overleaf)

not irritant and no treatment is necessary. It will resolve spontaneously after a few months. However, referral is necessary if the condition becomes infected or the child scratches the lesions.

Napkin dermatitis

Most babies develop napkin rash at some stage and it is a condition that often causes more distress to the parents than to the baby. Classically, it appears as a confluent red rash over the napkin area. In some cases it may take the form of papules or vesicles, and there may be fissuring. The condition is caused by a contact dermatitis from the ammonia released from the urine, by faecal organisms, and from other constituents of urine and faeces. It may be worsened by constant soaking of the skin in the napkin area. This contact dermatitis spares the intertriginous areas of skin (between skin folds) where there is no contact with the irritant urine, and thus it can be distinguished from candidal infection, seborrhoeic eczema and psoriasis, in which the intertriginous areas are affected.

Treatment includes more frequent nappy changes, gentle cleansing of the skin (no soap), and barrier agents applied at each change. Such barrier agents include zinc cream, zinc ointment, zinc and castor oil ointment, and various proprietary products containing zinc, titanium and dimeticone. Whenever possible, the skin should be exposed by removing the nappy to allow drying and healing. At night nappies can be placed like sheets under and above – but not around – the trunk, so facilitating some circulation of air. The use of powders may cause irritation of the skin.

Candidal napkin dermatitis

The wet, warm environment under a nappy provides an ideal place for the growth of *Candida* and bacteria. Candidal infection of the napkin area causes a bright red eruption with pinpoint papules or pustules covering all the skin, including intertriginous areas. It may also be associated with oral candidiasis (thrush) and can be a sequela to antibiotic treatment.

Candidal infection should be suspected when a napkin rash fails to respond to simple symptomatic remedies. Treatment with topical imidazole creams should be tried for 7 days; if there is no improvement, or if the rash spreads to the trunk, referral to the GP should be considered.

Staphylococcal napkin dermatitis

If a nappy rash appears pustular there may be bacterial infection. The pustules may rupture and produce scaling. If suspected, the patient should be referred for consideration of antibiotic treatment.

Seborrhoeic napkin dermatitis

This may appear as a red scaling eruption, especially in the intertriginous areas. Often the infant also has seborrhoeic eczema of the scalp (cradle cap), face, trunk, and behind the ears.

Psoriatic napkin dermatitis

Psoriasis in the nappy area, which is rare, occurs initially as a red eruption. There may be some scaling, but not as much as is found in psoriasis that occurs elsewhere on the body. The condition may later spread to the trunk and limbs. Failure of nappy rash to resolve after several weeks of standard treatment may raise the possibility of napkin psoriasis and requires referral.

Seborrhoeic eczema

Seborrhoea may affect the intertriginous zones of the napkin area and spread to the trunk. It appears as a confluent papular red rash. On the scalp (cradle cap), forehead and behind the ears, seborrhoeic eczema appears with characteristic scaling. Cradle cap can be treated by softening the scales with olive oil or emulsifying ointment and then washing the scalp with a baby shampoo. Intertriginous seborrhoea may require topical steroids and referral is therefore indicated.

Head lice

Head lice are most commonly found in children, but adults can have them too. Head lice cannot jump and they can only spread by children touching heads, usually for some time. Head lice found on pillows, hats and other locations are generally thought to be incapable of infecting a person and usually die within 24 hours. The head louse, *Pediculus capitis*, is 1–3 mm long and has three pairs of legs (Figure 14.1). It clings to hair with its claws and feeds on blood from the host's scalp. The female lays five or six eggs per day (up to 300 eggs in her lifetime), which attach to hair shafts by means of a glandular discharge that she secretes. After 7–10 days the eggs hatch and leave white, shiny cases (nits) on the hair (Figure 14.2). Within 10 days, fully developed adult lice form. Lice live for 1–2 months. The eggs (nits) are laid close to the scalp and are found further from the scalp as the hair grows.

Nowadays, most children's heads will be infected with as few as 10–20 lice. Such small numbers will be difficult to find with the naked eye, and this is why inspection by the school 'nit nurse' is a thing of the past. Infection may be asymptomatic in some children, whereas in others there will be an itchy scalp, especially behind the ears. This itch can take a few weeks to develop after infection, as it is a manifestation of an allergic response to the lice, and by the same token the itch may persist for some time after successful eradication with insecticidal lotions.

Infection can only be reliably diagnosed when a louse is found, and this can only be successfully done by detection combing.

Technique for detection combing

1. The hair should be wetted and dried to dampness to prevent lice moving when combed. Many sources recommend wetting the hair with a conditioner, but this can produce a foam on the hair shaft which makes visualisation of the lice or nits difficult. The use of an oil such as olive or coconut is said to be better.
2. The hair is then combed with a normal comb to remove tangles.
3. The hair should then be combed using a plastic detection comb, starting at the roots and combing along the length of the hair. This process should be repeated several times.
4. The comb should be tapped on white paper to dislodge any lice, which can then be seen. Each louse is about the size of a pinhead.
5. Any lice found should be stuck to the paper with a piece of sellotape and taken to the pharmacy or nurse as proof of infection.
6. The comb should be washed under the tap.
7. Detection combing is best performed on all contacts and family members to discover who is infected. Family members should not be routinely treated unless lice have been detected.

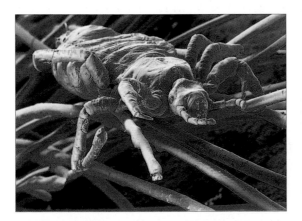

Figure 14.1 Head louse. Scanning electron micrograph of *Pediculus humanus capitis* among hair. Actual size is approx 2–3.5 mm. The louse's three pairs of legs can be seen directly behind the head. (Reproduced with permission from Eye of Science/Science Photo Library.)

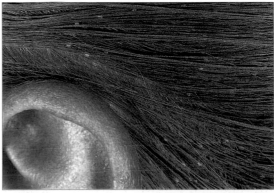

Figure 14.2 Head louse eggs (nits). (Reproduced with permission from Dr Chris Hale/Science Photo Library.)

Treatment of head lice

Treatment with insecticidal lotions should only be carried out when lice have been found by detection combing. If no lice have been seen, treatment is unnecessary. The use of insecticidal lotions as a preventative measure is not recommended. Insecticidal products should not be used for babies under 6 months old.

OTC topical insecticides available include malathion, permethrin and phenothrin (the latter combined with piperonal butoxide as a synergist). Although good clinical trials are few in number, the evidence in the literature shows that all these agents appear to be equally effective. At the same time, resistance exists to varying extents in different regions, and patterns vary in different countries. Although these agents are effective in killing the lice, their ovicidal efficiency is unreliable and thus a second treatment is necessary 7–14 days after the first in order to kill the lice that have hatched from eggs not killed by the first application. There have been no good-quality trials comparing different formulations or vehicles, but the view is generally held that insecticidal shampoos have too short a contact time to be maximally effective, and thus lotions and liquids are to be recommended.

No evidence exists of the efficacy of other chemical control methods, such as herbal treatments or aromatherapy. Published clinical trials showing the effectiveness of non-chemical methods such as wet combing ('bug busting') or dimeticone lotion have generally received a mixed reception (see below).

Lotions and liquids should be applied as follows. Failure to apply products properly will often result in treatment failure, which may be perceived as resistance to the agent used. This may result in a second course of treatment with another chemical, which may produce the same results for the same reason that the first treatment failed.

1. Approximately 50–100 ml of insecticidal lotion will be needed per head, depending on the amount of hair.
2. The lotion must be applied to dry hair. This is because lice can close down their respiratory airways for a short time when immersed in water. It is thought that insecticides enter the louse (at least in part) through the respiratory airways to exert their effect. Thus the presence of water, particularly combined with the use of an insecticidal shampoo, may reduce the efficacy of the agent used. The hair should be separated with the fingers to expose the scalp, and then a small amount of lotion rubbed in until the scalp is wet. Special attention must be paid to the nape of the neck and behind the ears, where lice are usually found in greater abundance. For long hair the lotion should also be applied to the first 1 or 2 inches of the hair, which is the distance the lice may move from the scalp.
3. It is advisable for the child to hold a towel over the face and eyes to avoid spillage while the parent applies the insecticide.
4. The hair should be allowed to dry naturally and the lotion left on, preferably overnight.
5. The lotion should be shampooed off the next day.
6. The application should be repeated after 7 days to kill the lice that have hatched from eggs not killed by the treatment.
7. The hair can be inspected by detection combing a few days after the second application.
8. Where there is still evidence of infection (and only when the evidence is presented on a piece of paper beneath a square of sellotape), consideration must be given to the possibility of inadequate application before considering the use of another insecticide. Friends and family should also be investigated for infection. If a second agent fails, despite proper application, wet combing may be considered before referring the patient to the GP, when a prescription for carbaryl may be considered.

The treatment of head lice requires a huge commitment from both patients and parents. Resistance to insecticides can occur, and in the past health authorities implemented a policy of rotating use of particular agents, but this is no longer justified. Most apparent treatment failures are due to poor technique, use of inadequate quantities of lotion, or forgetting that a persistent itch is not necessarily a sign of continued infection. Sometimes young lice, which have hatched from eggs after the first application, may be found after the first application of insecticide, but they should not survive the second application (see Table 14.1).

Adverse effects are usually minor, such as irritation and erythema of the scalp and irritation of the hands.

The practice of 'bug busting' or wet combing has been advocated, and is especially favoured by parents who consider chemical treatment undesirable. This technique involves wet combing of the hair with a detection comb until no more lice are found. Combing is carried out first after the application of hair conditioner and then repeated on rinsed hair. Combing is done every 3 or 4 days for 2–3 weeks and continued until no further lice are found, and then for another 3–4 days. The process should take 2 hours each time. There is, however, controversy about the effectiveness of this method, and it is generally not recommended as first-line treatment of infection. However, because it requires time and dedication on the part of parents the reasons for failure in many cases may be due to poor methodology, and thus in particular limited circumstances it may have a role. Clinical trials comparing the cure rates of 'bug busting' with those of treatment using pediculicides are difficult to evaluate and the results are controversial. There are potential flaws in study design, such as a lack of blinding, inappropriate regimens, alleged differences in comb design and the methods of assessment of cure. The interested reader is referred to the bibliography at the end of this chapter.

Scabies

The intense itching of scabies is caused by an allergic reaction to the excreta of the mite *Sarcoptes scabei*, and it sometimes takes several weeks after infection before the pruritus begins. The pruritus is sudden in onset, severe, and worse at night. The rash is papular but not always obvious. The presence of a pruritic rash in other family members will provide a clue to its diagnosis. In infants and toddlers the head and neck, trunk, wrists, palms, soles and insteps are particularly affected. This distribution is slightly different from that seen in adults.

Suitable scabicides for children are malathion and permethrin, but the latter is more suitable because it can be left on the skin for only 8 hours, rather than 24. Treatment should be applied to the whole body, and details are given in Chapter 13. Children under 2 years should be referred for treatment under medical supervision, and up to this age the face (up to and around the hairline), neck and ears should also be treated. If the hair is thin or fine, the scalp should be treated too. In older children with more dense hair, as well as in adults, the application of lotion is difficult, and in any case infection on the scalp is less likely unless the child is immunocompromised. In children over the age of 2 the treatment should be applied only on the body and not on the head and neck. Particular attention should be paid to finger and toe webs. Lotions containing permethrin should be left on for 8 hours and care taken that children do not wash or put their hands in water during that time. The allergic reaction responsible for the pruritus may take 2 weeks to disappear, and during this time calamine lotion or crotamiton cream should be used to relieve symptoms.

Bedding and clothing should be washed at temperatures above 40°C.

Table 14.1   Reasons for failure of treatment of head lice

- No proven initial infection (as evidenced by detection of live lice)
- Insufficient quantities of product applied to the scalp, especially in patients with long hair
- Repeat application not done after 7 to 10 days
- Resistance to insecticide
- Short contact time of insecticide with scalp (e.g. shampoo for ten minutes)
- Use of permethrin after failure of a course of pyrethrin due to cross resistance. (However there may be some cases where pyrethrin may be successful after permethrin has failed)
- Poor understanding of the need for careful application of the treatment by the parent

Impetigo

Impetigo is caused by a staphylococcal or streptococcal infection of the skin. The rash occurs most commonly on the face, chiefly around the nose and mouth, but sometimes also affects the limbs. It begins as vesicles which rupture and weep, with the affected skin beneath becoming very red. The exudate then dries to form yellow-brown, sticky crusts. The skin is sore, and scratching the lesions can cause the infection to spread. The condition is contagious and children should be kept from school until the lesions have dried up (usually only a few days).

Referral is necessary for topical or systemic antibiotic therapy.

Measles

Measles has become uncommon nowadays because of widespread immunisation. The virus is spread by droplet infection from the respiratory tract, and the incubation period (time between exposure and symptoms) is 7–14 days. The condition begins with a fever and symptoms of an upper respiratory tract infection. Conjunctivitis and small red spots on the buccal mucosa will often be present (Figure 14.3). After about 4–5 days the blotchy, flat rash appears, starting on the face and then spreading down to the trunk and limbs. It lasts about 7 days. The child should be kept away from school for a minimum of 7 days from the appearance of the rash.

Children who have been vaccinated may still have measles in a mild form. Standard treatment includes paracetamol for fever, and promethazine syrup if there is pruritus.

Chickenpox

Chickenpox is now the most common infectious disease of childhood. It spreads readily among school and family contacts, either by droplet infection from the respiratory tract or by contact with the vesicular exudate. The incubation period is between 10 and 24 days. Children may catch chickenpox from an adult with shingles, but not vice versa. The child should be excluded from school until the rash is dry and crusted, with all vesicles gone. Viral particles can be isolated from the vesicle fluid, increasing the infectivity. The period of infectivity lasts for about 7 days from the appearance of the vesicles.

The chickenpox rash appears as characteristic tiny vesicles (small blisters) surrounded by reddened areas, mainly on the trunk rather than the face and limbs (Figure 14.4); it may also appear on the scalp. The rash develops over 2–5 days

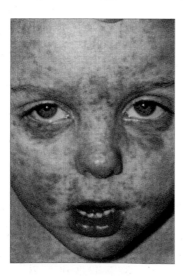

Figure 14.3   Measles. (Reproduced with permission from the Wellcome Trust Medical Photographic Library.)

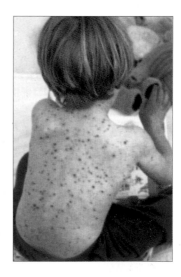

Figure 14.4   Chickenpox. (Reproduced with permission from Mark Clarke/Science Photo Library.)

and the vesicles eventually burst and form crusts or scabs, which disappear after about 10 days. Early on both forms of the rash, i.e. vesicles and scabs, will be found simultaneously.

The condition is very irritant, but patients should be persuaded not to scratch the lesions as this may cause scarring and also releases the virus from the vesicles.

Complications are rare in children, although immunocompromised patients must be referred to the GP. Standard treatment is with calamine lotion and oral antihistamines.

Gastrointestinal

Oral candidiasis

Oral candidiasis (thrush) commonly occurs in babies as white patches on the tongue and buccal mucosa. It may be treated with an oral gel containing an antifungal agent such as miconazole. If it follows a course of antibiotics, or there is also evidence of candidal infection of the skin in the napkin area, referral is needed for treatment with an oral agent, such as nystatin, to eradicate the infection from the gut.

Vomiting and diarrhoea

Vomiting and diarrhoea, either together or alone, are usually mild, benign symptoms in babies and older children.

Gastroenteritis, in a mild or severe form, is more common in bottle-fed than in breast fed infants. Mild or short episodes will resolve spontaneously, as in adults. However, symptoms lasting more than 24 hours in babies less than 6 months old or more than 48 hours in children under 2 years should be referred if there is no sign of improvement. Similarly, any baby who has vomited at least half of its feed on three occasions in the last 24 hours should be referred. If there has been a reduction in normal fluid intake by more than 50 per cent, this is also a reason for referral.

Diarrhoea alone should be reviewed after 2 or 3 days to see whether there are signs of improvement. There is no need to discontinue either breast- or formula milk feeding in babies with diarrhoea alone. If the baby appears ill or listless after this time, referral should be considered.

The major complication of vomiting or diarrhoea is dehydration, resulting in electrolyte and water imbalance. This can lead to severe illness. It would be extremely rare for a child to become significantly dehydrated within the timespan referred to above without appearing obviously ill and in need of referral. However, electrolyte replacement mixtures are available and may be recommended by pharmacists. Any unusual signs, such as excess drowsiness or the parent thinking that the baby looks paler than usual, should be referred.

Some babies have a habit of bringing up small amounts of milk after a feed (posseting). Provided that weight gain is normal, this is of no significance and the parents can be reassured that this is a perfectly normal occurrence.

Pyloric stenosis

Pyloric stenosis is a congenital defect of the pyloric sphincter in the stomach that prevents some of the ingested food passing into the duodenum, with the result that it is vomited. The condition can become symptomatic within a few weeks of birth. It may be differentiated from the more common causes of infantile vomiting (such as virus infections) by its projectile nature. Large quantities are ejected with considerable force and travel some distance from the patient. Constipation frequently accompanies pyloric stenosis, and in severe cases there may be dehydration. If suspected, the baby should be referred.

Colic

A baby that cries after a feed has usually been underfed or has swallowed an excessive amount of air. In bottle-feeding the latter may be caused by the baby sucking too hard on a teat with a small hole, or a gulping action while trying to keep pace with the rapid flow of milk from a teat with a large hole. Large quantities of air cause damp and cool, and by giving them cold drinks. Paracetamol can also be given.

Respiratory tract

Infections

Respiratory tract infections can cause distress to babies and young children out of proportion to the severity of the infection because of their narrow airways. Usually no treatment is necessary, although symptomatic relief is often given by inhalant balms or capsules. These should not be put on a baby's skin and generally are not recommended in infants under 3 months. When used, the inhalant should be dabbed on a handkerchief and placed out of reach, as a high concentration of volatile oils close to the airways has been thought to induce reflex apnoea in a few cases.

If a baby stops feeding, is febrile, or appears generally unwell or different from normal, then a referral should be made.

Benign coughs are often worse at night, but persistent night-time coughs, wheezing or breathlessness are signals for referral to exclude such conditions as asthma.

Some children between the ages of 4 and 8 years develop a chronic catarrhal syndrome comprising recurrent colds, coughs and earache. Provided that other possible conditions have been excluded and a doctor has been seen, the parents require only reassurance that no treatment is necessary, and that the condition will eventually resolve.

Tonsillitis

A sore throat is often thought by parents to be tonsillitis, but this is rarely the case. The tonsils normally appear as oval, fleshy red glands at either side of the back of the throat. White (pus-filled) patches speckled on their surface indicate acute tonsillitis, and this requires referral to the doctor. There is otherwise no need for referral unless the child appears ill in any other way, such as with feverishness, headache or earache.

In children, especially adolescents, a sore throat that persists for longer than 1 week or is recurrent and follows a week or two of malaise, or is accompanied by enlarged cervical lymph nodes, requires referral to exclude complications such as glandular fever.

Croup

Croup refers to the cough associated with partial airway obstruction in the larynx. It is more common at night, and in babies and young children. The breathing is noisy and there is a characteristic high-pitched wheezing, which can be heard during the cough on expiration. The child will be distressed and appear ill. Croup is caused by oedema and narrowing of the airway resulting from inflammation around the larynx, epiglottis and vocal cords. It is rare and requires instant medical referral.

Whooping cough

Although most children are vaccinated against whooping cough, the disease can still occur in a mild form. It may present as a dry, irritating cough leading to continuous bouts of coughing, terminated by the characteristic whooping noise when the child takes a long, deep inspiration. In its mild presentation the whoop may be absent. If a cough continues for 10 days without improvement, and is accompanied by general malaise, anorexia or weight loss, the patient should be referred.

Teething

The eruption of the first teeth can be accompanied by a syndrome of inflamed painful gums, fever and irritability, and often the symptoms of a mild upper respiratory tract infection. Mothers will usually have diagnosed the problem themselves. Treatment is with paracetamol for the fever and pain, and this is generally more effective than a teething gel.

Earache

Ear pain in children always warrants referral to determine whether there is an infection (otitis media) and to consider appropriate treatment. Not all doctors will automatically prescribe antibiotics, and it may be wise to advise parents that they need to seek the doctor's opinion about the condition but not necessarily to expect a prescription for antibiotics, at least in the first instance.

Headache

After a fall or head injury, children should be observed over the next 24 hours for signs of concussion, such as drowsiness, lack of coordination, nausea or vomiting. Any of these symptoms require referral.

In the same way as adults children will suffer headaches that are short in duration, of no consequence and responsive to paracetamol. However, severe or recurrent headaches, those with other symptoms such as visual disturbances, and those that are terminated by vomiting should be referred for exclusion of conditions such as migraine.

Meningitis is an inflammation of the membranes enveloping the brain and spinal cord. The cardinal symptoms are headache (although some children will be too young to verbalise this), neck or back stiffness, fever, photophobia, nausea and vomiting, irritability or drowsiness. These symptoms are non-specific and a high index of suspicion is necessary. Meningitis usually occurs secondarily to bacterial infection elsewhere, following upper respiratory infection, or viral infection, including mumps and measles. The potentially rapidly fatal form is caused by a meningococcus. This form is associated with a purple purpuric rash (haemorrhagic, bruise-like spots of varying sizes) and is characterised by its extremely fast onset and rapid deterioration of the patient. Although all epidemics have to start somewhere, meningococcal meningitis is rare, particularly in the absence of other locally reported cases. However, the seriousness of the diagnosis means that every pharmacist should bear it in mind as a possibility.

Second opinion

Children are one of the most common groups presenting to GPs. Elsewhere in this book we are reminded how important it is to establish who the patient is, and to be wary when taking a history from a third party, although this is common when the patient is young. It is important to listen to the parents' description of the problem and to try to hear their concerns and expectations, but it can be very useful to spend time with the child as well, as soon as they are old enough to give their own account.

Childhood illnesses are common, although major problems are, thankfully, rare. For most doctors the management contains a large element of reassurance, the occasional intervention with drugs or referral to secondary care, and constant vigilance for serious and urgent disorders. Thus vomiting in babies is common, whereas pyloric stenosis is rare. Abdominal pain is thought to be appendicitis far more frequently than it occurs, but it does happen. For the most part a global view of the child can be very helpful. A child who looks well and whose bodily functions are relatively unaltered can usually be observed. One that has deteriorated requires a full assessment, often with considerable speed.

Doctors are reluctant to investigate children unless it is necessary to affect management decisions. Even venepuncture may be traumatic, and all doctors see children who scream upon entering the room. Thus children requiring blood tests are often referred to the paediatric ward at the nearest hospital, and those in whom the doctor feels further investigation may be required to a consultant paediatrician at an early stage.

The management of children in general practice is considered by many to be one of the most satisfying parts of the job, watching and encouraging children as they develop from birth into adults. Major disease is rare, so a high index of suspicion is essential.

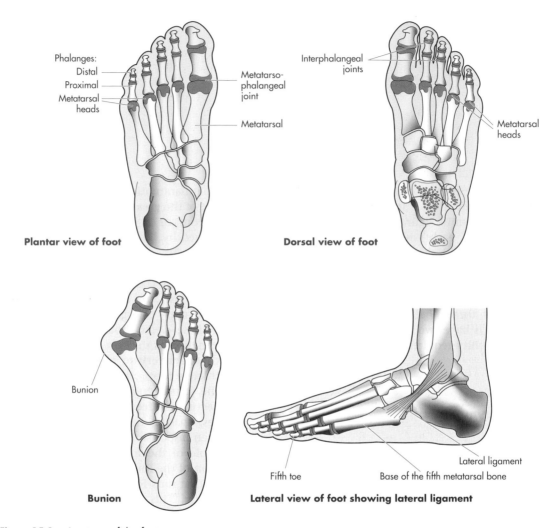

Plantar view of foot

Phalanges:
  Distal
  Proximal
Metatarsal
heads

Metatarso-
phalangeal
joint

Metatarsal

Dorsal view of foot

Interphalangeal
joints

Metatarsal
heads

Bunion

Bunion

Lateral view of foot showing lateral ligament

Fifth toe

Lateral ligament
Base of the fifth metatarsal bone

Figure 15.1   Anatomy of the foot.

of the great toe, suggests an ingrowing toenail. In this condition, a spicule of nail is trapped by and later grows into the nail fold, i.e. the ridge between the side of the toe and the nail bed.

A yellow discoloration of a toe nail, often that of the big toe, indicates a fungal infection caused by the same fungus responsible for athlete's foot. The nail thickens and may crumble and becomes unsightly. Although judged by some doctors to be a cosmetic problem requiring no treatment, it can be treated with oral antifungals, and if it is causing distress to the sufferer it should be referred.

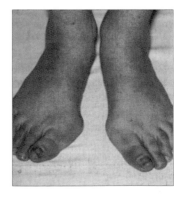

Figure 15.2   Bunions. (Reproduced with permission from the Wellcome Trust Medical Photographic Library.)

Pain in the heel from bursitis is discussed in Chapter 11.

Severity

Patients with severe pain in the foot or ankle will be unable to walk easily and thus will present comparatively rarely to the pharmacist. Differentiation should be made between pain that is constant and that brought about by or greatly aggravated by weightbearing. A constant pain around the first metatarsophalangeal joint, at the base of the great toe, may be an attack of gout, whereas a similar distribution of pain present all the time but made worse on walking is more descriptive of an inflamed bunion (hallux valgus).

The conditions most frequently brought to the attention of the pharmacist will be less acute and may be pain free. Foot infections, often fungal or viral in nature, cause irritation rather than frank pain; minor deformities, with their resulting corns and calluses, usually cause most pain on walking and when there is friction with the inside of footwear. Corns produce a sharper pain than calluses, which may present more as a burning sensation over a wider area of skin.

Verrucae, like corns, are usually painless until pressure is applied on walking.

Duration

It is convenient to consider most conditions of the feet as either of short duration (acute) or long lasting (chronic). Into the former category will come those based on, or aggravated by, trauma, such as strains, sprains and friction injuries, as well as the potentially more serious thromboembolic problems and bony injuries. Repeated but low-grade trauma to the bony prominences of the feet in the elderly or those with ill-fitting footwear will result in a callus or corn; acute trauma to these areas, arising from sporting pursuits, after walking long distances, or when fashion takes precedence over practicality, will result in a simple but painful blister.

For the most part, pharmacists will be asked for advice on chronic conditions. Athlete's foot, a fungal infection, can be present for months,

if not years, and is often recurrent, even after treatment.

Verrucae that are not treated, as well as some that are, can persist for similar lengths of time, as can minor but distressing orthopaedic conditions, including plantar fasciitis and metatarsalgia. However, these conditions will often resolve spontaneously.

Onset

The speed of onset can give clues to the aetiology of many foot problems. Obviously, a fracture will be immediately painful after the causative injury. A severe ligamentous strain can produce as much pain, swelling and disability as a fracture, but may have a slower onset. This means, for example, that a sportsman may return to the field after the injury, only later feeling the full effect of the insult.

Thromboses of either the arterial or the venous systems of the foot or leg are extremely rare, but a sudden unexplained and severe pain should trigger consideration of this possibility.

Accompanying symptoms

Pain and inflammation

The predominant symptom accompanying an injury to the foot is pain. This is usually felt maximally at the point of damage, although sometimes the pain may radiate to where the tissues are under greatest strain, or to the weightbearing point of contact. Thus, an inflamed plantar fasciitis at the calcaneum may produce pain in the longitudinal arch of the foot, although when examined the tenderness will be further back.

The inflammatory exudate associated with injury produces swelling, and rupture of blood vessels adds discoloration. Because the foot is largely comprised of muscles and tendons held in lubricating sheaths, supported by less elastic ligaments and bones, these fluids may be unable to expand freely where they originate, or find their way to the subcutaneous spaces locally, and instead track down the sheaths to appear as swelling or bruising.

With inflammation, areas of the foot may become hot and red. During an attack of gout the area around the base of the great toe becomes visibly reddened and swollen, and hot to the touch, as well as painful. This is rarely true of trauma.

Infection

Infections of the feet must be regarded with some caution. Although minor tineal infections are irritating but of no serious significance, bacterial infections can spread rapidly and cause both local and systemic effects. Through an abrasion or small laceration, the organisms enter the foot and an ascending cellulitis begins. The area is hot, painful and swollen. The same sheaths that allow tracking of extracellular fluids are colonised by the bacteria, with rapid upward spread. These cramped structures are particularly vulnerable to damage and subsequent scarring, and treatment must be provided quickly and vigorously.

Coldness and discoloration

Some conditions can produce areas of cold in the feet. Chilblains start as white, cold, avascular patches of skin before developing into the typical hot, red, flame-shaped areas, usually on or around the toes. A potentially more serious and generalised embarrassment of the arterial circulation is seen in Raynaud's phenomenon, a constitutional tendency to vasoconstriction that causes painful cold feet, usually with similar signs of vasoconstriction elsewhere, typically the fingers.

Thromboses of blood vessels within, or supplying, the foot will produce marked and severe symptoms. Arterial blockage results in pain and in a loss of blood supply, leaving the foot cold and white, whereas venous thrombosis causes congestion, the painful foot being swollen and blue or even black in colour. Such acute events are rare. More chronic disruption of the circulation is common. Atherosclerosis will produce a pale and cold extremity; if unchecked, this may progress to an area of local gangrene, the skin turning blue and finally black, while the affected part (usually a toe) withers and dies. Such lesions should be suspected in smokers, patients with diabetes, those with other forms of arterial disease, and with increasing age.

Rashes

Rashes that affect the feet can similarly affect other parts of the body. Fungal infections may occur as part of more widespread disease, with similar lesions in other areas, especially the groin.

Eczema on the feet, which is often aggravated by contact irritants in footwear, may be reflected in more generalised eczema. In chronic forms, especially on the sole, the condition produces hyperkeratosis and the patient will complain of hard skin. If the skin is not hydrated it may crack and cause pain, especially where pressure is applied on walking, such as on the heel and the metatarsal heads.

Arthritis

Bunions are common in patients with rheumatoid arthritis, as are calluses. The latter are often caused by deformity of the joint alignment, such that the metatarsophalangeal joints become subluxed and the patient walks on the metatarsal heads.

Aggravating factors

Ill-fitting shoes can cause or aggravate a number of foot problems, particularly bunions and corns. Sport shoes, including trainers, tend to be worn a size too small. There should be a half-inch gap between the end of the big toe and the end of the training shoe. Patients who suffer hyperhidrosis (excessive perspiration) or bromhidrosis (odorous perspiration due to bacterial breakdown of sweat) and wear training shoes should be encouraged to wear two pairs on alternate days to allow them to dry out.

Incorrect nail cutting may lead to ingrowing toenails. This happens when the nail is cut too short or tapered at the sides, instead of being trimmed straight across.

Incidence and recurrence

Verrucae are extremely common in children, although by no means restricted to them. It is assumed that one method of spread is by barefoot contact, and infected school children are often banned from physical training and swimming, or condemned to wear unsightly occlusive rubber socks. There is in fact little evidence for this type of spread, and experiments allowing free contact have shown little consequent increase in the incidence of these infections. Some authorities believe that the child's immunological status and their ability to resist infection are more important in both the acquisition and the duration of the infection.

Verrucae may be difficult to differentiate from corns: the latter are more common in middle age and beyond, whereas verrucae are seldom seen in this age group.

Fungal infections have a tendency to recur, even after apparently adequate treatment. Again, resistance to the infection may be a factor. Also, these organisms have the ability to spore and to lie dormant for long periods; once established, even enthusiastic and protracted treatment may leave sufficient spores to await a more favourable opportunity.

Special considerations

Care should be taken when known diabetic patients present with certain foot problems. Such people often have reduced sensation in the feet because of neuropathy, and poor blood circulation can affect the rate of healing. They may also have poor vision owing to retinopathy. Thus small cuts, corns and calluses may go unnoticed and untreated for some time, and then develop into serious lesions that can become infected. In most cases it will be appropriate to refer diabetic patients to a podiatrist.

Management

Ill-fitting footwear is a common cause of corns and calluses, and advice in this area is a good place to start treatment.

Injuries

After an injury to the foot first-aid treatment can be helpful, comprising rest, ice, compression and elevation of the foot (RICE) (see Chapter 11). Bandages and padding materials of foam or felt are useful in supporting strains, sprains and sporting injuries during recovery, and in limiting the movement of affected parts. This will reduce pain, rest damaged tissues, speed recovery and help prevent further injury. Even if used improperly, such products will do little harm. Some, however, such as arch supports and metatarsal pads, although efficacious, may not immediately be comfortable to use.

Stubbing the foot against an unforgiving surface, or dropping a heavy weight on the toes, can give rise to swollen, bruised and very tender toes, which may even be fractured. If there is no apparent deformity, and no question of injury to the metatarsal bones, an X-ray of the foot is of doubtful value as it will not influence the management. The patient can be advised to place a support of gauze or something similar between the toes to preserve the space and stop them rubbing, and then to bind the injured toe to the next largest one.

Corns and verrucae

Many OTC preparations are available for the treatment of corns and verrucae, and are often purchased without advice. However, impregnated corn plasters, corn pastes and verruca treatments used indiscriminately or over a protracted period can be harmful, and it might be wise to situate them close to the pharmacy counter so as to be in a position to offer advice to potential purchasers.

Most medicated corn and callus plasters contain not less than 40 per cent salicylic acid, in a variety of bases, and verruca dressings contain a minimum of 10 per cent salicylic acid. Other liquid and ointment formulations contain at least 10 per cent salicylic acid. The surrounding normal skin should be protected. A traditional treatment for verrucae was to soak the foot in a formalin solution for 10–15 minutes, but this can cause irritation of soft skin, such as between the toes.

All OTC packs carry health warnings for those with diabetes; it should be remembered, however, that one complication of diabetes is a deterioration in vision.

Some products carry a warning against use in those with circulation problems and an age range for treatment of between 16 and 50 years. However, an assessment of vascular efficiency is probably beyond most people. The results of over-liberal application can be quite severe, especially in those with impaired circulation. Treatment can produce pain and inflammation or, in more severe cases, tissue maceration and occasionally ulceration.

It would be worth considering medical referral before the use of high-strength salicylic acid preparations in the elderly or those taking certain other medications, such as anticoagulants or oral steroids, in whom the consequences of ulceration could be particularly severe.

Fungal infections

Tinea infections such as athlete's foot can be treated effectively with terbinafine or imidazole creams, such as clotrimazole, miconazole and econazole. The user should be advised to continue administration until several days after all traces of the infection have gone. Benzoic acid ointment is also effective, although cosmetically less acceptable. The undecenoates are probably less effective, and have largely been superseded.

More rarely, candidal infection may be found in the toe clefts, especially in the elderly, in patients with diabetes and in the immunocompromised. Again, imidazole creams are effective. Dusting the toe clefts with antifungal powders is useful in addition to, but not instead of, the application of cream. If fungal infection cannot be excluded, topical hydrocortisone preparations are contraindicated unless in combination with an antifungal agent.

The only reliable treatment for fungal nail infections is a prescribed oral antifungal drug. Unless the nail becomes detached from the nail bed or infection of a single nail spreads to others, it may not be necessary to treat, although cosmetically it is not particularly attractive. Women can paint their nails to cover up the problem,

and with time (usually several months) the infection often resolves itself. If it is painless, an antifungal spray or nail paint may be effective in some cases, but the condition is likely to last for several months or more.

Ingrowing toenails

Ingrowing toenails are best treated by doctors or chiropodists. The offending spike of nail needs to be resected carefully under local anaesthetic, shaping the nail to prevent a recurrence.

Second opinion

Conditions of the feet may be somewhat arbitrarily divided into those requiring medical treatment, such as dermatological and orthopaedic problems, and those that may be best dealt with by podiatry. Podiatry is usually available as part of the NHS, although many people attend privately for convenience and speed. Podiatrists will treat disorders of toenails, corns and callosities, and give general advice to people with special needs, including the elderly, who may find it difficult to cut their own nails safely, and diabetics.

They will also treat ingrowing toenails with partial or complete removal, and sometimes avulsion of the nail bed. Some GPs offer these services too. Many minor ingrown nails will grow out and resolve themselves, particularly if left unclipped, but the discomfort they cause, particularly if infected, may make intervention urgent.

Hallux valgus is another example of a condition shared between general practice and chiropody. Ultimately orthopedic surgery may be needed to correct the deformity, although doctors treat the early stages with both analgesics and anti-inflammatory drugs. Podiatrists may be able to reduce the discomfort by treating any overlying callosity, and with advice about suitable footwear. Indeed, inappropriately narrow shoes may aggravate or even cause early deformities, and present an opportunity for health education to both groups of professionals, as well as to pharmacists.

Special care is needed when assessing the elderly, or people with diabetes, whose circulation may be impaired, making otherwise simple problems both prolonged and potentially more serious. Infection must be treated early and vigorously, and infections deep in the tissues of the foot represent a medical emergency.

SUMMARY OF CONDITIONS PRODUCING FOOT DISORDERS

Bunion

A bunion (hallux valgus) is a lateral displacement of the first metatarsophalangeal joint, causing a swelling of the bursa that lies above it (see Figure 15.2). It results in a marked increase in the prominence at the base of the toe, and a compensatory inturning of the toe itself, with bunching and compression of the other toes. Tight shoes and high heels aggravate it. If severe or disabling, **refer.**

Callus

A callus is a hardening or thickening of the skin over joints and areas of weightbearing and friction (Figure 15.3). It is similar in appearance to a corn, but larger.

Cellulitis

Cellulitis is an infection of the subcutaneous or deeper tissues, often streptococcal in origin. It may spread rapidly and needs an early medical assessment and treatment – **refer.**

Chilblains

Chilblains are produced by a localised area of ischaemia. They are induced by cold and are common when the peripheral circulation is impaired. The affected area of skin is initially white, later becoming red, and finally bluish. Chilblains are often multiple and painful. Susceptible patients should be advised to dress warmly. Serious cases should be referred.

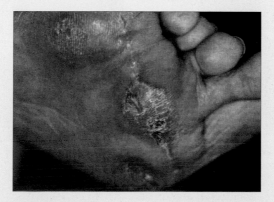

Figure 15.3 Callus. (Reproduced with permission from the Wellcome Trust Medical Photographic Library.)

(continued overleaf)

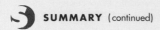 **SUMMARY** (continued)

Corns
Corns are hardened areas of skin (Figure 15.4) produced in response to trauma. They occur when the skin over bony prominences is irritated by ill-fitting footwear or deformities of the feet, such as hammer toes or bunions.

Fungal infections
Athlete's foot is caused by tineal infection, and is commonly seen as maceration between the toes. From this site, the infection may spread to adjacent parts of the foot and can cause considerable irritation. It can usually be treated with OTC preparations. If the diagnosis is in doubt or the toenail is affected (Figure 15.5), **refer.**

Gout
Gout is an arthritis caused by the deposition of uric acid in the joint space, usually as a result of a metabolic failure to excrete this waste product. The first metatarsophalangeal joint is involved – **refer.**

Ingrowing toenail
Tight-fitting shoes and the temptation to cut the toenail too short (or with rounded rather than square edges) can result in the nail edge turning into the nail fold (Figure 15.6). The toe will be swollen and painful, and may become infected. If unchecked, the nail bed granulates, producing a lump of fleshy tissue around and over the nail – **refer.**

Metatarsalgia
Metatarsalgia produces pain across the ball of the foot on weightbearing. It is a somewhat vague term applied to a variety of conditions. Chronic strain of the ligaments supporting the forefoot, with consequent loss of the lateral arch, is the most common explanation. It may be treated with rest, analgesia or anti-inflammatory drugs; if severe, **refer.**

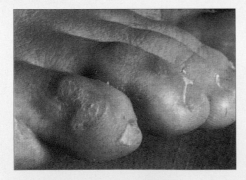

Figure 15.4   Corn. (Reproduced with permission from the Wellcome Trust Medical Photographic Library.)

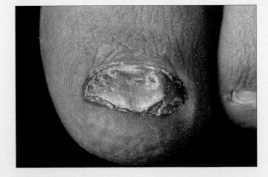

Figure 15.5   Fungal infection in the big toenail. (Reproduced with permission of Custom Medical Stock/Science Photo Library.)

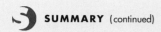 **SUMMARY** (continued)

Plantar fasciitis

The plantar fascia comprises two arch ligaments and a band of fibrous tissue overlying them and runs over the calcaneum (heel bone) to the toes. Plantar fasciitis is a chronic strain of the posterior attachment of the longitudinal arch ligament at its insertion into the calcaneum. It is also known as policeman's heel, a reference to the time when policemen were on their feet all day. The condition may be relieved by rest, but often recurs and requires treatment – **refer.**

Thrombosis

Occlusion of the arterial system can happen acutely or gradually. The usual clinical picture affects the elderly. There is a history of increasing vascular insufficiency, with claudication and cold extremities. The acute episode is of sudden severe and constant pain, the foot and lower leg becoming white and pulseless. It is a medical emergency – **refer.**

Venous thrombosis affects a wider age range. It may particularly be suspected in younger patients taking oral contraceptives, and postoperatively, although with the move to low-dose oestrogens and the use of surgical anticoagulation both these causes are infrequent. Again, the foot and (often) calf are painful, with oedema and, in very severe cases, a blue venous congestion of the skin – **refer.**

Verrucae

Verrucae are viral infections caused by the wart virus (the human papilloma virus). Usually affecting pressure areas of the foot, the lesion is constantly pushed into the epidermis, giving rise to the typical hard plaque of dry skin, with a small central ulcer revealing several black roots, which are In fact blood vessels (Figure 15.7). Verrucae may be treated with topical applications, or attempts can be made to destroy them with local cautery or freezing with liquid nitrogen.

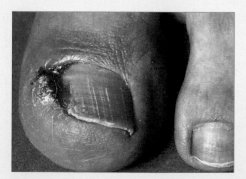

Figure 15.6   Ingrowing nail of the big toe.
(Reproduced with permission from the Science Photo Library.)

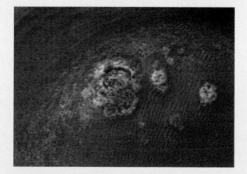

Figure 15.7   Verrucae. (Reproduced with permission from the Wellcome Trust Medical Photographic Library.)

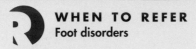

WHEN TO REFER
Foot disorders

- All diabetic patients with foot problems (refer to either the doctor or the podiatrist)

Refer to the chiropodist
- Bunions
- Calluses
- Corns
- Ingrowing toenail

Refer to the GP
- Pain on weightbearing
- Severe sudden pain, with or without obvious inflammation in the first metatarsophalangeal joint of the big toe
- Foot colour and appearance abnormal, e.g. cold and white, swollen and blue/black (unless a healing sprain)
- Severe and lasting pain of sudden onset with no apparent cause such as trauma – urgent referral

CASE STUDIES

Case 1

A man in his 20s presented his pharmacist with a repeat prescription for a moderately potent topical steroid and emulsifying ointment. In addition he was buying a number of cosmetics, including deodorants and antiperspirants.

Is any comment appropriate?

There are possible risks with any topical preparation and a pre-existing dermatitis. Sensitisation may aggravate, or even cause an eczematous reaction.

This man suffers from eczema, mostly on his face, hands and axillae. He is a keen athlete, and it appears to be consequent on sweating during and after exercise. The antiperspirant was intended for his feet. As it appeared he had not discussed his foot problem with his GP, further enquiry would have been useful.

Proper footwear is essential for sport, but may encourage perspiration and irritation. Eczema on the feet may be provoked by the prolonged use of trainers and sports shoes.

Further history disclosed moist macerated areas between the toe clefts, made worse by training. He is a keen long-distance runner and had noticed dermatitis on his feet.

This history is almost diagnostic of tinea pedis (athlete's foot). His sporting activities and his eczema will both have contributed to it, and make it more difficult to treat.

The use of steroids on the feet must be carefully monitored, as they may promote the spread of any fungal infection.

→

Case 2

A man in his mid-40s returned from a holiday in Greece and asked for his pharmacist's opinion on medication he had been supplied while away. He had developed severe pain in one foot after a long walk, and was given two medicines containing diclofenac and allopurinol. He has no other medical reports.

What advice can he be given?

The use of a specific medication suggests a diagnosis of gout has been made, which is compatible with his clinical history.

Gout may be a difficult diagnosis to make in a single visit to a doctor, and may need confirmation.

Further questioning revealed that he was examined by the doctor he visited, and his foot was extremely tender to touch. A blood test was suggested, but as he was returning home it was deferred.

Measurement of serum uric acid during an acute attack of pain may not show an elevation. It is not usual to start long-term uric acid reduction before a definitive diagnosis is established, or during the first attack.

This man was referred to his doctor. With rest and the anti-inflammatory drug, but without the allopurinol, his pain settled to the point where re-examination isolated the tenderness to the metatarsal area of the forefoot. Gout can present in many joints, but is most common in the metatarsophalangeal joint of the great toe. Estimation of the serum uric acid 2 weeks later was normal, as was an X-ray to exclude a 'march' fracture. A diagnosis of acute metatarsalgia following exercise was finally made, and the condition resolved over the next month.

Case 3

A man in his mid-60s asked the pharmacy assistant for a tube of verruca gel, which he has purchased before. As she could not recall this she referred him to the pharmacist. Verrucae are uncommon in people of this age. It emerged that this man's daughter had been buying a gel for him. As this treatment appears to have failed, a clinical examination is appropriate before proceeding.

The pharmacy had a consultation area and the man preferred to resolve the diagnosis immediately without reference to his doctor.

On examination the heel was tender, with dry flaking skin on the sole, fissured along the sides, but no discrete lesion suggesting a verruca. It seemed likely that the original lesion was a callosity, in which case the treatment may have been aggravating rather than helping it.

After 10 days with no treatment he was re-examined. The skin on the heel was then dry and hyperkeratotic, but remained tender and painful to walk on. Emulsifying ointment was recommended to soften the skin, with soaks in warm water to which a little of the ointment could be added.

As the condition was unilateral, an ill-fitting shoe might have been responsible.

If the condition had not improved, a medical opinion would have been needed.

16

Oral and dental disorders

Guest contributor: Robin A Seymour BDS, PhD, FDSRC(Ed.)

Oral and dental disorders can be categorised into those affecting the teeth and the supporting structures (i.e. the gums and periodontal tissues; Figure 16.1) and disorders of the oral mucosa and associated structures (e.g. the lips, tongue, salivary glands and temporomandibular joint). The mouth is also often the site of adverse drug reactions and manifestations of systemic disease.

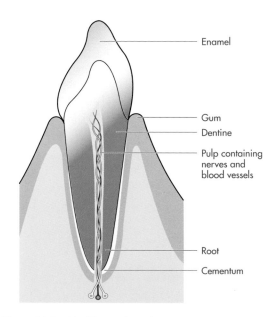

Figure 16.1   Healthy tooth and supporting structures.

Assessing symptoms

The tooth

The most common dental complaint presenting to pharmacists is toothache. The patient will typically complain of continuous pain, usually throbbing in nature. The pain may be exacerbated by hot, cold or sweet foods or drinks. Some patients have difficulty discerning which tooth is causing the pain. In many instances there may be an obviously carious or broken tooth. Toothache may also arise as a result of a lost restoration (filling), or from a heavily or recently restored tooth.

Pain arising when hot, cold or sweet stimuli are applied to the teeth may be due to dentine sensitivity arising as a consequence of gingival recession. This is invariably a localised sharp pain of short duration. Examination of the teeth will often show an area of gingival recession and exposed dentine.

Severe continuous pain may be caused by a dental abscess, which often arises from an infection of a necrotic dental pulp. Pain is often accompanied by localised swelling that can spread to parts of the face. The tooth is often slightly extruded from the socket. The commonest cause of pulpal necrosis is dental caries, although trauma and periodontal disease can compromise a tooth's vitality (i.e. its nerve and blood supply). Caries can sometimes be recognised readily either by an obvious hole in the tooth, often on the occlusal (biting surfaces) or by an area of discoloration (usually brown).

Pericoronitis is a specific infection that arises in the soft tissue covering impacted third molars (wisdom teeth; Figure 16.2). Because these teeth erupt between the ages of 18 and 25 years, such infections are often seen in young adults. The infection is nearly always associated with lower third molars. A localised soreness in the soft tissues overlying an impacted or erupting tooth will develop into pain and swelling if untreated. Swelling is often buccal and, as with dental abscesses, can spread and potentially compromise the airway. It is very rare for pericoronitis to affect both lower third molars at the same time.

A localised continuous pain arising in a tooth socket some 3–4 days after tooth extraction may be due to dryness of the socket (alveolar osteitis). The precise cause is uncertain, but fibrinolysis of the blood clot appears to be important in the pathogenesis. The socket will be tender, show signs of breakdown of blood clots and poor healing, and there may be exposure of bone. Referral to a dental surgeon is necessary as the socket will require a dressing.

Supporting dental structures

The periodontal tissues are the supporting structures of the tooth in alveolar bone. They comprise gingiva (gums), periodontal ligament, root surface cementum and the lamina dura of the alveolar bone. Periodontal diseases are caused by bacterial plaque and compromise the supporting structures. Essentially these diseases can be classified into gingivitis, where plaque-induced inflammatory changes are confined to the gingival tissues, and periodontitis, where these changes have involved periodontal ligament and alveolar bone. Gingivitis is reversible, but periodontitis is not and treatment is aimed at preventing further loss of tissue.

Bleeding gums, especially on tooth-brushing, is the most common symptom of gingivitis (Figure 16.3). The patient may also complain of swelling and soreness of the gums, particularly in the interdental area, and bad breath (halitosis). Plaque-induced gingival inflammatory changes can be exacerbated during pregnancy and at puberty, and in some patients taking oral contraceptives.

Periodontitis is characterised by loss of periodontal attachment and resorption of alveolar bone. The condition is chronic and many patients are unaware that they have anything wrong with their teeth. The loss of supporting structures can result in gingival recession, pocket formation and an increase in tooth mobility. In advanced forms of periodontitis the teeth may become very loose and drop out. As with gingivitis, the causative agent is bacterial plaque. Periodontitis is exacerbated by smoking and certain systemic diseases, in particular diabetes, osteoporosis and rheumatoid arthritis.

A localised swelling adjacent to a tooth may be a periodontal abscess. Such abscesses are often chronic in nature and discharge pus into the

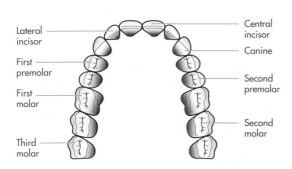

Figure 16.2   Permanent dentition of the upper dental arch.

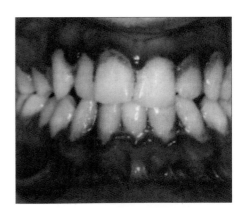

Figure 16.3   Gingivitis. (Reproduced with permission from the Newcastle Dental School.)

mouth. Most periodontal abscesses are caused by Gram-negative microorganisms. Occasionally they may be due to a foreign body lodged between the tooth and the gum.

A specific infection of the gingival tissues is acute necrotising ulcerative gingivitis (ANUG). In this condition there is pain, swelling and ulceration of the gingival tissues, particularly in the interproximal area. ANUG is much more prevalent in smokers, and is also associated with HIV infection.

Gingival overgrowth is a well documented unwanted effect associated with phenytoin, ciclosporin and calcium antagonists, particularly nifedipine. The prevalence of gingival overgrowth varies from drug to drug. For phenytoin, approximately 50 per cent of dentate patients are affected; this figure decreases to 30 per cent for ciclosporin and 10 per cent for nifedipine. Drug-induced gingival overgrowth (Figure 16.4) impedes mechanical plaque removal, and the subsequent gingival inflammation further distorts the tissue.

Herpetic infections in the mouth are of two types: primary acute herpetic gingivostomatitis and herpes labialis (cold sore). The initial herpetic infection often occurs in children and can be confused with teething. The child is unwell, pyrexic and irritable. The gingival tissues are usually fiery red and very painful; vesicles may be present throughout the mouth, but these will usually have burst, leaving ulcerated areas. Acute herpetic gingivostomatitis is usually self-limiting,

but the viral infection can recur in the form of cold sores. These usually start as a vesicle on the surface of the lips which bursts and the raw area becomes crusted over. Healing occurs within 7–10 days. Cold sores can be precipitated by trauma to the lips, sunlight or cold. They tend to occur when patients are run down or suffering from other viral infections.

Oral mucosa

Dry mouth (xerostomia) can have a variety of causes, including mechanical obstruction of the salivary gland, drug therapy (Table 16.1) and Sjögren's syndrome. This is a connective tissue disease of unknown aetiology. Features include dry mouth, dry eyes and rheumatoid arthritis.

A dry mouth is more prone to candidal infections and the reduced salivary flow increases the patient's susceptibility to caries, especially if there is gum recession causing exposure of the root surface. Apart from dryness of the mouth, patients with xerostomia will complain of difficulties in eating, swallowing and talking.

Aphthous ulceration of the oral mucosa is a troublesome, often recurrent problem that affects a large proportion of the population. Ulcers can occur in small crops, usually on the tongue, the floor of the mouth or the base of the buccal fold (Figure 16.5). Once there is a break in the continuity of the epithelium the site becomes readily infected from the oral bacterial

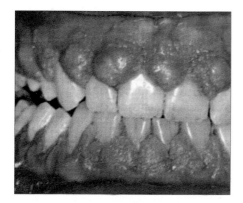

Figure 16.4 Drug-induced gingival overgrowth.
(Reproduced with permission from the Newcastle Dental School.)

Table 16.1 Drugs commonly implicated as causing xerostomia

Amphetamines
Antineoplastic drugs (occasionally)
Antiparkinson drugs, e.g. benzhexol (trihexyphenidyl), benztropine, orphenadrine
Antihistamines (H_1 blockers), atropine and atropine-like antispasmodics
Clonidine
Levodopa
Phenothiazines
Tricyclic and tetracyclic antidepressants

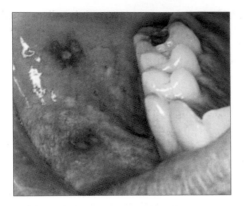

Figure 16.5   Aphthous ulceration. (Reproduced with permission from the Newcastle Dental School.)

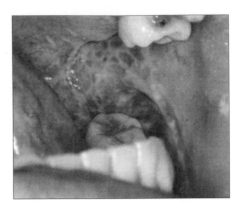

Figure 16.6   Erosive lichen planus. (Reproduced with permission from the Newcastle Dental School.)

flora. Such infections delay ulcer healing. Some patients experience a burning or tingling sensation in certain parts of their mouth just before an outbreak of ulceration. Most patients tend to respond well to topical medication. The aetiology of aphthous ulceration is uncertain, but may be related to diet, hormonal changes, blood disorders or other causes.

Patients suffering from aphthous ulceration will complain of mouth soreness that is exacerbated by foods (especially spicy food). Ulcers often appear covered with a yellowish slough. They heal in 7–10 days.

Lichen planus is a dermatological disorder that frequently involves the oral mucosa (Figure 16.6). Patients will complain of a sore mouth which is exacerbated by strong or spicy foods. The oral mucosa and gingival tissues are often ulcerated and show characteristic white striae (Wickham's striae).

Common candidal infections include thrush, denture-induced stomatitis and angular cheilitis. Such infections are characterised by a soreness of the mouth (Figure 16.7), a bad taste and discomfort on eating. This last problem is particularly likely if the patient wears dentures.

Candida albicans is an opportunistic commensal of the oral flora. Thrush infections are more common in babies and may be related to systemic antimicrobial therapy. Other types of candidal infection are frequently seen in elderly people wearing ill-fitting dentures. This so-called den-

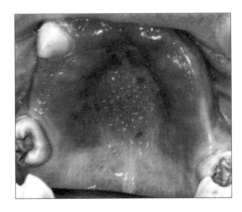

Figure 16.7   Oral candidiasis. (Reproduced with permission from the Newcastle Dental School.)

ture stomatitis is characterised by a fiery red palatal mucosa, which can exhibit hyperplasia. If there has been excessive wear on the dentures the patient becomes 'overclosed', i.e. the dentures do not provide sufficient support for the facial tissues. This exacerbates the creases at the angles of the mouth, which become infected with both *Candida* and staphylococci (angular cheilitis). All candidal infections cause soreness of the oral mucosa. There is a tendency for the inflamed mucosa to bleed. Candidal infections are also likely to occur in patients who are immunocompromised, either due to drug therapy or to an underlying systemic disease.

Lips

Cheilitis (inflammation of the lips; Figure 16.8) may be secondary to xerostomia, related to a systemic disease, or caused by trauma or a hypersensitivity reaction. Symptoms can be sudden in onset, and apart from being disfiguring, cheilitis will be associated with pain, soreness and problems with both eating and speech.

Tongue

Glossitis (inflammation of the tongue) can be caused by an obvious pathology, such as ulceration or trauma, but in many cases it is difficult to establish a cause. Iron and vitamin deficiencies (B_{12} and folate) are associated with glossitis, but haematological screening often reveals no abnormality. Glossitis is often associated with burning mouth syndrome. In some cases allergic reactions to denture materials may be implicated.

A black hairy tongue is due primarily to a change in the tongue surface, notably an elongation of the filiform papillae, which is associated with the overgrowth of pigment-producing bacteria and fungi. The latter probably arises as a consequence of a disturbance in the normal oral flora. Drugs are the main cause of black hairy tongue, and those commonly implicated include penicillin and tetracyclines. The condition has also arisen following the use of oxygenation mouthwashes, such as those containing sodium perborate or hydrogen peroxide.

Black hairy tongue should be distinguished from black staining of the tongue, which can follow the use of certain iron preparations, or the use of mouthwashes containing chlorhexidine.

Accompanying symptoms

Facial swelling may arise from a dental abscess, often with discharge of pus into the mouth, and should be regarded as serious, requiring referral to a doctor or dentist. Swelling in the soft tissue overlying an impacted or erupting third molar may be accompanied by difficulty in opening the mouth (trismus). The swelling is often buccal and potentially can compromise the airway – refer.

A haemorrhage following a tooth extraction can arise within a few hours or 2–3 days after extraction. It is necessary to take a detailed history to ascertain whether there is any underlying cause, e.g. recent aspirin consumption, patient taking anticoagulant drugs or a haemorrhagic disorder. Early post-extraction haemorrhages are often due to a tear in the overlying gum (mucoperiosteum) and hence require suturing. Haemorrhage occurring 2–3 days after extraction is invariably due to infection, and this requires appropriate treatment.

An unpleasant taste in the mouth and bad breath may accompany a dry socket or gingivitis. A foul halitosis is also often associated with ANUG. There are many causes of halitosis, some of which relate to gastrointestinal diseases, others to chronic infections of the sinuses

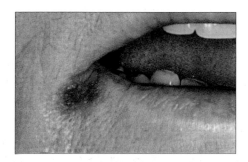

Figure 16.8 Angular cheilitis. (Reproduced with permission from the Newcastle Dental School.)

Table 16.2 Drugs commonly implicated as causing disturbances of taste

Aspirin	Imipramine
Carbimazole	Lithium carbonate
Chlorhexidine	Lincomycin
Clofibrate	Levodopa
Ethambutol	Metformin
Griseofulvin	Metronidazole
Gold salts	Penicillamine

or tonsils. Taste disturbances may also be associated with a dry mouth. Some drugs cause taste disturbances (Table 16.2).

Onset and trigger factors

The pain of toothache and that associated with dentine sensitivity resulting from gingival recession is invariably exacerbated by hot, cold or sweet stimuli. Sensitivity to hot and cold stimuli can also arise in restored (filled) teeth. The latter may be due to a leaky (defective) filling that is poorly adapted to the tooth, or to a lack of an insulating lining under the filling.

The pain of aphthous ulceration is stimulated by foods (especially spicy foods).

Pain arising 3–4 days after a tooth extraction may be due to a localised infection in the socket (dry socket or alveolar osteitis).

Gingival changes caused by drugs can start within 3 months of commencing therapy; the gums of the upper and lower anterior teeth seem to be most affected (see Figure 16.4).

Special cases

Children

Teething is a common disorder associated with the eruption of the primary dentition. It is characterised by a localised inflammation of the gum overlying the erupting tooth and is associated with an increase in daytime restlessness, finger sucking, gum rubbing and drooling, sometimes with a temporary loss of appetite. Localised eruption cysts can occur during teething, but these burst of their own accord. There is conflict as to whether teething produces any systemic disturbance. The child may be pyrexic, suffer from diarrhoea, and be prone to upper respiratory tract infections while teething. Whether there is a link between tooth eruption and these constitutional disturbances has not been established.

Management

Tooth problems

Temporary fillings

A lost filling or other restoration (e.g. a crown) requires dental treatment for replacement. Temporary filling kits are available. These contain zinc oxide and eugenol, which the patient mixes to a thick paste and places into the cavity. A weaker mixture can be used to re-cement crowns, purely for cosmetic purposes. However, the emphasis must be placed on the temporary nature of the restoration provided by these kits. They are no substitute for appropriate treatment from a dental practitioner, but are useful in an emergency. Extreme care should be taken by patients re-cementing crowns, as they are easily displaced during fitting and readily swallowed. They can also be lodged in the airway and cause respiratory obstruction.

Dentine sensitivity

A variety of proprietary toothpastes contain active agents to reduce dentine sensitivity. These agents work by blocking the permeability of dentine to stimuli such as heat, cold and sweetness. Desensitising agents include strontium chloride, formaldehyde, and stannous and sodium fluoride. The last two agents are also useful for preventing dental decay on exposed root surfaces. Toothpaste containing a desensitising agent should be used on a regular basis, giving relief that occurs gradually over a period of days. Excessive dentine sensitivity may be indicative of caries, and therefore the patient should be advised to seek dental treatment. Dentists and hygienists can also treat dentine sensitivity by applying varnishes that contain a high fluoride concentration to the exposed root surface.

Toothache

There is little effective treatment for toothache apart from extraction or a new filling and/or removal of the tooth pulp. Analgesics appear to afford little or no pain relief and the so-called toothache tinctures can cause burns to the gums.

Furthermore, there is little evidence to suggest that such solutions actually relieve toothache.

Some patients believe that an aspirin tablet placed against the gum of the offending tooth will provide pain relief. However, this will cause an aspirin burn on the oral mucosa and the patient should be warned accordingly. As with most tooth disorders the patient should be encouraged to seek dental treatment.

Dental abscesses require drainage and, if necessary, appropriate antibiotic therapy. If there is a discharge of pus the patient should be advised to use a hot saline mouthwash (e.g. one teaspoonful of salt in a cupful of water) to encourage further drainage. Severe infections should be referred to the Accident and Emergency department of a hospital.

Pericoronitis likewise often requires antibiotic therapy and subsequent removal of the impacted tooth. NICE guidelines require at least one acute episode of infection before an impacted third molar can be removed. Hot saline mouthwashes are of some value in reducing swelling, and simple over-the-counter (OTC) analgesics may afford some degree of pain relief.

Teething

There are many proprietary OTC teething gels available. Their active ingredient is usually a local anaesthetic agent (often lidocaine hydrochloride) or an anti-inflammatory drug such as choline salicylate. Although both types of product are claimed to reduce the local symptoms of teething, there is little clinical evidence to substantiate their use. Teething is often accompanied by pyrexia, and sugar-free paracetamol elixir should be recommended.

If teething is accompanied by diarrhoea, the child must be encouraged to take plenty of fluids.

Post-extraction conditions

Some post-extraction haemorrhages respond to simple pressure, achieved by the patient biting on to a clean gauze pad. If this does not arrest the haemorrhage the patient should be referred back to the dental practitioner or to an Accident and Emergency department, because the socket will need packing and suturing.

Dry socket (alveolar osteitis) responds to local irrigation and the application of a proprietary dressing. Examples include bismuth iodoform paste, Whitehead's varnish impregnated into ribbon gauze, or a proprietary preparation containing butyl paraminobenzoate (a topical anaesthetic), iodoform (an antiseptic) and eugenol, which provides further pain relief. Such local medicaments can only be applied by a dental practitioner. Occasionally the patient may require a systemic antibiotic. There is little evidence that OTC painkillers are of any value in this condition.

Periodontal disorders

Periodontal disease is caused by the accumulation of bacterial plaque at the margin between tooth and gum and in between teeth. Most plaque can be removed mechanically using an appropriate tooth-brushing technique, interproximal cleaning aids and dental floss. However, many patients lack the motivation and dexterity to obtain zero or low plaque levels. Regular use of dental floss is particularly challenging in the vast majority of patients. It is against this background that there has been a considerable expansion in the development of agents to control plaque and periodontal disease.

Gingivitis is the early stage of periodontal disease and results from poor oral hygiene. Poor plaque control may have caused the problem, and this needs to be rectified. However, because the gums are inflamed and bleed readily (see Figure 16.2), patients may be reluctant to clean their teeth thoroughly, especially with a new toothbrush. For these patients, a plaque-inhibitory agent (usually an antiseptic) may be of benefit. Many commercial plaque-inhibitory agents are available either as a mouthwash or incorporated into toothpaste. Of the mouthwashes, chlorhexidine and those containing phenolic mixtures appear to be the most efficacious. These agents will only destroy or inhibit the formation of supragingival plaque, and should be used in conjunction with mechanical plaque removal. There is now convincing evidence that when antiseptic mouthwashes are used as adjuncts to tooth-brushing and flossing there is a significant reduction in plaque scores and gingival inflammation (gingivitis). Mouthwashes that contain chlorhexidine do stain the teeth, however, and many patients find the taste unacceptable. Mouthwashes containing either phenolic compounds or essential oils do not have this unwanted effect and hence may be more appropriate for long-term use.

There are a variety of commercially available pre-brushing rinses that facilitate plaque removal by mechanical means. However, there is little evidence to support the efficacy of these agents in reducing gingival inflammation, and their regular use will not resolve bleeding and inflamed gums.

More advanced periodontal disease is characterised by movement of the teeth and an increased propensity to abscess formation. This condition requires specialised dental treatment and patients should be referred accordingly. Mouthwashes will not have a significant effect on advanced periodontal disease, but they will help to control plaque, which is an important requisite for successful treatment.

It is helpful if pharmacists stock a full range of oral hygiene aids to enable patients to optimise their plaque control efforts.

Electric toothbrushes are of value where there is a problem handling a conventional toothbrush, for example in patients with rheumatoid arthritis or other musculoskeletal disorders. They do seem to be more useful at reaching those parts that are difficult to access with an ordinary brush. Interproximal cleaning aids, e.g. brushes, wood sticks and various types of floss, are also of value.

It is thought that anaerobic bacteria play a significant role in the pathogenesis of ANUG. Most cases require referral for antimicrobial therapy, and metronidazole is the drug of choice. Early and mild cases of ANUG may respond to an oxygen-releasing mouthwash (e.g. sodium perborate).

Pharmacists should be aware of drugs that cause gingival overgrowth, if only to reassure the patient. Excessive gingival overgrowth is treated by surgical means, but in many patients the recurrence rate is high. If an alternative medication exists it may be worth contacting the patient's GP to consider such a change.

This policy may be particularly relevant for those patients who undergo repeated surgical procedures to correct their gingival overgrowth.

Disease of the oral mucosa

Dry mouth in the dentate patient will cause an increased susceptibility to dental caries. Fluoride mouthwashes will reduce this problem and these may be recommended. Salivary substitutes will certainly – albeit temporarily – reduce some of the oral discomfort associated with xerostomia. Preparations that are currently available are based on mucin, methylcellulose or carboxymethylcellulose. Various proprietary brands are available as aerosol sprays or pastilles. Dentate patients suffering from xerostomia may also obtain some relief by chewing sugar-free gum.

For the edentulous patient, xerostomia poses the additional problem of poor denture retention. In such cases a denture fixative will be helpful. Salivary substitutes are also useful for these patients, together with lemon and glycerine pastilles or mouthwashes. These pastilles are unsuitable for dentate patients as the low pH value will increase the risk of dental caries. Patients with xerostomia are more prone to candidal infections, which should be treated with an appropriate antifungal agent (see below).

All patients with a history of recurrent aphthous ulceration require a full blood screening. The ulceration may be due to deficiencies in iron, vitamin B_{12} or folate. Symptomatic relief can be obtained with chlorhexidine mouthrinses (0.2 per cent w/v) or topical corticosteroids. Chlorhexidine reduces the incidence of secondary infection, which occurs shortly after the ulcer has formed. Topical corticosteroids in the form of pellets (hydrocortisone) and dental paste (triamcinolone) are available OTC. A range of topical preparations exist for the management of aphthous ulceration. Some contain a salicylate, others a topical anaesthetic. There is little evidence to suggest that either is of value in reducing either the soreness arising from aphthous ulcers or in promoting healing. The major problem with all topical medicaments is compliance.

Patients will find it difficult to apply the preparations, and there is the obvious problem of retention and displacement that arises with eating and talking. Some patients experience a burning sensation in their oral mucosa just prior to the outbreak of an ulcer. In these situations the local application of a corticosteroid can abort the outbreak.

Lip conditions

Aciclovir is the treatment of choice for herpetic infections. For primary herpetic gingivostomatitis referral for oral aciclovir is necessary. Herpes labialis (cold sores) should be treated with aciclovir cream 5 per cent, applied four to five times a day starting at the tingling phase, i.e. as early as possible. If sunlight is a causative factor in herpes labialis the patient should be prescribed a sunblock.

Treatment of cheilitis is often unsatisfactory and is dependent on the underlying cause. A lip salve will prevent further drying of the lips, and this should be applied regularly. If the cheilitis is thought to be due to a hypersensitivity reaction, then a topical antihistamine cream may help to reduce symptoms.

Mouth disorders

The aetiology of glossitis and burning mouth syndrome is often multifactorial. The condition can be associated with vitamin B complex deficiency, hypersensitivity to denture materials, haematological deficiency, diabetes mellitus, reduced salivary function or psychological factors. Vitamin B therapy may be of some value, together with the use of salivary substitutes. It is obvious that these patients need a thorough appraisal to ascertain the cause of their symptoms.

Lichen planus requires treatment with topical corticosteroids (see aphthous ulceration) and severe cases may require systemic corticosteroids. If the lesions involve the gingival tissues this will impede mechanical plaque removal. Regular use of a plaque-inhibitory agent such as chlorhexidine or a mouthwash containing essential oils will help to alleviate this problem.

Candidiasis is the most frequent fungal infection affecting the oral mucosa. If the patient is dentate an antifungal oral gel may be tried. Severe candidal infections require systemic antifungal agents. In edentulous patients the fungal infection is often confined to the fitting area of the denture. For these patients, the denture should be thoroughly cleaned with a 1 per cent sodium hypochlorite solution at night and miconazole gel applied to the fitting surface of the denture four times a day.

Angular cheilitis (see Figure 16.8) is often caused by both *Candida* and *Staphylococcus aureus*. Miconazole gel is the treatment of choice for this condition since it possesses both antimycotic and antibacterial properties.

There is no treatment of black hairy tongue apart from reassurance. The condition will usually resolve on cessation of any causative drugs. Brushing the tongue with a toothbrush may help to disperse the pigment-producing bacteria and reduce the length of the filiform papillae.

Staining and discoloration of the teeth

There are many causes for staining or discoloration of the teeth, ranging from rare genetic defects in tooth formation, dental caries, excessive fluoride intake (fluorosis) and dietary factors. Simple extrinsic staining arising from smoking, excessive coffee intake or chewing betel nut can be removed in part by short-term use of an abrasive toothpaste. Resistant stains need professional cleaning.

Defects in the tooth surface will require repair and coverage with a veneer. Similarly, tetracycline staining of the teeth can be covered using thin porcelain veneers. Chlorhexidine mouthwashes stain the teeth, and the staining potential is enhanced by foods and beverages rich in tannins. Because of this unwanted effect the use of chlorhexide should be limited to just a few weeks.

Prevention of dental caries

Over the past 20 years there has been a significant decline in the prevalence of dental caries.

Fluoride has been mainly responsible for this, through either the water supply or its incorporation into toothpastes. In spite of these measures, however, there is still a need for further action to maintain the decline in dental caries.

Dietary advice is paramount in any caries prevention programme. Particular attention should focus on the intake of refined carbohydrates and snacking between meals. Confectionery eaten between meals causes a significant drop in the pH of the oral environment, rendering the teeth more prone to acid attack. Chewing gum stimulates salivary flow, which buffers the oral environment to this acid attack and helps promote remineralisation of the tooth surface.

Fissure sealants applied professionally do reduce the incidence of dental caries on the occlusal (biting) surface of posterior teeth. However, such sealants should not be an excuse for overindulgence in confectionery or the avoidance of regular tooth-brushing. It is important for the maintenance of oral health that these measures are attended to.

Bacterial plaque is the main aetiological agent in dental caries. Regular tooth-brushing (at least twice daily) will remove most plaque deposits and hence reduce the bacterial challenge on the tooth surfaces.

SUMMARY OF ORAL AND DENTAL DISORDERS

Lost filling or other restoration
Fillings and other restorations can be lost following fracture of a tooth cusp secondary to recurrent dental caries or, in the case of a crown or a bridge, fracture of the dental cement. Eating sticky foods such as toffee can readily displace a restoration – **refer.**

Sensitivity of the teeth
Sensitivity arises as a result of either gingival recession or periodontal disease. The exposed root surface is sensitive to hot, cold or sweet stimuli, which produce pain, often short and sharp in nature. Dentine sensitivity responds to toothpastes that contain active agents such as sodium fluoride, strontium chloride or formaldehyde. Intractable cases may require a permanent restoration.

Teething
Soreness of the gums often accompanies the eruption of the primary dentition. Local application of gels containing lidocaine or choline salicylate may afford relief until the tooth erupts through the mucosa. Teething is often associated with pyrexia, for which paracetamol elixir is recommended.

Dental abscess
Dental abscesses often arise from a necrotic dental pulp. They can present as a localised swelling associated with the tooth, or with marked facial swelling. The latter requires urgent treatment with antibiotics and drainage – **refer.**

→

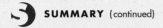

SUMMARY (continued)

Pericoronitis

Pericoronitis is an infection associated with the eruption of third molars (wisdom teeth). It may present initially as a localised soreness over the erupting tooth, but can progress to cause severe facial swelling and restriction in mouth opening (trismus). Antimicrobials are the treatment of choice, followed by extraction of the third molar. Hot saline mouthwashes may provide some temporary relief in mild cases – **refer.**

Toothache

Toothache (pulpitis) can present as severe pain, often throbbing in nature. The pain is exacerbated by hot and cold stimuli, and may be accompanied by abscess formation. Analgesics afford little or no relief – **refer.**

Post-extraction haemorrhage

Most post-extraction haemorrhages are caused by a tear in the gingival tissues. Some can be arrested by biting on a gauze pad. If this fails the socket needs to be packed and sutured – **refer.** It is important to check that the patient has no bleeding disorders and is not taking drugs that interfere with haemostasis.

Dry socket

Dry socket (alveolar osteitis) is a localised infection arising in the tooth socket some 2–4 days after tooth extraction. The pain is localised, continuous, and can radiate along the jaw. Treatment involves debridement of the socket, followed by the insertion of a local dressing. Antibiotics may be required in severe cases – **refer.**

Periodontal disorders

Periodontal diseases are caused by bacterial plaque. Gingivitis is the early manifestation of periodontal disease and is characterised by bleeding, sore gums (see Figure 16.2), and often bad breath. Treatment is aimed at improving oral hygiene with particular attention to tooth-brushing and interproximal cleaning. Plaque-inhibitory agents have a significant effect on bacterial plaque and help to resolve the inflammatory changes in the gingival tissues.

More advanced periodontal disease (periodontitis) is characterised by loss of the supporting dental structures (the periodontium) and the resorption of alveolar bone. The condition is chronic. Smoking is now recognised as a significant risk factor for periodontitis and also affects the outcome of treatment. Pharmacists can offer advice on smoking cessation. Periodontal disease can result in gingival recession, movement and spacing of the teeth, and an increase in tooth mobility. Local abscess formation can occur. Plaque-control measures are essential for the successful management of periodontitis, but such measures do not remove plaque from beneath the gingival margins – **refer.**

Acute necrotising ulcerative gingivitis

This is a condition of uncertain aetiology characterised by soreness and local ulceration of the gingival tissues. It is accompanied by a foul smell and may be generalised or localised to a few teeth. Poor oral hygiene, smoking and general debilitating illness (especially HIV infection) predispose patients to this infection. Mild cases may respond to a mouthwash containing an oxygen-releasing agent. More established cases require antimicrobial therapy – **refer.**

(continued overleaf)

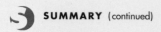

SUMMARY (continued)

Gingival overgrowth

This is an unwanted effect associated with phenytoin, ciclosporin and some calcium antagonists. Gingival overgrowth can be severe, disfiguring, and interfere with both speech and eating (see Figure 16.4). Gingival changes also impede mechanical plaque removal, which exacerbates the condition. Drug-induced gingival overgrowth is treated by surgery, but the recurrence rate is high. Alternative medication (if available) may be appropriate for those patients who experience recurrence of this unwanted effect. In such cases, **refer.**

Dry mouth

The causes of dry mouth (xerostomia) are many and varied, e.g. following radiotherapy to the head and neck, secondary to Sjögren's syndrome and certain drugs. The consequences include soreness of the oral mucosa, lips and tongue, difficulty in eating and speech, and an increased propensity to oral infections (especially candidiasis) and caries. Artificial salivas, sugar-free chewing gum and, for edentulous patients, lemon and glycerine pastilles are useful.

Aphthous ulceration

Recurrent ulceration of the oral mucosa is a common condition causing localised soreness and pain (see Figure 16.5). Patients require thorough investigation to elucidate and treat any underlying cause. The ulcers occur in crops, and in some patients their outbreak is preceded by a tingling/burning sensation in the oral mucosa. Local antiseptics such as chlorhexidine reduce the incidence and severity of secondary infection and promote healing. Topical corticosteroids are the treatment of choice; their efficacy is related to use as early as possible in the course of the ulceration. There are problems with delivering any topical medication to the mouth, as active ingredients are washed away by saliva. If severe or recurrent, **refer.**

Herpetic infections

Acute herpetic gingivostomatitis (AHGS) and herpes labialis are the two principal oral herpetic infections. AHGS is more likely to occur in children and is sometimes confused with teething. The condition is very painful and is characterised by vesicles on the tongue, gingiva and hard palate. These burst to leave ulcers, which readily become secondarily infected. The infection is often accompanied by pyrexia and lymphadenopathy. Patients will complain of marked pain and soreness of the mouth that is exacerbated by eating and swallowing – **refer.**

Cold sores are a recurrent form of herpetic infection that break out on the borders of the lips. A vesicle may form, which bursts to leave a small raw area. Aciclovir cream is the treatment of choice.

Glossitis and burning mouth

These two conditions often occur together and are difficult to treat. Patients need thorough investigation to identify any predisposing cause – **refer.**

Lichen planus

Lichen planus is a condition of unknown aetiology that is characterised by bouts of disease activity followed by periods of quiescence. Erosive, ulcerated lesions occur, usually on the gingival tissues and buccal mucosa (see Figure 16.6). Treatment involves topical and occasional systemic corticosteroids – **refer.**

→

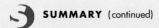

SUMMARY (continued)

Candidal infections
Candidal infections (see Figure 16.7) cause soreness of the mouth and occur more frequently at the extremes of age. They are particularly common in denture wearers. Treatment is with a topical antifungal gel in the first instance, and this can also be applied to the fitting surface of the denture.

WHEN TO REFER (TO EITHER A DOCTOR OR A DENTIST)
ORAL AND DENTAL DISORDERS

Teeth and gums
- Continuous pain that does not improve
- Swelling of the gums
- Sharp pain of short duration, aggravated by hot or cold stimuli, that does not respond to treatment with a desensitising toothpaste
- Lost filling
- Soreness and pain over impacted third molars (wisdom teeth) in a young adult
- Post-extraction pain
- Bleeding or painful gums
- Gum recession, together with movement of the teeth within the socket

Oral mucosa and lips
- Persistently inflamed, sore or painful tongue
- White patches on the buccal mucosa or tongue
- Mouth ulcers that do not respond to OTC local steroid treatment
- Dry mouth

Other
- Facial swelling
- Trismus (limited mouth opening)
- Haemorrhage from a tooth socket
- Severe halitosis
- Taste disturbance
- Inflammation of the tongue
- Hairy black tongue

CASE STUDIES

Case 1

A young woman, well known to her pharmacist, calls early one morning.

Her child of 6 months has been teething again and they have both had a sleepless night. She asks for a further supply of the teething medicine she had found so successful before.

The pharmacist should evaluate any signs or symptoms.

The pharmacist commiserates and notices that both mother and child seem more distressed and agitated than expected.

Coming round the counter, the pharmacist finds the child to be hot, with sores on the edge of her mouth. Closer inspection reveals her to be dribbling profusely and her gums are fiery red.

It seems possible that the child has something more than simple symptoms of teething, and a stomatitis, possibly herpetic, could be causing the distress. The pharmacist explains that on this occasion the doctor should see the child, adding that there is nothing very serious and that the doctor might well not prescribe for the condition.

The pharmacist should remind himself that occasionally people need encouragement even to ask for advice. Most problems are minor, although vigilance is always necessary for the rare occurrence of something unusual.

In this case, the doctor concurred with the diagnosis, advised fluids, rest and paracetamol, and saw the child again 3 days later, when she was already recovering.

Case 2

A young man asks for a large pack of paracetamol, unless the pharmacist can recommend anything stronger. He is obviously in considerable pain, holding one side of his face and having difficulty speaking. There is a noticeable swelling and he has felt feverish. He has taken almost 20 paracetamol in the last 36 hours.

The pharmacist is reluctant to supply either a further large quantity of paracetamol or a combination analgesic, and advises the man to seek an urgent dental opinion. The young man is hesitant, put off by the anticipated cost and the fact that he is very overdue for a check-up.

The pharmacist explains that he probably has a dental infection, and if not treated promptly it might progress to an abscess and require draining, as well as threatening his teeth.

The advice is taken and the man returns the following morning with a prescription for amoxicillin. An old filling has been removed, the pressure relieved, and the pain is subsiding. In this case the man had probably feared that the consequences were going to be worse than they actually proved to be. His request for symptomatic treatment was a tactic to avoid what he perceived to be an unpleasant experience at the dental surgery. In this case his symptoms would not be self-remitting and the advice to seek further expert assistance was sound.

Case 3

A woman in her mid-20s asks the pharmacist to recommend something for her sore mouth. She has been advised she could have cold sores, and is embarrassed to think she might pass them on to other people.

On closer questioning it is found that she has no sores around her lips, but instead they take the form of ulcers on her tongue and the floor of her mouth, and the diagnosis is aphthous ulceration.

The pharmacist is happy to make a recommendation for a topical steroid formulation.

The woman states that this condition often occurs premenstrually and can be predicted – 'Like so many things around that time,' she adds.

→

CASE STUDIES (continued)

The pharmacist is prompted to ask about her headaches, fluid retention and heavy periods as well.

The pattern thus emerged of a range of hormonally related problems. Medication was recommended for her mouth ulcers, as her next period was imminent, and a consultation with her GP was recommended to review the broader symptoms.

This patient was amused to think a change of her contraceptive pill might help mouth ulcers: the pharmacist reflects on how often one seemingly minor problem is part of a distant but more significant condition.

Part B

Preventative self-care

17

Smoking cessation

Since the 1970s smoking rates in the UK have declined because of the association between cigarette smoking and serious illness. Nevertheless, there are still large numbers of adults who smoke, and the proportion of young people doing so has increased. In 1998 there were 13 million adult smokers in the UK. In England, smoking prevalence dropped from 28% in 1998 to 26% in 2002 according to the General Household Survey. Cigarette smoking causes over 100 000 deaths per year in the UK. It causes 80% of the deaths due to lung cancer, and also causes respiratory and heart disease.

Apart from the clinical consequences of smoking there are economic implications too. Over 34 million working days are lost per year in England and Wales due to smoking-related illness. The latter costs the National Health Service about £2 billion per annum.

The health benefits of quitting smoking increase with time (Figure 17.1). The quality of life increases and health improves.

Cigarette smoking leads to an addiction to nicotine. Nicotine gives a feeling of pleasure, and withdrawal or attempts to withdraw from the habit result in unpleasant symptoms, including

20 minutes	Blood pressure and pulse return to normal
8 hours	Oxygen concentration in the blood increases to normal Nicotine and carbon monoxide concentrations in the blood are reduced by 50 per cent
24 hours	Carbon monoxide has been eliminated from the body Lungs begin to clear mucus and debris Risk of myocardial infarction decreases
48 hours	Nicotine has been eliminated from the body Sense of taste and smell improve
72 hours	Breathing is easier Bronchi begin to relax Energy levels begin to increase
2–12 weeks	Circulation improves, making physical activity easier
3–9 months	Lung function has increased by 10 per cent Cilia in airways regrow Coughing, shortness of breath and wheeziness improve
5 years	Risk of myocardial infarction falls to half that of a smoker Risk of cancer of the mouth, throat and oesophagus is half that of a smoker
10 years	Risk of lung cancer is half that of a smoker
15 years	Risk of myocardial infarction falls to the same as someone who has never smoked

Figure 17.1 A timetable of the benefits of smoking cessation.

anxiety, irritability, lack of concentration and low mood. Smokers who have attempted to give up smoking find that there are also other unwanted sequelae, such as an increase in appetite and weight gain. There is therefore a problem in motivating people to give up smoking.

Passive smoking

For many years the problems associated with cigarette smoking were confined to those that affected smokers themselves, i.e. active smokers. In more recent times the effects of smoking on non-smokers who share the same environment as smokers have been elucidated. For example, passive smoking increases the risk of coronary heart disease in non-smokers by as much as 30 per cent. Mortality is increased by 15 per cent in 'never smokers' who live in the same household as a smoker. Smoking harms the unborn child and increases the risk of reduced fetal growth, premature birth, miscarriage and perinatal death.

Smoke-free policies in public places reduce the health hazard caused by exposure to cigarette smoke. Several countries have adopted a policy of smoke-free zones in places such as restaurants and bars.

Who benefits from stopping smoking?

From the above it is obvious that health benefits from stopping smoking accrue to both those who smoke and those who do not. Many non-smokers, i.e. passive smokers, cannot control and do not have the freedom of choice to alter their environment. This is especially true of children and those as yet unborn.

Smoking-related diseases cause much absenteeism from work, and the economic implications for industry, services and the country in general are enormous.

Interventions designed to stop smoking are very cost-effective – the National Institute of Clinical Excellence (NICE) estimated a cost of £1,000–2,400 per life saved for an intervention that consisted of nicotine replacement therapy combined with supporting services.

Why is smoking bad for you?

The association of cigarette smoking with chronic respiratory and cardiovascular disease has already been referred to.

There are financial reasons why patients will benefit if they quit smoking. In the current climate, 20 cigarettes per day can cost over £1,500 per annum (equivalent to over £50,000 in a lifetime). This latter figure puts into perspective the relatively low cost of a course of nicotine replacement therapy over 10 or 12 weeks. Besides being a health hazard to smokers themselves, cigarette smoke is harmful to non-smokers. Smoking may be regarded therefore as an antisocial behaviour.

Cigarette smoke contains over 4000 chemicals, including carbon monoxide, hydrogen cyanide and others (Box 17.1). At a personal level, an individual can expect to reduce his life by 11 minutes every time he smokes a cigarette.

Box 17.1 Some of the chemicals in tobacco smoke
Acetone
Ammonia
Arsenic
Benzene
Cadmium
Carbon monoxide
Cyanide
Formaldehyde
Shellac
Tar

Why do people smoke?

Young people experiment with cigarettes for various reasons, including pure curiosity, as a symbolic act of rebellion against advice given by adults, or in the belief that smoking is a ritual that gives them recognition as an adult. Girls in particular may start smoking to control their weight, appreciating the suppression of appetite that smoking brings.

Pressures and stimulants in the environment cause people to smoke cigarettes. For example, in households where the parents smoke it is more likely that the children will themselves become smokers. Peer pressure will have an influence. There are more smokers in deprived areas, and in young people it has been postulated that feelings of low self-esteem and poor recognition of achievement in schools and in society provide an incentive for rebellious behaviour.

Social factors that may be instrumental in taking up the habit then give way to the pharmacological effect of nicotine, and addiction follows shortly afterwards.

Pharmacology of nicotine

It is thought that nicotine stimulates dopaminergic pathways in the brain, which results in the stimulation of the mesolimbic system that gives rise to feelings of pleasure.

The absorption of smoke from the lungs is rapid and gives rise to high concentrations of nicotine in the brain within a few seconds.

Nicotine has a terminal half-life of 2 hours, and thus withdrawal effects are seen within a short time. Withdrawal is evidenced by a change of mood and performance which is reduced or eliminated by the next cigarette.

Other effects of nicotine withdrawal are irritability, increased appetite, poor concentration and insomnia. These effects occur fairly rapidly and are most pronounced during the first week after withdrawal.

Public perceptions and myths

The following are some popular beliefs among the general public.

'Cutting down the number of cigarettes smoked will reduce harm.'

There is no evidence that this is true, but it is a controversial area. The issue is complicated by the fact that many smokers who reduce the number of cigarettes they smoke per day tend to compensate by taking more puffs per cigarette and inhaling more deeply.

'Switching to low-tar cigarettes reduces harm.'

This is largely untrue because again smokers tend to change their method of smoking, as low-tar cigarettes deliver less nicotine. Smokers therefore take deeper puffs, or occlude the ventilation holes in the cigarette filters with their fingers or lips. These holes are designed to prevent or reduce the intake of smoke. This change in smoking method therefore results in little or no change in the actual intake of nicotine and tar.

'Switching to cigars or pipes reduces harm.'

This is a controversial belief, but many authorities state that former cigarette smokers will still inhale the smoke and therefore do not gain any perceived benefit.

'Smokeless tobacco is better than smoking.'

Other means of using tobacco may reduce the health risks of smoking. However, in India, chewing tobacco is associated with an increased risk of oral cancer.

Nicotine replacement therapy

In the UK, nicotine replacement therapy (NRT) products may be purchased over the counter as well as obtained on prescription, or they may be obtained through specialist smoking cessation clinics funded by the NHS. It should be used within a support framework of advisors who can offer behavioural support.

NRT delivers nicotine to the individual by a different route or method, such that equivalent doses do not attain the same rapid high blood concentrations that occur when smoke is inhaled. Thus a lower blood concentration initially, followed by a tapering of the dose over 10–12 weeks, can reduce or totally eliminate the effects of withdrawal and the development of a withdrawal syndrome.

The different types of product available are described briefly below.

- NRT products were formerly licensed in the UK for short-term use, but can now be used for up to 9 months to allow resistant smokers to reduce the amount smoked before undertaking the final quit attempt.

- NRT can be used safely in smokers who have cardiovascular disease (except for a short period after a myocardial infarct), and relatively safely in pregnancy.
- All forms of NRT have an equal chance of success. The actual type of product used depends on the level of dependence and the personal preference of the user.

Transdermal patches

The transdermal patch is popular because of its convenience. It is simple and discreet and requires the least effort of all the formulations available. The patch allows continuous dosing of nicotine and is normally changed once daily. Its onset of action is within about 2 hours and will continue as long as the patch is left in contact with the skin. The patch may be left on for 24 hours, or may be removed at bedtime and a new one applied the following day. Patches left on for 24 hours can cause sleep disturbance in some patients. Such patients would prefer to remove the patch before retiring.

The 24-hour patch is useful for those who crave a cigarette immediately upon waking. The patches usually come in three strengths and are designed to follow a step-down programme. The recommended duration of treatment is 10–12 weeks.

Nicotine gum

Nicotine gum is suitable for chewing when necessary to control the craving to smoke. The gum should be chewed slowly (to release nicotine), and then when the taste changes it should be rested between the cheek and gums to allow the nicotine to be absorbed. It is then chewed again when the taste has faded. This is known as the 'chew–rest–chew' technique. This sequence should be carried out for 30 minutes. The onset of action is 10 minutes, and for optimal effect the average usage would be about 15 pieces of gum per day.

The gum is provided in two strengths, depending on the number of cigarettes smoked per day.

Nasal spray

The nasal spray may be used up to a maximum of twice per hour during a 16-hour period. This may be used for a period of 8 weeks and then reduced over the next 4 weeks to zero. Peak blood concentrations of nicotine are produced between 5 and 10 minutes after inhalation. The nasal spray may cause some local irritant effects, such as a sore throat, but these usually resolve within a few days.

Nicotine lozenges

Nicotine lozenges are provided in three strengths: 4 mg for those who smoke shortly after waking, 2 mg for those who wait more than 30 minutes after waking for their first cigarette, and 1 mg to be sucked every hour on the urge to smoke. The lozenge is sucked on a 'suck–rest–suck' regime, like that for gum. This is continued until the lozenge has dissolved.

Treatment can be continued for 3 months and then reduced, with a maximum period of treatment of 6 months. Maximum dosage should not exceed 15 lozenges per day.

No food or drink should be taken while the lozenge is in the mouth; some drinks may decrease the absorption of nicotine and are best avoided for 15 minutes before sucking a lozenge.

Nicotine sublingual tablets

These tablets are provided in a strength of 2 mg. They are allowed to dissolve under the tongue for about 30 minutes and one or two tablets per hour can be used as required. Use may be continued for up to 6 months, reducing the dosage after 12 weeks to one or two tablets per day.

The Inhalator

The Inhalator or inhaler consists of a mouthpiece and a holder containing a replaceable nicotine cartridge. It provides a source of nicotine in a format that simulates the behavioural habit of the hand-to-mouth action of the smoker. Nicotine is absorbed through the buccal lining and the onset of action is 15 minutes. Up to 12 cartridges per day may be used for 8 weeks before reducing to zero over the last 4 weeks of treatment.

A smoking cessation service

In the UK community pharmacists can set up a smoking cessation service as part of their contribution to public health. Nicotine replacement products can be provided over the counter or via a patient group direction (PGD), whereby local arrangements allow government funding to pay for the cost of the products. Pharmacists should be trained as 'intermediate advisers' along with other health professionals such as nurses.

Requirements for the service:

- Time
- A designated consultation area suitable for a one-to-one interview
- Appropriate training

Approaching the smoker

Pharmacists should take the opportunity to raise the issue of smoking cessation in such a manner that the individual does not feel pressurised. The approach should be one of questioning the willingness of the smoker to give up, and offering them help to do so. The first milestone in the process may just be to achieve a state of mind where the smoker will at least consider quitting. This can be achieved by offering to work with the smoker and monitor their progress ('support' may be a wrong choice of words and appear patronising, whereas 'working together' may sound better).

If the pharmacist has not already done so, it is pertinent at this stage to discuss the risks and benefits of quitting smoking. If the individual does not accept the reasons for giving up then they will not stop.

The second milestone is to agree a timeframe and a date to stop. Some means of reinforcement may be helpful here. For example, the pharmacist could provide the smoker with a diary,

which might also contain a table of benefits for the smoker to refer to, and at this stage an action plan can be drawn up and summarised in the diary, with an outline of the time intervals for monitoring the number of cigarettes smoked during the treatment period.

The process should be taken one step at a time, both at this stage and later, when monitoring or reviewing progress. A timescale can be worked out for each step of the monitoring plan, which must be agreed by both parties and be realistic.

Assessment of the smoker's motivation

There is no doubt that the success of a smoking cessation programme depends largely on the individual's motivation to give up. Motivation varies with time, and smokers may not always be honest about their real feelings. Surveys indicate that about 70 per cent of smokers want to quit, and motivation can be judged by asking a number of questions:

- Has the individual made an attempt to stop smoking on a previous occasion?
- Do they want to stop smoking for good?
- Do they want to start the smoking cessation programme very soon?
- Would they like someone to work with them as an adviser during the treatment period?

However, even a high degree of motivation at this stage does not predict the success of the attempt. Success in quitting also depends on the degree of dependence on nicotine.

Dependence can be judged by the degree of difficulty a smoker has in refusing a cigarette at times when they would normally smoke, for example on awakening or on social occasions.

A commonly used measure of dependence is the Fagerstrom Test, which assists in predicting the outcome of an attempt to stop (Table 17.1). A high score (greater than 9) suggests a high level of dependence.

Starting the programme

The choice of products to be used in the cessation plan should be agreed and a start date suggested

Table 17.1 The Fagerstrom Test for nicotine dependence

Questions	Answers	Points
1. How soon after waking do you smoke your first cigarette?	a) Within 5 minutes b) 6–30 minutes c) 31–60 minutes d) After 60 minutes	a) 3 b) 2 c) 1 d) 0
2. Do you find it difficult to refrain from smoking in places where it is forbidden (e.g. cinemas, restaurants)?	a) Yes b) No	a) 1 b) 0
3. Which cigarette would you hate most to give up?	a) The first in the morning b) Any other	a) 1 b) 0
4. How many cigarettes per day do you smoke?	a) 31 or more b) 21–30 c) 11–20 d) 10 or fewer	a) 3 b) 2 c) 1 d) 0
5. Do you smoke more frequently during the first few hours after waking than during the rest of the day?	a) Yes b) No	a) 1 b) 0
6. Do you smoke if you are so ill that you are in bed most of the day?	a) Yes b) No	a) 1 b) 0

A score of 9 or above indicates high dependence
       4–8 indicates medium dependence
       3 or less indicates low dependence

within the next 2 weeks unless the plan is to reduce first, then quit later. At this stage the smoker should be reminded that it may be necessary to make some changes in lifestyle or habits, even temporarily, such as not attending social gatherings in places where others may be smoking. The next step is to agree follow-ups, and the pharmacist should stress the need to maintain the effort. It may not be appropriate to put negative thoughts into the individual's mind, but it should be remembered that relapse is not uncommon, and that although 4-week quit rates may be 50 per cent this can decline to less than 20 per cent over a longer period. Weekly support reviews for the first fortnight, followed by every 2 weeks, and then monthly, would be a suitable programme.

If patients do not attend for a follow-up interview they should be contacted by telephone and several attempts made before they are designated as 'lost to follow-up'.

Monitoring

At each follow-up patients can be monitored by, for instance, measuring their carbon monoxide output to validate any claims they make about quitting. The carbon monoxide reading should be fewer than 10 parts per million to indicate that they are not smoking. The basal level for a non-smoker will vary according to the location and pollution (e.g. by traffic) of the environment.

How successful is NRT treatment?

NRT doubles the cessation rates achieved by any other non-pharmacological method of intervention. Maximum effect is gained when it is part of a programme that includes behavioural support (Table 17.2).

Adverse effects

Besides the adverse effects of individual product formulations, smoking cessation may result in weight gain.

NRT is safer than smoking because there is no exposure to harmful smoke and the chemicals it contains. NRT can be used in those with cardiovascular disease, because although nicotine is a vasoconstrictor the lower levels of concentration produced by NRT, together with the lack of smoke, mean that patients should come to less harm than if they were smoking. If a patient has recently suffered a myocardial infarction or a stroke then it is advisable that they be offered advice about NRT by their doctor, if this has not already happened.

In pregnancy NRT is again safer than cigarettes, and 20 per cent of women who smoke in the UK continue to do so throughout pregnancy. Carbon monoxide binds to haemoglobin and reduces the availability of oxygen to the fetus. Smoking causes fetal growth retardation. However, concentrations of cotinine in the blood of pregnant women who are being treated with NRT are lower than those in pregnant women who smoke.

Patients may ask if they will become addicted to NRT and can be assured that this is extremely rare, because the blood concentrations of nicotine that occur with NRT are much lower than with cigarette smoking.

Bupropion

Bupropion is a prescription-only medicine in the UK. Without a support service its success rate in smoking cessation is about 20 per cent. Local arrangements can be made for non-medical health professionals such as pharmacists and nurses to supply bupropion through a patient group direction.

If the latter arrangement does not exist but a pharmacist feels that this drug may be the best option for a smoker, he or she may refer the individual to their GP, perhaps with a note to verify that there are no contraindications for this individual.

Adverse effects include weight gain and rarely seizures, and therefore patients with a low threshold for seizures, such as those with diabetes, eating disorders, head trauma or alcohol misuse, should not be treated with this drug. Also, patients who are concurrently taking theophylline, antipsychotic drugs, antidepressants or steroids should not take bupropion. Pregnancy and breastfeeding are also contraindications to its use.

Table 17.2 Outline of supporting service provided by a pharmacist

- Give support both during the time the smoker expresses an interest to give up as well as during the treatment period
- Give advice on the choice of method/formulation, in keeping with the patient's lifestyle
- Monitor progress using diary cards, regular follow-ups, telephone calls
- Provide feedback using carbon monoxide monitors
- Maintain motivation, e.g. calculate the financial savings of smoking cessation to the individual on a weekly basis and record in the diary card
- If a course of NRT fails, then encourage the individual to try again
- Encourage quitting with a friend to provide motivation and encouragement
- Plan ahead, especially in the initial stages, but take a practical day-to-day approach

Second opinion

Smoking is for most people the most important risk factor in respiratory and cardiac disease, and stopping is therefore the single most effective act of health promotion. GP surgeries have run smoking cessation clinics for many years, and these became very popular under the NHS Contract of 1990. Despite this, success rates have been variable, with a high degree of motivation and persistence required from both doctor and patient; the doctor should also avoid patronising the patient by simply stating the obvious, i.e. that smoking is dangerous.

Smoking cessation is now largely in the hands of practice nurses, who have more time, see patients more often, and incorporate advice and support into general health education. The use of nicotine replacement and bupropion is structured and monitored, and success appears to be improving.

Many doctors have felt the frustration of patients with smoking-related diseases who, perhaps right to the end of their lives, are unable to resist the powerful addiction of nicotine. The pharmacology of smoking cessation has improved, as has the organisation of services and the associated communication skills. No one initiative will reduce the mortality attributed to smoking, but possibly for the first time there is a guarded feeling of optimism.

Bibliography

Britton J (ed) (2004). *ABC of Smoking*. Oxford: Blackwell.

PharmacyHealthLink (2003). *Improving local access to smoking cessation therapies by using Patient Group Directions*. www.rpsgb.org.uk/phshome.htm (accessed 9 March 2006).

 CASE STUDIES

Case 1

A teenage girl comes into the pharmacy for a follow-up after an initial supply of NRT skin patches was given to her a few weeks ago.

The pharmacist is aware that only 2 weeks' supply of patches was given, and that several weeks have elapsed since the last visit.

The pharmacist should enquire about general progress and her reasons for not reattending at an earlier date. It seems that there has been a lack of concordance and the girl has not kept her side of the agreement. This has been caused by her developing a rash on her arm where she applied the patches; her friends telling her that she is putting on weight; and a general lack of motivation to continue.

Lack of compliance because of the skin irritation can be overcome by either advising her to position the patches on a different site each day or suggesting that another product be used – either a different brand of patch that might have a different adhesive, or another route of administration, such as chewing gum.

→

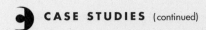 **CASE STUDIES** (continued)

Weight gain is a possible adverse effect of smoking cessation. Positive counselling about the benefits of giving up cigarettes is required, as well as the need for a sensible diet and exercise. The weight problem should be monitored, but the priority is to stop her smoking, and this is where attention should be focused for the time being.

The carbon monoxide monitor showed a slight improvement in the amount of gas in her breath, but some encouragement by the pharmacist was needed. This could be followed up by telephoning the girl every few days to ensure her compliance and to check her progress before the next follow-up.

Case 2

A man in his 40s has asked for a further supply of nicotine replacement therapy. He has purchased it before and tells the pharmacist he believes it to be helpful.

Is any further enquiry needed before supplying it?

Support is probably as important as medication. Any success should be encouraged, any failures understood. An appreciation of his achievements, even if limited, will assist.

Most people will respond positively to a sympathetic review of their situation, an understanding of the problems they have had, and a repeat of the benefits they have identified.

On questioning, the man is clearly still smoking and has only been able to reduce rather than to stop. Also, his last request for NRT was sufficiently recent to indicate that he is substantially overusing it.

To criticise is unlikely to be helpful, but honesty on both sides is also important, and the pharmacist should be sure to have an accurate history.

The addictive effect of nicotine should not be underestimated. NRT is always safer than smoking, and easier to stop with time.

There is a case here for continuing the NRT, at least in the short term. If it fails he should be counselled to abandon it, but if he has reduced his smoking he may be able to cease with firm encouragement and a realistic timescale.

Case 3

A woman attends the pharmacy in the company of her daughter with a repeat prescription for bupropion. She asks if the pharmacist can supply additional help for her daughter, as she also smokes. Her daughter is 17 years old.

Smoking cessation is rarely achieved without motivation. The girl's perceptions, pressures and motivation need to be identified, if necessary without her mother present. A discussion of the health risks may have little relevance at her age.

She tells the pharmacist that she smokes 'because she enjoys it', and that many of her friends smoke. She has made up her mind to smoke for about 10 years, when it will be socially acceptable, and then to give up. Her perception is that smoking is for the young, that older people look unattractive with a cigarette, and that she will place herself in no danger by following this strategy.

She is probably correct in thinking that giving up in her 20s is likely to reduce her risk of disease before it becomes a reality. The problem she will encounter is that of quitting when addicted, and the consequences if she fails.

Health education seems unlikely to succeed at this time in her life. A better approach might be to mention the effects of smoking on the values she holds dearest, such as her looks, by reminding her of its ageing effects on the skin.

18

Cardiovascular disease

Cardiovascular disease is the major cause of death in the United Kingdom, being responsible for over one-third of deaths. Cardiovascular disease comprises heart disease, stroke and circulatory disease, of which coronary heart disease (CHD) is the main form. The mortality rates for coronary heart disease in England have fallen by about 50 per cent in the last 25 years. The UK government has set a target to reduce death rates from myocardial infarction and stroke for under-75-year-olds by at least 40 per cent from the 1997 baseline by 2012.

The risk factors for cardiovascular disease that can be influenced are listed in Table 18.1.

There are some risk factors that cannot be altered, such as age, male gender, pre-existing cardiovascular disease, family history and ethnicity.

The reduction of modifiable risk factors in individuals who are at low to moderate risk of CHD should be undertaken as a holistic approach aimed at promoting 'healthy living'.

Table 18.1 Risk factors for cardiovascular disease

Modifiable risk factors	Non-modifiable risk factors
High blood cholesterol concentration	Age
Smoking	Gender
Obesity/overweight	Family history
Diet	South Asian ethnicity
Physical inactivity	
Diabetes	
Hypertension	
Alcohol intake	
Stress	

The use of statins

In the UK, the National Institute for Health and Clinical Excellence (NICE) has recommended that statins be used for the secondary prevention of cardiovascular disease and also for primary prevention in people with a 10-year risk of cardiovascular disease greater than 20 per cent (i.e. > a two in 10 chance of having an event in the next 10 years), equivalent to a 10-year risk of CHD greater than 15 per cent.

Over-the-counter (OTC) statins, such as simvastatin, are intended to improve the primary prevention of cardiovascular disease in people with a 10–15 per cent 10-year risk of CHD (this is equivalent to a 15–20 per cent 10-year risk of cardiovascular disease). It is important to remember that the thinking behind the use of statins in this way includes the evidence that blood lipids, including total cholesterol, are independent risk factors for CHD. That is, lowering total cholesterol will reduce the risk of CHD in any individual regardless of their risk profile. It could then be extrapolated that all adults would benefit from the use of a statin.

There are of course a number of flaws in this conclusion. Without measurements of blood cholesterol concentration the dose used in the OTC product is arbitrary, and the benefit gained may be considerably less than optimal. The use of long-term or even lifelong self-medication must be carefully considered and the risks weighed against the potential benefits, including compliance, cost, side effects and interactions. In attempting to lower risk we are considering communities before individuals. In any group taking statins, the majority will derive no benefit because they would have no cardiovascular event anyway if left untreated. Some will suffer such an event in any case, and for some this will be delayed or the risk removed. It is because we cannot individualise within the group that we rely on the perception of risk.

There is a cardinal rule that should not be forgotten when using statins, i.e. that they only modify one risk factor for cardiovascular disease – that of raised lipids. Other risk factors should not be forgotten, however, and the approach should be to modify all risk factors.

Pharmacology of statins

Statins inhibit an enzyme, 3-hydroxy-3-methyl-glutaryl coenzyme A (HMG-CoA) reductase, which catalyses the conversion of HMG-CoA in the biosynthetic pathway of cholesterol in the liver. This results in an increase in the number of low-density lipoprotein (LDL) receptors and thus lowers the levels of LDL cholesterol and increases high-density lipoprotein (HDL) cholesterol levels in the blood.

It is claimed that 10 mg of simvastatin daily reduces LDL cholesterol by about 25 per cent, and this equates to a fall of one-third in cardio-vascular events such as angina attacks and myocardial infarctions.

There may be other effects besides their choles-terol-modifying activity exerted by statins that contribute to the reduction in cardiovascular risk.

Modifiable risk factors for CHD

Smoking

The incidence of cardiovascular and coronary heart disease is about 50 per cent higher in smokers than in non-smokers. Passive smoking is said to increase the risk by about 25 per cent. Five years after cessation of smoking the risks of CHD are said to be equivalent to those of non-smokers (see Chapter 17, Smoking cessation).

Weight

Clinical trials have shown that a weight loss of 10 kg can reduce systolic blood pressure by 10 mmHg and diastolic blood pressure by 20 mmHg. Blood concentrations of HDL choles-terol are increased and those of LDL cholesterol reduced by weight loss, although the magnitude of this effect is sometimes quite small.

However, weight loss does reduce morbidity and mortality. One definition of the term 'over-weight' is a body mass index (BMI) of 25–30 kg/m², and the term 'obesity' refers to a BMI of more than 30 kg/m². BMI is the weight of an individual in kilograms divided by the square of his or her height in metres. The risk of morbid-ity increases as BMI increases. The risk is also greater in men with a waist greater than 102 cm (40 inches) and women with a waist greater than 88 cm (35 inches).

Overweight people are also at increased risk of developing an abnormal glucose tolerance, which may lead to type 2 diabetes.

Exercise

A lack of exercise is a risk factor for cardiovascu-lar disease, and it has been shown that increas-ing exercise is beneficial against CHD and stroke. The amount of exercise required is controversial, but it may be as little as 1 hour's walking per week to achieve measurable benefits. Ideally 30 minutes of moderate aerobic exercise on most days is the quoted norm. Exercise is bene-ficial in achieving weight loss, reducing blood pressure and reducing blood lipids, by small amounts.

Diet

A normal healthy diet should be low in fat and should be encouraged in everyone. The total amount of fat ingested should be low, and the total amount of saturated fat should be relatively low compared with unsaturated fats.

A healthy diet should also have a high content of fruit and vegetables (fibre) to help reduce fat absorption and promote gut transit. Oily fish con-tains omega-3 fatty acids, believed to be beneficial in reducing cardiovascular disease, and current recommendations are two portions of fish, such as mackerel, sardines or salmon, per week.

Olive oil contains monounsaturated fatty acids and is believed to be beneficial, being a component of the Mediterranean diet. Antioxidants, for example flavonoids, such as those occurring in red wine, are believed to have a beneficial effect on atherosclerotic plaques in arteries.

Changes in the diet will usually only produce a modest reduction in total blood cholesterol (of the order of 10 per cent), but components such as olive oil and antioxidants may have beneficial effects that are not directly related to cholesterol levels.

A moderate intake of alcohol is beneficial, but ingestion of more than 2–3 units per day is detrimental to health and causes increases in blood pressure, body weight and blood triglycerides levels, and an increased risk of CHD and liver disease.

Clinical trials have shown that reducing salt intake reduces blood pressure. Although these reductions will be small in the majority of people, a reduction of 5 mmHg can be critical for someone whose blood pressure lies around a critical threshold for treatment. The public should be educated that salt is present in many convenience and frozen foods, particularly soups, and reducing the intake of this kind of food may be easier than attempting to alter the habit of adding salt at the table.

Blood pressure

A raised systolic or diastolic blood pressure is a risk factor for cardiovascular disease. This risk increases with age, and treatment of a raised blood pressure, particularly in the elderly, can result in significant reductions in morbidity and mortality. Blood pressure can be reduced by manipulating the diet, taking exercise, reducing stress and stopping smoking.

Cholesterol

It has been shown that lowering blood cholesterol levels reduces the morbidity and mortality of cardiovascular disease, and this appears to be unrelated to the baseline or pretreatment level.

OTC statins are being marketed with the aim of reducing risk in individuals with a 10–15 per cent 10-year risk of CHD. This equates to a 1 in 10 or a 1 in 7 chance of having a cardiovascular event in the next 10 years. However, it should be noted that raised blood cholesterol levels alone do not increase the risk of cardiovascular disease in the majority of patients unless there are also other risk factors. It is very important to convey this message to the public. The national service framework target in the UK for total blood cholesterol is 5.0 mmol/litre, but this does not mean that every person who has a blood cholesterol above this level should be given treatment. The average total cholesterol in men in the UK is approximately 5.8 mmol/litre, and over 75 per cent of men will have a total cholesterol greater than 5.0 mmol/litre.

Again, it should be stressed that any attempts to lower blood cholesterol levels should be made as part of a lifestyle programme to reduce all risk factors for cardiovascular disease.

Non-modifiable risk factors

These are listed in Table 18.1 and are those that individuals cannot change.

Age

CHD increases with age in both men and women, becoming particularly significant in those over 55 years of age.

Gender

The risk of CHD increases in women after the menopause, when the protective effect of the female sex hormones declines. The average age of the menopause is 51 years. An earlier menopause is associated with a higher risk of CHD than for other women of the same age. Hormone replacement therapy is not protective against cardiovascular disease.

Family history

CHD tends to run in families, and families with a number of members affected by cardiovascular disease at an early age have a higher risk than others. The increased risk of an individual with a close family member who has had CHD is estimated to be one and a half times greater than an individual who has not.

South Asian family origin

People from the Indian subcontinent (India, Pakistan and Bangladesh) are at an increased risk of CHD, estimated to be about one and a half times that of an individual who is not from that part of the world.

Evaluation of the risk

The overall absolute risk of CHD is an important criterion when deciding how to make an intervention for an individual. The interaction of some of the risk factors is complex.

On average, statins reduce the risk of cardiovascular events by about one-third. Thus a person with a 20 per cent 10-year risk of CHD can expect to have the risk reduced to 14 per cent after using a statin. This is an absolute risk reduction of 6 per cent. If someone begins with a 10 per cent 10-year risk then an equivalent reduction in absolute risk would reduce the risk to 7 per cent.

OTC simvastatin

As has already been said, the reduction of blood cholesterol levels should be part of a programme aimed at reducing as many other risk factors for CHD as possible. Simvastatin 10 mg is claimed to reduce the risk of CHD by about one-third in people who have been taking it for more than 3 years.

Risk assessment

The following factors should be assessed:

- Age
- Gender
- Ethnicity
- Smoking history
- Family history of premature coronary disease
- Level of activity
- Diet and alcohol history
- Obesity
- History of diabetes
- Blood pressure
- Cholesterol measurement in the last 12 months
- Familial hypercholesterolaemia

Who is not at increased risk?

- Men under 45 years of age
- Men under 55 years without risk factors
- Women under 55 years
- Women over 55 years without risk factors

Who is at increased risk?

People with a 10–15 per cent 10-year risk (described as moderate) over 10 years will fit into the following categories. They are eligible for OTC statins.

- Men 55 years of age or over
- Men between the ages of 45 and 54, or postmenopausal women over 55 years with one of the following risk factors:
  - Family history of CHD (father or brother having had an MI or angina before the age of 55, or mother or sister before the age of 65 years)
  - Smoker – current or in the last 5 years
  - Overweight/obese – waist more than 102 cm (40 inches) for males; 88 cm (35 inches) for females, or a BMI greater than 25 kg/m^2
  - South Asian family origin

An OTC statin should not be sold to:

- Individuals who have cardiovascular disease
- Individuals who have diabetes
- Those who have a risk of CHD greater than 15 per cent over 10 years
- Men over 70 years or women over 55 with a family history of CHD plus one other risk factor
- Those with familial hyperlipidaemia
- Those with high blood pressure (>140/90), or any patient who is being treated for hypertension by their doctor

- Women who are pregnant
- Those with liver or kidney disease
- Those with hypothyroidism
- Those with a family history of muscle disorders
- Those with unexplained chest pain
- People who have a high alcohol intake
- People who drink grapefruit juice

It is imperative that pharmacists and GPs discuss the protocol to be used by the pharmacist, and ascertain whether the doctor will require to know which patients are being advised to take OTC statins.

An example of a simple questionnaire to aid pharmacists in collecting the appropriate data is shown in Figure 18.1.

Blood pressure measurement

Guidelines issued by the Royal Pharmaceutical Society of Great Britain make recommendations on the measurement of blood pressure by community pharmacists and should be followed wherever pharmacists offer this service. Of particular importance is the requirement to measure the blood pressure of an individual on three separate occasions (i.e. at three separate visits) when the initial reading appears to be raised above normal. As stated above, it is advisable that pharmacists and GPs discuss protocols and blood pressure measurement services, and the implications of referral by pharmacists to doctors.

1 ABOUT YOU...

Are you:
- Male and aged 45 to 54? ☐   Male and aged 55 to 70? ☐
- Female and aged 55 to 70? ☐
- If you are female, have you reached the menopause? Yes ☐ No ☐
If none of these applies to you, talk to the pharmacist before going further.

Do any of the following risk factors apply to you?
- Current smoker, or a smoker within the last five years   Yes ☐ No ☐
- A family history of early heart disease:
  – your father or brother had a heart attack or angina before the age of 55
  – your mother or sister had a heart attack or angina before the age of 65   Yes ☐ No ☐
  Angina is heart pain in the chest brought on by exercise or exertion.
- Overweight   Yes ☐ No ☐
  Your pharmacist can help you with this if you know your height, weight and waist measurement.

Height ☐ ft/in or m/cm   Weight ☐ stone/kg   Waist ☐ in/cm

- Family origin from South Asia*   Yes ☐ No ☐
  (for example, India, Pakistan, Bangladesh or Sri Lanka)
  Being of South Asian origin means your risk of heart disease is higher.

2 ABOUT YOUR MEDICAL HISTORY...

Has your doctor told you that you have or have had any of the following?
- **Diabetes**   Yes ☐ No ☐
- **Heart problems** (for example, heart attack or angina), a stroke or peripheral vascular disease (for example, poor blood flow to the legs with pain on walking)   Yes ☐ No ☐

- A condition called '**familial hypercholesterolaemia**'   Yes ☐ No ☐
  (FH), (a very high cholesterol level that runs in families)
- **High blood pressure** that your doctor has prescribed medicine for   Yes ☐ No ☐
  If you haven't had your blood pressure checked within the last six months, your pharmacist may be able to offer you a check.

Do you have any of these conditions?
- **Liver disease** or abnormal liver tests in the past
- Muscle problems that run in your family (for example, muscular dystrophies)
- An underactive thyroid gland
- Kidney problems   Yes ☐ No ☐
  If you are not sure about any of these, please ask the pharmacist.

- Have you recently had unexplained heart or chest pain brought on by exercise or exertion?   Yes ☐ No ☐

- Do you drink an average of more than four units of alcohol a day (if you are a man), or three units (if you are a woman)?   Yes ☐ No ☐
  1 unit is 1/2 pint of beer, one small glass of wine or one pub measure of spirits.

- Do you drink more than one litre of grapefruit juice a day?   Yes ☐ No ☐

- Have you been prescribed cholesterol-lowering medicine in the past?   Yes ☐ No ☐

- Are you taking medicine prescribed by your doctor?   Yes ☐ No ☐

  Please write down the name of any medicines you are taking. If you are unsure of the names, please ask the pharmacist.
  ....

Figure 18.1   Example of a questionnaire to assess risk factors for OTC simvastatin. (This consumer questionnaire was published prior to evidence which suggests that smaller quantities of grapefruit juice can affect blood concentrations of simvastatin).

Measurement of total cholesterol concentrations in the blood

Advice about OTC statins currently states that cholesterol testing is not considered to be essential before recommending OTC simvastatin, although it may be good for feedback and motivation of individuals.

Where a measurement is made, a fasting blood sample is not necessary for cholesterol (either total or HDL and LDL) and the patient need only be fasting when triglycerides are going to be measured.

Current UK recommendations are that the blood concentration of total cholesterol be kept at less than 5.0 mmol/litre for high-risk patients and that of LDL cholesterol less than 3.0 mmol/litre. HDL cholesterol should be more than 1.0 mmol/litre. However, in other parts of Europe the advice is to keep total cholesterol less than 4.0 and LDL cholesterol less than 2.0 mmol/litre. The product licence for OTC simvastatin states that individuals with an LDL cholesterol greater than 5.5 mmol/litre or a total cholesterol above 7 mmol/litre should be referred to their GP, because OTC statins would not be potent enough to bring the cholesterol within the target range.

This therefore raises problems in a situation where a pharmacist recommends simvastatin 10 mg to a person whose blood cholesterol has not been measured, but whose levels of total cholesterol are higher than those mentioned, which would require them to seek a medical opinion.

Similarly, if only blood concentrations of total cholesterol were measured, this would give only a limited amount of information about a patient's cardiovascular risk. For a complete picture, LDL and HDL cholesterol also need to be measured.

Adverse reactions to statins

Statins generally have a high benefit to risk ratio. The most serious (although rare) adverse effects are myositis and rhabdomyolysis, which will manifest as muscle pain. These will be rare at the OTC recommended dose and are more common in higher doses. Other side effects complained of may be abdominal pain, constipation or diarrhoea, nausea and vomiting, flatulence, headache and peripheral neuropathy (such as a sensation of pins and needles).

Problems

- Measurement of total cholesterol levels alone can overestimate the risk of CHD. Hospital laboratories measure LDL cholesterol and the ratio of total to HDL cholesterol levels, which give a better estimation of risk.
- For low- to moderate-risk patients it is assumed that taking a history from an individual would be sufficient to estimate the degree of risk for that person, although in higher-risk groups it is not consistently possible to do this, even for doctors, without the assistance of risk tables or calculation tools. However, like any tool, a risk calculator is only useful if it is used appropriately.
- Thus any kind of approach to calculating risk has its limitations and pharmacists should be aware of this and be particularly careful not to over- or underestimate risk, based on one factor alone.
- There is a natural variation within patients for measured blood cholesterol levels, and this, together with measurement errors, can lead to cholesterol measurements varying by over 10 per cent from the actual blood concentration.
- External quality control is mandatory to give confidence and credibility to the method of measurement used.

Conveying information to the patient

Individuals must be educated about the nature of their risk and to take measures themselves to reduce it. This means following a healthy lifestyle. However, this should not be misinterpreted as spartan, nor anything requiring hard work except for the effort involved in making some adjustments to daily routines. Any changes made will in the end make an individual healthier, both now and, more importantly, in 10–20 years' time, when age-related illnesses begin to take their toll.

Individuals should be told how they can help themselves and what can be changed and what cannot (see Table 18.1). Changing modifiable factors will help reduce the risks posed by the non-modifiable ones. If an individual has one risk factor, education will be necessary to reinforce the message that this will not increase the overall risk significantly if no other factors are apparent.

OTC statins are relatively expensive to purchase. Their benefits only come after long-term use (at least 3 years), but they need to be taken consistently for a lifetime and this requires great commitment and compliance. Statins are very effective, as many clinical trials and years of clinical use have shown.

It cannot be overemphasised that pharmacists and GPs should agree a protocol for recommendations about OTC statins and lifestyle advice given to patients with a moderate risk of cardiovascular disease.

Second opinion

Cardiovascular diseases – commonly hypertension and cardiac ischaemia – have long been a vital part of primary care and now, with their relationships with renal disease and type 2 diabetes, are even more important and occupy many working hours for both doctors and practice nurses. The new General Medical Services contract of 2004 put further emphasis on the recording of blood pressure, smoking habits and lipid levels, and most practices have found that their use of drugs in this therapeutic area, including statins, has risen considerably. Although each risk factor should be considered in its own right, a global evaluation of risk is estimated for each patient and a holistic mix of lifestyle and drug interventions often results. This will include repeated measurement of blood pressure, blood lipids and other parameters such as renal function or, where appropriate, glycaemic control. The health promotion aspect of the contract also highlights the importance of recording blood pressure, smoking history and BMI, as well as the non-modifiable risk factors in all adults, which in turn will identify still more of the population at appreciable risk.

Bibliography

British Heart Foundation website: www.heart statsorg/homepage.asp

National Institute for Health and Clinical Excellence (2006). Statins for the Prevention of Cardiovascular events. Technology Appraisal 94. London: National Institute for Health and Clinical Excellence.

National Prescribing Centre (2004). *Updating Local Policies for Reducing the Impact of Cardiovascular Disease: Where does OTC Simvastatin Fit In?* (obtainable at www.npc.co.uk)

Practice guidance (2004). OTC Simvastatin 10 mg. *Pharm J* 273: 169–170.

Royal Pharmaceutical Society of Great Britain (2003). *Practice Guidance on Cholesterol Testing by Community Pharmacists.* www.rpsgb.org.uk/pdfs/choltestguid.pdf

Royal Pharmaceutical Society of Great Britain (2003). *Practice Guidance on Blood Pressure Monitoring by Community Pharmacists.* www.rpsg.org.uk/pdfs/bpmonitguid.pdf

Royal Pharmaceutical Society of Great Britain (2004). *Practice Guidance on the Sale of Over-the-Counter Simvastatin.* www.rpsgb.org.uk/pdfs/otcsimvastatinguid.pdf (accessed 9 March 2006).

CASE STUDIES

Case 1

A middle-aged man asks for advice about lowering his cholesterol and wishes to know how the OTC statin will affect his chances of having coronary heart disease.

The pharmacist should take a history from the patient in a quiet private area. The use of an *aide mémoire* such as that shown in Figure 18.1 will be helpful. If the man fits the profile of someone who would benefit from a statin, clear concise messages about risk reduction should be conveyed to him. This can be done in a number of ways:

- You have a 15 per cent risk of CHD in the next 10 years and this will be lowered to 10 per cent if you take a statin.
- Fifteen people in every 100 like you will have a coronary event (such as a heart attack or angina) and an OTC statin will reduce this to 10.
- For every 100 people who take a statin, five will benefit by not having a coronary event in the next 10 years which they otherwise would have had if they had not taken a statin.
- Without a statin, one in seven people would have a coronary event, but with a statin only one in 10 will do so.
- Your chance of having an event is at present 1 in 7, and this will decrease to 1 in 10 in the next 10 years if you take a statin.

The message should be conveyed that the patient will only benefit when he has taken the statin consistently for about 3 years. Taking it for 1 year, for instance, will only reduce the risk from a 1 in 7 to a 1 in 8 chance of having an event.

The pharmacist must choose which of the above explanations suits both himself and, more importantly, the patient for the message to have maximum impact.

The pharmacist should take the opportunity to discuss a variety of lifestyle factors that will be helpful for particular individuals.

Case 2

A man reports that he has had his blood cholesterol level measured recently and it was found to be 5.8 mmol/litre. On further questioning it transpires that he is less than 40 years old but is a heavy drinker and smoker. He has heard that his total cholesterol should be less than 5.0, and asks whether he should see his doctor, or what else can be done.

The pharmacist should ascertain whether he has other risk factors. If he does not, then it should be pointed out to him that his total cholesterol is probably about average for someone his age in the UK.

In this particular case the pharmacist ascertains that lifetime compliance with OTC statins is a remote possibility. The plan, therefore, should be to try and persuade this man to reduce some of his other risk factors by cutting down his alcohol consumption and stopping smoking. Although these may be equally difficult lifestyle factors to change, they do have the added advantage that they involve no further expenditure and the financial savings may be used as an incentive.

If the man drinks more than the recommended levels of alcohol (more than 28 units per week) he should be encouraged to reduce this. High alcohol consumption is associated with cardiovascular and liver disease, and would exclude him from using statins because of the potential for liver problems. He should be given brief and supportive advice about smoking cessation, and guidance on this aspect is available in Chapter 17.

→

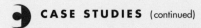 **CASE STUDIES** (continued)

Case 3

A 50-year-old professional man has type 2 diabetes which is controlled by diet. He is fit and very health conscious, and is asking about OTC statins.

It is likely that this man has a higher risk of CHD because of his type 2 diabetes, but his GP should have checked his risk factors at some point in one of his visits to the practice.

An enquiry as to whether his blood pressure has been measured recently (in the last year) should be made, as should the date of his last medical check and whether his lipids have ever been measured. If he has not had any of these done they should be measured by the practice nurse at a time convenient to him. The pharmacist could measure the blood pressure too. If the man has had measurements taken, then it should be assumed that the doctor is aware of this man's risks and there is no need to refer. It is necessary to check local protocols for prescribing lipid-lowering drugs with GPs, as many authorities regard diabetes as an indication for prescribing statins.

The pharmacist should take this opportunity to give lifestyle advice to this man, as he would with anyone else.

19

Emergency hormonal contraception

Emergency hormonal contraception (EHC) has been available over the counter in pharmacies in the United Kingdom since 2001. Often referred to as 'the morning-after pill', EHC is available in a preparation that provides a single dose of 1500 µg of levonorgestrel. This allows community pharmacists to play a significant role in contraception services. It is not intended for regular use as a contraceptive, but is for emergency situations when a contraceptive method has not been used or has failed (see below).

EHC is a means by which pharmacists contribute generally to the public health agenda and specifically to one of the objectives of the National Strategy for Sexual Health and HIV.

Unwanted pregnancies and the subsequent abortions are a significant public health problem in the UK. EHC is an effective means of preventing accidental pregnancy and the related anxiety it causes in a woman who has had unprotected sex. Pharmacists should be able to offer a non-judgemental, discreet and helpful service in a private area (preferably a consulting room) in the pharmacy.

The sexual health charity fpa (the Family Planning Association) has supported the use of EHC as a bathroom preventative. That is to say, a woman may be able to obtain the EHC pill before having unprotected sex. Surveys have shown that the majority of women would prefer to be given the pill in advance, and some family planning clinics and doctors already provide it on this basis. It is thought that women will be more likely to use EHC if they have been provided with it beforehand, although such use would not motivate them to use contraceptives in the normal way. However, the Royal Pharmaceutical Society of Great Britain does not at present recommend that pharmacists supply EHC in advance of clinical need.

Surveys have reported that 12 per cent of 16-year-olds and 16 per cent of those aged 18–19 have used the morning-after pill, with one in 25 using it more than once. About a quarter of these women bought the pill from a pharmacy.

Indications for EHC

1. Unprotected sex
   - No contraception
   - Rape
2. Contraceptive failure
   - Barrier method failure
   - Failure of an intrauterine contraceptive device (IUCD)
   - Missed oral contraceptive pills

Pharmacology of EHC

Levonorgestrel, when taken in a large dose in the morning-after pill, is believed to act by preventing ovulation or fertilisation in the follicular stage and preventing implantation in the luteal phase of the menstrual cycle. (In the normal menstrual cycle the follicular phase is variable in length but usually lasts for the first 14–15 days. If the cycle is longer or shorter than the average 28 days then it is usually the follicular phase that changes. During this phase a number of follicles grow in the ovary and the most mature will produce an ovum capable of being fertilised. The luteal phase has a fairly constant length of 12–16 days and is the second phase of the cycle, beginning after ovulation has taken place. The follicle that releases the ovum is transformed into the corpus luteum and produces progesterone.) There is no effect on established pregnancy or on a fetus.

Approximately 85–95 per cent of expected pregnancies can be prevented by a morning-after pill containing a single dose of levonorgestrel 1500 µg when taken within 24 hours of unprotected sex. Between 24 and 48 hours it is expected to be 85 per cent effective, and between 48 and 72 hours the efficacy is about 58 per cent.

Setting up a service

EHC is relatively expensive to purchase over the counter in the UK. However, many women do obtain it in this way. Some pharmacists participate in a scheme by which the pill is provided under a patient group direction (PGD) protocol, whereby the drug is paid for by a primary care organisation. Ideally, a supply of EHC should be accompanied by counselling regarding sexually transmitted infection and methods of contraception.

A pharmacy service has the advantage that no appointments are necessary, and in many circumstances pharmacists are available on Sundays and in the evenings (extended hours) when GPs are not normally available. Not all out-of-hours services carry supplies. In addition, Monday mornings appear to be the time when women will frequently require advice and/or EHC, and this may be easier to obtain in a community pharmacy, without appointment and without taking time off work, than obtaining an appointment with the GP, which may mean taking time off work.

Requirements

- Privacy – pharmacists should provide a private consulting area where conversations cannot be overheard.

- Training – pharmacists should be trained so that they can take an appropriate history to determine whether EHC is appropriate. As indicated above, some training will be necessary to give a background on sexually transmitted disease and contraceptive methods.

- Time – pharmacists must be prepared to have time available to consult with women who are requesting EHC. Such consultations will be required without prior appointment, and because the woman may be embarrassed by the sensitive nature of her enquiry the consultation cannot be delayed to a more convenient time for the pharmacist.

Questions for pharmacists to ask

A number of questions are necessary before a decision can be made about the appropriateness of EHC. These can be asked by the pharmacist or, if the woman prefers, a questionnaire can be completed to relieve any initial embarrassment on her part. A template for a suitable questionnaire is given in Figure 19.1.

- *Is the woman 16 years of age or older?*
  Some PGDs may allow the supply of EHC to girls under 16.
- *Is the EHC for the woman who is requesting it?*
  EHC should only be supplied to a third party in very exceptional circumstances.
- *Has there been unprotected sex in the last 72 hours?*
  This question should be asked because the product licence for EHC requires it to be used within 72 hours of unprotected sex.
- *Has the woman had intercourse since the last period before this time?*
  This question should be asked to ascertain whether there is a possibility of the woman already being pregnant as a result of previous intercourse. Although EHC will not harm a woman who is in the early stages of pregnancy, it will obviously not be effective at this stage and pregnancy is a contraindication.
- EHC can be used more than once in the same menstrual cycle, but in such cases women should be directed to seek advice about con-

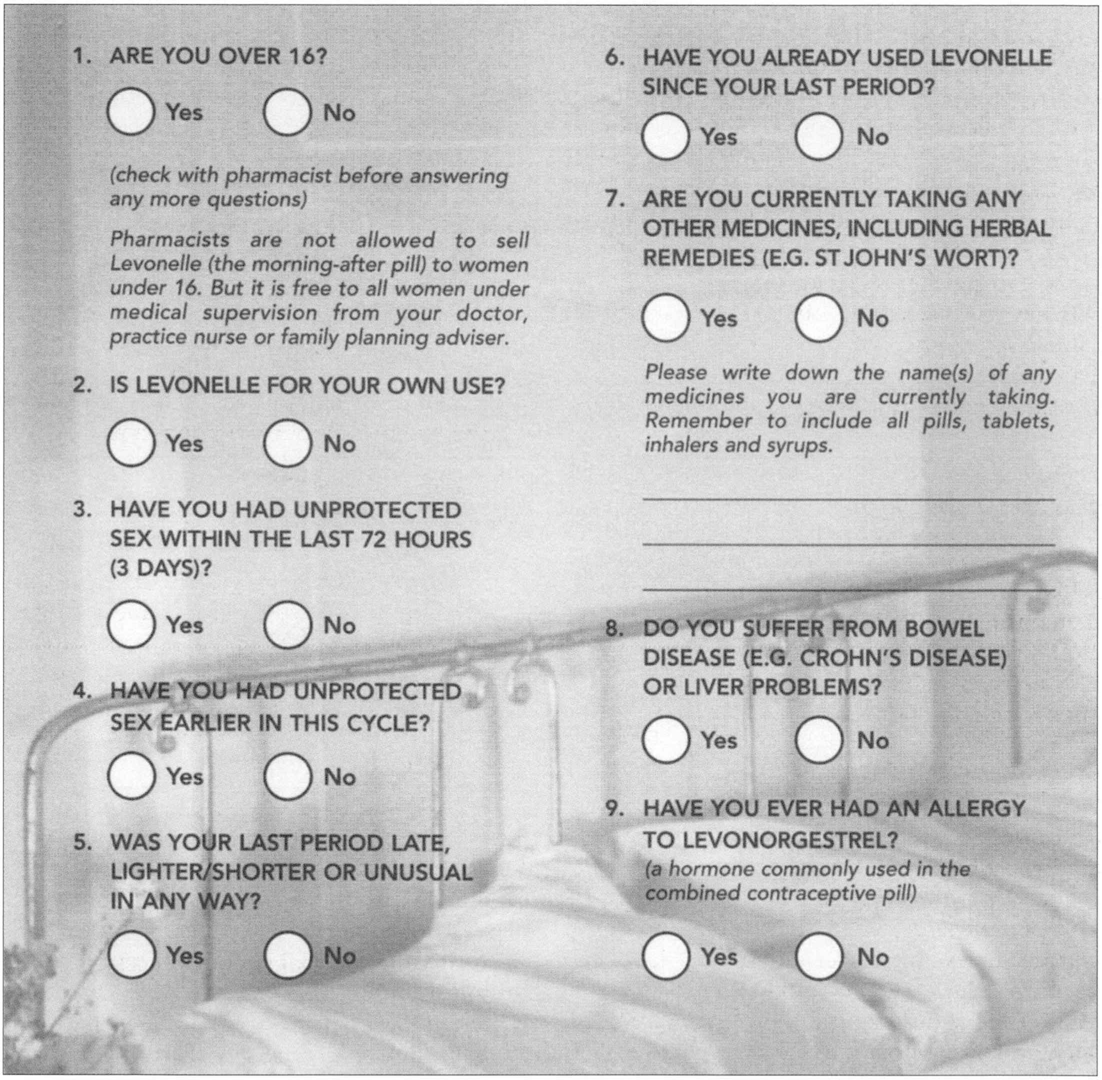
1. ARE YOU OVER 16?

Yes No

(check with pharmacist before answering any more questions)

Pharmacists are not allowed to sell Levonelle (the morning-after pill) to women under 16. But it is free to all women under medical supervision from your doctor, practice nurse or family planning adviser.

2. IS LEVONELLE FOR YOUR OWN USE?

Yes No

3. HAVE YOU HAD UNPROTECTED SEX WITHIN THE LAST 72 HOURS (3 DAYS)?

Yes No

4. HAVE YOU HAD UNPROTECTED SEX EARLIER IN THIS CYCLE?

Yes No

5. WAS YOUR LAST PERIOD LATE, LIGHTER/SHORTER OR UNUSUAL IN ANY WAY?

Yes No

6. HAVE YOU ALREADY USED LEVONELLE SINCE YOUR LAST PERIOD?

Yes No

7. ARE YOU CURRENTLY TAKING ANY OTHER MEDICINES, INCLUDING HERBAL REMEDIES (E.G. ST JOHN'S WORT)?

Yes No

Please write down the name(s) of any medicines you are currently taking. Remember to include all pills, tablets, inhalers and syrups.

8. DO YOU SUFFER FROM BOWEL DISEASE (E.G. CROHN'S DISEASE) OR LIVER PROBLEMS?

Yes No

9. HAVE YOU EVER HAD AN ALLERGY TO LEVONORGESTREL?
(a hormone commonly used in the combined contraceptive pill)

Yes No

Figure 19.1 Example of a consumer questionnaire to assess suitability for EHC.

traception from a family planning clinic or practice nurse, and told that EHC can disrupt the cycle and cause intermenstrual bleeding or 'spotting', which may lead to confusion about the timing of the last menstrual bleed.

- *Is the woman taking other medicines or herbal remedies?*
  Various drugs will interact with levonorgestrel, and these are indicated in Table 19.1.

Further questions should be asked to ascertain whether levonorgestrel may be inappropriate. If the answer to any of the following questions is positive, the patient should be referred to a GP or family planning clinic.

- *Does the woman have any known allergy to levonorgestrel?*
  Some contraceptive pills contain levonorgestrel, and previous intolerance should be enquired for.

Table 19.1 Drug interactions with EHC (levonorgestrel)

Interacting drug	Consequence
Barbiturates Carbamazepine Phenytoin St John's Wort Rifampicin Ritonavir Rifabutin Griseofulvin	These drugs increase the metabolism of levonorgestrel and may reduce its efficacy
Ciclosporin	Levonorgestrel inhibits the metabolism of ciclosporin and increases the risk of ciclosporin toxicity. Refer to GP

- *Is there any small bowel disease (including Crohn's disease) or any liver problems?*
  Such conditions may interfere with the absorption or metabolism of the pill.
- *Are there any problems that may affect absorption of the pill, such as vomiting or severe diarrhoea?*

Adverse drug reactions

The adverse effects of levonorgestrel are listed in Table 19.2.

Advice for missed combined oral contraceptive pills

EHC can be used in some circumstances when a woman has missed her contraceptive pills. The

Table 19.2 Adverse drug reactions to EHC

Nausea
Vomiting
Abdominal pain
Headache
Breast tenderness
Irregular menstrual bleeding (bleeding may be earlier or later than usual, and lighter or heavier)
Spotting (mild, intermittent bleeding during cycle)

following guide can be used to determine whether EHC will be necessary or effective.

Combined oral contraceptives

- If the contraceptive pill is less than 12 hours late the missed pill can be taken immediately and subsequent pills taken as usual. No EHC is necessary.
- If one contraceptive pill has been missed and it is more than 12 hours but less than 24 hours late, the missed pill should be taken immediately and further pills taken as usual. Extra precautions should be taken for 7 days. EHC is not appropriate.
- If one pill is more than 12 hours late and a woman has fewer than seven pills left in the pack for that cycle, she should take the rest of the pills as usual and extra precautions as above, but she must also start the next pack of pills without a break. EHC is not necessary.
- If more than one contraceptive pill is missed from the first week or more than four pills from the second week, EHC is necessary. In addition, extra precautions are necessary for the next 7 days.
- If more than one contraceptive pill is missed at the end of a pack and there are fewer than seven pills left, EHC is not necessary. However, further pills should be taken as usual, extra precautions taken and the next pack started without a break.

Progestogen-only pills

If one or more progestogen-only pills have been missed and it is more than 3 hours since the last pill was due (or 12 hours for desorgestrel), then EHC is necessary as well as extra precautions for the next 7 days. If fewer than seven pills remain, then another pack should be started without a break.

If the time since intercourse is more than 72 hours the woman should be referred to her GP, when the insertion of an IUCD may be considered. The woman should also be referred if the next period is different from usual.

Second opinion

People requiring contraceptive advice have several sources to choose from, and doctors and nurses in general practice are often unaware of those who purchase condoms or who use the family planning clinic services. With the possible delay in making appointments and the unpredictability of which clinician will be available, many women seeking emergency contraception have chosen these options. Increasingly GP appointments can be offered on the same day or even advice given by telephone, and this, together with the service offered by pharmacists, has further increased the choice available. Protocols such as those mentioned above are now common in primary care, and EHC is usually supplied with the proviso that a more lasting solution to the problem should be sought.

Bibliography

Department of Health (2001). *The National Strategy for Sexual Health and HIV*. London: Department of Health.

Royal Pharmaceutical Society of Great Britain (2004). *Practice Guidance on the Supply of Emergency Hormonal Contraception as a Pharmacy Medicine*. www.rpsgb.org/pdfs/ehcguid.pdf (accessed 9 March 2006).

 CASE STUDIES

Case 1

A 17-year-old girl has returned from holiday and comes into the pharmacy the next day with her friend. It is a Saturday afternoon. She says that she has had sexual intercourse on several occasions while on holiday and fears that she may have forgotten to take her combined oral contraceptive on at least one day during that time. Her friend asks about the morning-after pill.

What should the pharmacist advise?

After questioning the girl, the pharmacist finds that although the last intercourse was within the previous 48 hours, there had been other occasions when she might not have been protected during the holiday.

Having confirmed that sex took place beyond the 72-hour limit, with the possibility of missed contraceptive pills, the pharmacist explains that EHC is not appropriate. He advises her to continue taking her contraceptive pills, to start a new pack without the usual 7-day break, and to take extra precautions until the end of her next cycle.

(continued overleaf)

CASE STUDIES (continued)

A referral is necessary and she should be advised to seek help at her medical practice or the family planning clinic. It is unlikely that she will be eligible for a coil to be fitted by a doctor, but she does need some education about contraception, the need to use condoms when having casual sex, and the need to have screening tests for sexually transmitted disease.

A few days later she presented a prescription for antibiotics to treat a chlamydial infection. The screening tests had shown white cells in the urine and *Chlamydia* was incubated from the vaginal swabs. Unfortunately, the partner who had transmitted the infection could be an asymptomatic carrier and unaware of his infectivity. The consequences of his ignorance and her lack of care had been explained to her by a sympathetic family planning nurse. The sequelae of chlamydial infection can be serious and can lead to pelvic inflammatory disease, resulting in infertility. Fortunately, the girl had the common sense to admit that she was having a relationship with a steady boyfriend at home, and she had persuaded him to go to the clinic with her and be screened to ensure that he had not contracted the infection from her. Nevertheless, the clinic had advised that he should be prescribed a course of treatment too.

The most pleasing outcome of this scenario was that the girl had gone through a learning process and had been educated not only about the risks of pregnancy, but also about safe sex and the need to avoid the transmission of infections.

Case 2

A young woman asks the pharmacist for the morning-after pill. It is known that she has already taken one course within the last 2 weeks. She is prepared to buy it over the counter and is requesting another supply.

What advice should be given?

The pharmacist should go through the usual line of questioning to determine whether EHC is suitable for this woman. He should ask which method of contraception she normally uses.

This woman is well known for her casual encounters, but after some rather obtuse answers to the questions she was asked it is revealed that she is planning 'for an emergency ahead' and has not had unprotected intercourse within the last 3 days. She is also forgetful with her oral contraceptive and uses the morning-after pill regularly as 'back-up'.

The pharmacist has to explain that he is not allowed to sell EHC in advance of clinical need. Some family planning clinics may do this, but he is unsure whether locally this is the case. However, it seemed a good opportunity to persuade this woman to go to the local clinic to enquire about the availability of this service, because the pharmacist knew that she might be also persuaded to try another mode of contraception, which would be more appropriate for someone with a bad memory.

A few days later, she returned several months' supply of oral contraceptives to the pharmacy, explaining that she was now having an injectable contraceptive at the clinic every 3 months and had also been given a free supply of condoms to support the advice she had been given by the clinic nurses about sexually transmitted infections.

20

Travel health

Global travel is increasing and, with it, access to more extreme destinations. The summer is the most popular time for continental travel from the UK for holidaymakers, and the USA and Mediterranean countries are favourite destinations. However, more people are taking holidays at other times of the year, and are also heading for less developed countries. Health problems await, and it is necessary to take simple precautions when travelling anywhere in the world.

Traveller's diarrhoea

This can be defined as three or more stools within a 24-hour period, plus one of the following: abdominal pain or cramps, nausea, vomiting, low-grade fever or tenesmus (a desire to empty the bowel, even when there is no stool present). The diarrhoea is usually watery and may contain mucus, but usually contains no blood or pus (except for *Shigella* infection, where this is more common). Traveller's diarrhoea is usually self-limiting and lasts 1–5 days. It is extremely common and can affect one in three travellers. Typically it begins within 1 or 2 weeks after the start of the holiday and results from the ingestion of microorganisms.

There are many causative organisms (Table 20.1), and many sufferers notice a transient change in bowel frequency associated with a change in their usual diet (sometimes including alcohol consumption) or due to a lack of fluid replacement in unaccustomed heat.

Sudden short-lived illness can result from improperly cooked or reheated foods. The symptoms are produced by chemical irritation rather than infection, the foods being allowed to act as culture media, with proliferation of the infection and the production of toxins. Subsequent heating may destroy the infection but leave the irritant toxins. The onset can be only a few hours after ingestion, clinically severe, but often resolving in around 24 hours.

Prevention

Sensible precautions such as good personal hygiene should be taken, as well as measures such as hand-washing, avoiding swimming in fresh water and avoiding swallowing water when

Table 20.1	Organisms that cause traveller's diarrhoea
	Principal mode of spread
Bacteria	
Escherichia coli	Faecal–oral, water, meat
Salmonella	Meat (especially chicken), dairy products
Campylobacter	Meat (especially chicken), milk
Shigella	Faecal–oral
Viruses	
Rotavirus	Food, faecal–oral, airborne spread
Norovirus (Norwalk virus)	Associated with cruise ships
Parasites	
Giardia	Fresh water
Cryptosporidium	Fresh water
Entamoeba histolytica (amoebic dysentery)	Fresh water, food

bathing. With regard to eating and drinking, water should be boiled for at least 3 minutes or treated with sterilising tablets containing chlorine-based preparations or tincture of iodine. Fruits should be peeled, and foods such as salads (which will be washed in tap water) and ice in drinks should be avoided. Where possible, food purchased from street vendors should be avoided too. Another precaution is to only drink bottled commercial water with an intact seal.

Treatment

The use of antibiotics in both the prevention and treatment of traveller's diarrhoea is very controversial. However, for travellers going to very remote areas, the pharmacist could advise that they might wish to purchase a course of quinolones such as ciprofloxacin on a private prescription from their doctor.

As with diarrhoea of any cause, the cornerstone of treatment of traveller's diarrhoea is adequate hydration. Generally traveller's diarrhoea is not a dehydrating disease, but obviously in hot climates it is necessary to maintain fluid levels. Oral rehydration solutions are not generally necessary but will do no harm. It should be remembered that fruits such as oranges and bananas are good sources of potassium. Alcohol and fats should be avoided.

There are a variety of proprietary products available for traveller's diarrhoea. The most effective symptomatic treatments are loperamide, a combination of diphenoxylate and atropine and bismuth subsalicylate. The latter is believed to inhibit enterotoxin activity and can also be used as a preventative measure. It interacts with anticoagulants and doxycycline (the latter may be being used as an antimalarial in some travellers). It also causes black stools.

Malaria

The increase in international travel has increased the risk of contracting malaria. Prophylaxis is the best policy, using antimalarial drugs and sensible avoidance measures. Concordance and compliance are essential, and the pharmacist can play a significant educative role with people travelling to areas where malaria prevails.

Malaria is spread by a protozoon called *Plasmodium*, which is transmitted by the bite from the female *Anopheles* mosquito in tropical climates (Figure 20.1). It is a potentially fatal disease. There are four species of *Plasmodium*, namely *P. falciparum* (the most common and the most dangerous species), *P. vivax*, *P. ovale* and *P. malariae*.

Prevention

- Wear sensible clothing – covering the arms, legs and neck, particularly at night, or when travelling or when near stagnant water, is an essential preventative measure.
- Use mosquito nets or plug-in antimosquito devices in rooms at night.
- Apply insect repellents – the most commonly used and efficacious agent is DEET (diethyltoluamide). Other repellents such as volatile oils, including citronella, have also been used, but may not be effective in all individuals. It is important to convey this message to travellers, as failure may result in painful bites at the very least. DEET is not suitable for children or for pregnant women. It should be remembered that DEET needs to be reapplied after several hours as it disappears from the

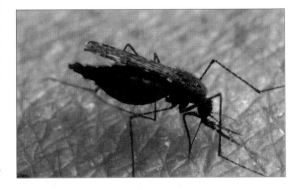

Figure 20.1   *Anopheles balabacenis* mosquito with proboscis inserted into the skin. (Reproduced with permission of Martin Dohrn/Science Photo Library.)

skin over a short period. It is wise to advise that it also melts plastic, such as spectacles.

- Chemoprophylaxis – the antimalarial agents most appropriate for individuals will depend upon the countries to which they are travelling. Chloroquine and proguanil are available over the counter. The appropriate regimen can be found from various sources, such as the *British National Formulary* and various websites (see Bibliography).
- Patients should be warned that no single measure, either of avoidance or of chemoprophylaxis, is adequate, and although 100 per cent protection is aimed for, even combinations of all the avoidance measures and antimalarial drugs cannot be guaranteed to give total protection.
- For pregnant women, a combination of chloroquine and proguanil has proved to be safe. However, the latter drug is a folate antagonist and must therefore be accompanied by folic acid supplements.
- Patients with epilepsy should avoid chloroquine (and also mefloquine on prescription). A combination of atovaquone and proguanil is safe in epilepsy.

Adverse effects of antimalarials

Chloroquine should be taken with food to avoid nausea and vomiting. It can cause headache, rash, and reversible blurred vision.

Proguanil can cause anorexia, nausea, diarrhoea and mouth ulcers. It may interact with warfarin.

Standby medication

Standby medication is a course of self-administered antimalarial treatment for use by travellers who may develop symptoms and signs of malaria but who are in a remote area at least 24 hours from medical facilities. Travellers should obtain advice from appropriate authorities or websites (see Bibliography) before the holiday starts. Various combinations of agents such as chloroquine, atovaquone, proguanil and qui-

nine may be used – quinine is the agent of choice for pregnant women.

Symptoms of malaria

Malaria presents as influenza-like symptoms, including headache, fever, and general aches and pains. It develops into cycles of shaking chills, fever and sweating that recur every 1–3 days. It may progress to haemorrhages, shock, kidney or liver failure, coma and death. Symptoms may take up to 1 or even 3 months after the mosquito has bitten before they appear.

General advice

It is essential that travellers understand the need to begin antimalarial treatment 1 or 2 weeks in advance of travel. The reasons for this are to identify any side effects and to allow blood concentrations to become high enough to be effective when they reach their destination. They should also be told to continue treatment for 4 weeks after returning from their trip. This is because the incubation period of the parasites in the blood can be up to 4 weeks.

Insect bites and stings

Besides an insect repellent such as DEET (see above), a cream containing an antihistamine or hydrocortisone for the treatment of insect bites and stings is essential to any traveller's first-aid kit (Table 20.2).

Vaccinations

Pharmacists may be asked about general advice for vaccinations. The main point to convey is that a course of vaccinations should be planned well in advance (up to 2 months is ideal) and that advice can be obtained from various websites and agencies as well as the local doctor's

Table 20.2   Contents of a travel first-aid kit

Paracetamol/ibuprofen

Antidiarrhoeal agent, e.g. loperamide, bismuth, subsalicylate or diphenoxylate with atropine

Antihistamine or calamine cream

Motion sickness remedy, e.g. hyoscine, cinnarizine, promethazine, ginger

Aciclovir cold sore cream

Sunscreen (SPR > 15)

Crepe bandage

Plasters

Insect-repellent cream

Condoms

Emergency malaria treatment (for travellers to remote areas only (check requisites with local experts))

Water-sterilising tablets (for emergencies if bottled water is not available)

surgery as to which vaccinations are appropriate. Generally travel outside Europe will require that the traveller is vaccinated against poliomyelitis (and tetanus, where not up to date), and where food and water hygiene and sanitation are of a poor standard, typhoid and hepatitis A, and possibly hepatitis B. For some destinations other precautions are necessary, such as vaccinations against diphtheria, rabies and yellow fever.

Travel sickness

Various products are available over the counter that are effective against motion sickness. These include anticholinergic drugs such as hyoscine and antihistamines such as cinnarizine or promethazine.

Sunburn

Protection of the skin from the radiation of the sun is essential for any visitor to a hot country, and for skiers. The effects of the sun on the skin increase with increased altitude.

The three types of ultraviolet radiation are UVA, UVB and UVC. UVA and UVB are the most damaging to the skin. UVA is responsible for the development of a quick tanning effect by oxidation of melanin. It is also responsible for skin cancer in the long term, and is the type of radiation present in sun beds. UVB produces burning and increases the amount of melanin in the basal layer of the epidermis. UVB causes skin thickening, and can cause skin cancers too. UVC is filtered out by the ozone layer and does not reach the earth. Some drugs can cause photosensitivity – see Table 20.3.

Treatment of sunburn

Cooling agents such as calamine cream or lotion offer symptomatic relief. Analgesics will relieve the pain and any fever. The cornerstone is prevention rather than treatment. This can be facilitated by avoiding exposure to the sun for an hour or two each side of midday, and the use of T-shirts, hats and sunscreens as appropriate.

Sunscreens

Sunscreens are of two types, organic and reflective. Organic sunscreens absorb UV radiation, mainly in the UVB range. Examples are para-aminobenzoic acid (PABA), octylmethoxycinnamate, oxybenzone, mexenone and avobenzone. The latter protects against UVA. Reflective sunscreens are a barrier to UVA and UVB light. Examples are titanium dioxide and zinc oxide. They act by deflecting the sun's rays by forming a physical barrier on top of the skin.

Table 20.3   Drugs that can cause photosensitivity

Amiodarone

Antihistamines

Griseofulvin

Non-steroidal anti-inflammatory drugs (NSAIDs)

Phenothiazines

Quinine

Quinolones

Tetracyclines

Thiazides

Tricyclic antidepressants

Sun-protection factor (SPF)

The SPF measures protection against UVB radiation. It is now recommended that all caucasians use a sunscreen with an SPF equal to or greater than 15. This means that the wearer can stay in the sun 15 times longer than he or she could with no skin protection. Current advice is that the use of a sunscreen can be stepped down to an SPF of about 10 if the wearer wishes to have a tan. Sunscreens should be applied generously and reapplied at frequent intervals.

Star system

The star system is a means of describing protection against UVA radiation.

Sunglasses

Sunglasses are necessary to protect against various eye problems, such as damage to the lens as may occur in cataract formation, conjunctivitis and snow blindness, resulting in temporary or permanent damage to the cornea. Sunglasses should comply with appropriate standards offering 100 per cent protection against UV light. For skiing holidays mirrored lenses are good for strong sunlight conditions, and goggles and wraparound sunglasses offer the best all-round protection.

Altitude sickness

Acute mountain sickness will affect people when they climb to a height of over 3000 metres. It has been quoted that at over 4000 metres about 50 per cent of people are affected.

Prevention

Commonsense measures such as ascending slowly and acclimatising are necessary. Dehydration should be avoided by drinking appropriate amounts of fluid and avoiding alcohol.

Symptoms usually occur within a day, but can be delayed. They consist of headache, dizziness, lethargy and loss of appetite. Sometimes more severe problems may occur, which will include pulmonary oedema with cough and dyspnoea (difficulty in breathing), or loss of consciousness and abnormal behaviour.

Polymorphic light eruption (PMLE)

PMLE is an itchy rash caused by exposure to sunlight. It occurs anywhere on the body and can take several weeks to clear. It may be treated with steroid creams or calamine cream and cooling.

Deep-vein thrombosis (DVT)

This condition can occur not only in air travel, especially long-haul, but also in car and coach journeys.

A DVT is a thrombosis (blood clot) in the deep veins, seen most often in the legs. It is caused usually by poor or sluggish circulation.

Symptoms

DVT may be felt as an ache or a pain in the calf, which is made worse particularly if the foot is turned upwards. There is also swelling and tenderness, and often the skin of the calf will appear red. DVTs in themselves are relatively harmless, but they can disperse, and if the clot goes to the lungs it can cause a pulmonary embolism, which may present as a cough, shortness of breath and blood in the sputum. If left untreated the condition is potentially fatal. Suspected DVTs should therefore be taken seriously and urgently referred for a medical opinion.

Risk factors for DVT are listed in Table 20.4.

Prevention

'Flight socks' are knee-length compression hosiery that improve blood flow in the lower limbs and reduce the incidence of DVT and ankle oedema. Various preventative measures

Table 20.4 Risk factors for DVT

Previous history of thrombotic conditions
Over 40 years of age
Pregnancy
Use of oral contraceptives or hormone replacement
  therapy
Obesity
Varicose veins
Malignancy
Recent surgery, especially hip or knee replacement
History of blood coagulation disorders

should be advised. For instance, on a journey of any kind the traveller should be encouraged to get up and walk around to stretch the legs as often as possible. It is necessary to keep hydrated, but drinks should be water and soft drinks, not alcohol, which has a dehydrating effect.

There is no evidence for the usefulness of low-dose aspirin, but this has been promoted as a preventative measure. Wearing sensible clothing – that is, loose-fitting and light – is advisable. While seated, travellers should be encouraged to perform various foot or leg movements to encourage the circulation in the lower limbs from time to time and, as mentioned above, if possible to get up and walk around. Legs should not be crossed because this restricts the circulation in the lower part of the leg.

Sexually transmitted infections

Holidays provide opportunities for increased sexual activity with new partners, often without condom use. Except for physical protection by using condoms, sexually transmitted infections are difficult to prevent, the only exceptions being vaccination against hepatitis.

Sexually transmitted infections include infection with *Candida, Chlamydia, Trichomonas,* HIV, genital herpes, genital warts, gonorrhoea and syphilis. The signs of sexually transmitted infection include vaginal or urethral discharge, dysuria, dyspareunia (painful intercourse) and

genital ulcers. The latter may take several weeks to develop. Some of these conditions are described in Chapter 9.

Anyone presenting or asking for advice on any of the above signs and symptoms after a holiday should be advised to contact their local genitourinary medicine clinic.

Prevention is always better than cure, and education about safer sex, hepatitis B vaccination and condom use will go far towards avoiding the risk of contracting sexually transmitted diseases.

Second opinion

Almost all GP surgeries will offer advice to intending travellers, an up-to-date list of vaccinations required or desirable, and provision of most of the common ones. Some of the more specialist vaccines, such as yellow fever, are given by practices that have been registered to provide them, but are also available at the travel health centres associated with ports and airports. As this is essentially a private service, travellers may choose sources other than their GP, especially if the provision is more extensive elsewhere.

Many people underestimate the time needed for effective immunisation, and courses are often rushed or left incomplete before travel. The usual philosophy is that whatever can be achieved will help in the prevention of what are potentially serious debilitating or life-threatening illnesses.

Bibliography

For advice on malaria regimes and travel vaccinations:
NHS advice for travellers – www.fitfortravel. scot.nhs.uk
Public Health Laboratory Service – www.phls. org.uk
For antimalarial regimens:
British National Formulary. London: British Medical Association & Royal Pharmaceutical Society of Great Britain.

Belcaro G, Cesarane MR, Shah SSG *et al* (2002). Prevention of edema, flight microangiopathy and venous thrombosis in long flights with elastic stockings. A randomised trial. The LONFLIT 4 Concorde Edema–SSL Study. *Angiology* 53: 635–645.

Goodyer L (2004). *Travel Medicine for Health Professionals*. London: Pharmaceutical Press.

Rogstad KE (2004). Sex, sun, sea and STIs: sexually transmitted infections acquired on holiday. *Br Med J* 329: 214–217.

Zuckerman JN (2004). Preventing malaria in UK travellers. *Br Med J* 329: 305–306.

CASE STUDIES

Case 1

A man returning from a 2-week holiday in the eastern Mediterranean reports to his pharmacist that, while there, both he and his wife had abdominal pain and diarrhoea which are still continuing. He requests advice.

A proper history should be taken, particularly of the symptoms and their duration, and the possible relation to any cause.

While abroad many people choose either to seek medical advice or to self-medicate, as prescription regulations may be relaxed. Any medications used should be noted.

For the last week they have both suffered episodes of watery diarrhoea and abdominal pain. Although uncomfortable, they were able to continue their travels. They have been taking medication purchased abroad, which seems to indicate codeine phosphate, kaolin and neomycin among its ingredients.

The history suggests an infective cause, and does not appear to be self-limiting. The medication may produce some symptomatic relief, but unless the cause of the illness is identified the medication cannot be relied on. Often foreign pharmacies are well versed in infections that are common locally, and may supply drugs such as metronidazole without investigation but with a high probability of success.

In this case, symptomatic treatment may be recommended but stool samples should be obtained to isolate the cause. The patients should therefore be referred to their GP.

Case 2

A young man presents a private prescription for malaria prophylaxis. He is then taken aback by the cost involved and declines.

Malaria is a serious condition, and all attempts must be made to prevent it.

Doctors are required to use private rather than NHS prescriptions for those drugs not available over the counter.

Part of the problem is a prolonged trip to Asia and the Far East, and the need for substantial supplies. He is travelling with companions from the countries to be visited, and will be staying with their families. They do not use antimalarial drugs, relying on insect repellents and mosquito nets at night.

Many people resident in malarial areas do not take prophylactic medicines, but the risk of infection still remains. This may be reduced if travel is exclusively in urban areas with little mosquito penetration, but higher when travelling in more remote and rural areas.

(continued overleaf)

CASE STUDIES (continued)

Case 3

A young woman asks for some confidential advice. About 3 weeks earlier she enjoyed the pleasures of a holiday romance, but with the benefit of hindsight is now concerned about what, apart from her memories, she may be harbouring.

A sexual history should be taken, including contraceptive use, and her reasons for seeking advice from the pharmacy must be identified. Information on any continuing contact with the man involved would be helpful.

It transpires that she uses oral contraception and thus the need for mechanical protection was not high in her mind. She had tried to contact the man involved, but without success.

At least the risk of pregnancy appears to be low.

Acute infections, such as gonorrhoea, would probably be evident by now, but not those such as *Chlamydia* or genital warts.

HIV transmission is low among solely heterosexual populations, unless they are intravenous drug users. It is too late for immediate immunosuppressive therapy, and too early for antibody testing.

Many people have reservations about the confidentiality of their GP, and seek independent or anonymous opinions.

This woman needs a full investigation for a number of potential infections. She may be tempted to 'wait and see', but referral to the local genitourinary medicine clinic will ensure early identification of any problems, the possibility of contact tracing, and the confidentiality that is so important to her.

Index

Page numbers in italics refer to tables; those in bold to figures. Alphabetical arrangement is letter-by-letter. When a subject appearing in the text gives a reference to an illustration on the same or adjacent page then only a reference from the text (in plain form) is given. 'vs' indicates the differentiation of two conditions.